Administering
Nursing Service

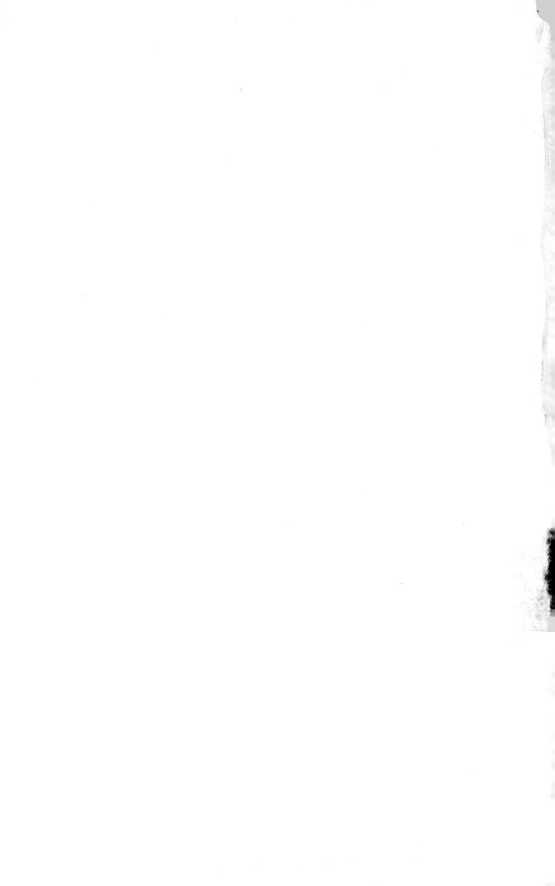

Administering Nursing Service

Second Edition

Marie DiVincenti, R.N., Ed.D.

Department Head, Master of Science in Nursing Program,
College of Nursing, Northwestern State University of Louisiana,
Shreveport

Little, Brown and Company
Boston

This book is dedicated to:

My mother and family for their support and devotion

Miss Helen Weber and Dr. Paul Bergevin, Indiana University,
whose teachings about people continue to be inspiring
and relevant in an ever-changing world

All individuals who are concerned with providing
quality nursing service to people

Contents

Preface *xiii*

Acknowledgments *xvii*

Part I. The Patient and His Needs

1. Trends in the Delivery of Health Care *3*
   Nurse Director Role *3*
   Trends and Issues *3*
   Professionals, Consumers, and Governmental Concerns *7*
   Comprehensive Health Care Needs *10*
   Hospital Role *12*

2. Patient Needs *15*
   Administration *15*
   Medical Care *15*
   Hospital Admission *16*
   Diagnostic Services *16*
   Drug Therapy *17*
   Patient Protection *17*
   Nursing Services *18*
   Spiritual Care *18*
   Dietary Requirements *19*
   Social Service *19*
   Recreational Service *20*
   Volunteers *20*
   Therapeutic Environment *20*
   Medical Records *21*
   Education and Teaching *22*
   Discharge Service *22*
   Continuity of Care *22*
   Patient Expectations *23*

   Part I References *25*

Part II. The Nurse Director's Role and Management Functions

3. Hospital Organization and the Nursing Service *29*
   Nursing Department *30*
   Trends in Nursing *31*
   The Nurse Director's Managerial Skills *33*
   Position of Nurse Director *34*

4. The Management Process *39*
   What is Management? *39*
   Nature of Management *39*
   Managerial Functions *41*

Planning *42*
Organizing *46*
Leadership *53*
Control *60*
Decision Making *63*
Systems Approach *67*

Part II References *77*

Part III. Management Tools

5. Organizational Philosophy *81*
Hospital Philosophy *82*
Nursing Service Philosophy *83*
Nursing Unit Philosophy and Objectives *90*

6. Management by Objectives *93*
Programming Objectives into Activities *97*
Progress Review *98*
Beginning of New Cycle *98*

7. Organizational Chart *101*
Organizational Structures *102*

8. Policies and Procedures *105*
Usefulness of Policies *105*
Policy Development *106*
Communication of Policies *107*
Legal Implications of Policies *108*
Nursing Policy and Procedure Manuals *109*

9. Budget *113*
Definition *113*
Advantages *114*
Prerequisites *114*
Types of Budgets *115*
Budgetary Factors *118*
Nursing Budget Committee *119*
Preparation of the Budget *120*
Budget Presentation *122*
Budget Review *123*
Budget Control *123*

10. Staffing and Scheduling *125*
Determining Personnel Requirements *125*
Staffing Objectives *127*
Factors Affecting Staffing *128*
Future Direction *129*
Master Staffing Plan *129*
Scheduling *131*

11. Standards of Performance *135*
    Definition of Nursing *135*
    Quality Assurance Program *137*
    Peer Review *147*

12. Methods of Assignment *149*
    Assigning Staff to Patient Care *150*
    Assignment Sheet *150*

13. Nursing Management *153*
    The Nursing Process *153*
    Nursing Care Plans *158*
    Nursing Rounds *160*
    Making Rounds with a Purpose *160*

14. Participative Administration and Records *163*
    Administrative Meetings *163*
    Committees *164*
    Records and Reports *166*
    Defining the Nursing Audit *176*

15. Job Organization and Appraisal *183*
    Job Evaluation Program *183*
    Wage and Salary Program *183*
    Job Analysis *184*
    Employee Performance Appraisal *189*

16. Staff Education Programs *195*
    Staff Education *195*
    Role and Responsibilities of the Nurse Director *196*
    Budget *198*
    Staff Education Program Areas *198*
    Program Planning *207*
    Identifying Educational Needs and Interests *208*
    Program Evaluation *210*
    Understanding the Adult as a Learner *212*
    Audio-Visual Instruction *214*
    Trends in Hospital Education *215*

17. Recruitment *217*
    Promotion Policies *217*
    Sources *217*
    Legislative Enactments *218*
    Staff Shortage *219*
    Turnover *221*
    Exit Interview *223*

18. Research *225*
    Meaning of Research *225*
    Scientific Base for the Practice of Nursing *226*
    Nurse Director's Role *227*

Human Rights *229*
Research Process *231*
Role of Nursing Personnel *231*

Part III References *235*

Part IV. Establishing and
Maintaining the Physical Environment

19. The Nursing Unit *243*
Size *243*
Shape *244*
The Patient's Room *244*
The Nurses' Station *246*
Special Rooms *247*

20. Review of Facilities *249*
Privacy and Efficiency *249*
Expansion and Maintenance of Facilities *250*

21. Safety *253*
Infection Control *255*
Occupational Safety and Health Act *257*
Getting Involved with OSHA *258*
Noise Control *259*

22. Supplies and Equipment *263*
Procurement Department *263*
Standardization Committee *264*
Establishing a System for Selection of Supplies and Equipment *265*

Part IV References *269*

Part V. Establishing and
Maintaining the Human Environment

23. Interactions of Nursing Service Administration *273*
Behavioral Science Concepts *273*
Communication *278*
Morale *282*
Discipline *284*

24. Unions *289*
Why Employees Join Unions *289*
Why Employees Reject Unions *291*
Union Objectives *291*
The Legal Framework *293*
Management-Union Relationships *295*

25. Present and Future Nursing Management *297*
    The Hospital Administrator *297*
    Hospital Departments *300*
    Medical Staff *303*
    Nursing Education *307*
    The Community *309*
    The Health Maintenance Organization *309*
    Change *310*
    The Nurse Director *323*
    Emerging Roles in Nursing *323*

    Part V References *327*

                                                      Appendixes

    1. Patient's Bill of Rights *331*

    2. AHA Chronology of Major Federal Health Planning
       Legislation *333*

    3. Philosophies of Nursing Service *335*

    4. Objectives *343*

    5. Items in Operating Budget *347*

    6. Items of Equipment, Capital Expenditure Budget *351*

    7. Hospital Calendar Budget *353*

    8. Nursing Calendar Budget *355*

    9. Nursing Definitions *359*

   10. Peer Review Guidelines *363*

   11. A Peer Review Tool for Directors of Nursing Service *375*

   12. Weekly Nursing Assignment *383*

   13. Individual Nursing Assignment *387*

   14. Nursing Care Plans *391*

   15. Standing Committees *401*

   16. In-service Education Program *415*

   17. Orientation Program *421*

18. Head Nurse Development Program *427*

19. Learning and Change *433*

20. Learning Experiences and Resources *435*

21. Nursing Research *437*

22. Nursing Service Committees *441*

23. Guidelines for Obtaining Approval for Nursing Studies *443*

24. Guide for Writing Study or Research Proposal *445*

25. Guidelines for Implementing Change *447*

Index *451*

The purpose of this book is to deal with concepts of administering nursing service and of the management necessary to implement them. The book was written to assist nurse directors who have had no formal preparation for the role of administrator, nurse directors with the required educational preparation but no experience, and nurse directors with no administrative background.

The text is divided into five parts. Part I presents an overview of trends in the delivery of health care and discusses patient needs in a hospital and the importance of sound nursing leadership in an increasingly complex situation. Part II considers the organization and administration of a hospital and how the nursing department relates to the whole. The functions and responsibilities of the nurse director are discussed. The concept of management and its functions of planning, organization, leading, and controlling are reviewed. Part III discusses certain managerial tools that contribute toward improving the administration of nursing service. Parts IV and V deal with the ways in which nursing administration can establish and maintain the environment of which it is a part. Part IV considers the physical environment; Part V, the human environment. As a supplement to the text, certain forms and lists of interest to administrators appear in the appendixes.

Nursing service administration is primarily concerned with making its share of the hospital organization effective through the process of management. Administration may be perceived as a vibrant, dynamic, challenging human activity or as a frustrating, unrewarding experience; or it can be viewed as a combination of these characteristics. The nurse director who wishes to participate in administration needs a well-thought-out philosophy of what she believes about administration. Administration is a human activity concerned with the survival and maintenance of an organization, the direction of the efforts of people working together in a relationship to accomplish the organization's purpose, and public relations, in the sense of obtaining material and moral support for an organization. Administration is generally responsible not for performing the work of an organization but for attending to its performance. As an organization becomes larger, administration becomes more distinguishable.

Administration is administrators; it is outstanding individuals, according to Dimock;[1] it is people who in their personalities and characters exhibit an integration of universal values such as wisdom, reverence, honesty, and integrity. These are the people who can most safely be entrusted with the governing function of a setting; they are the people who breathe life and spirit into the philosophy, goals, and structure of an organization.

It takes very special people to secure real unity and integration within a setting, and thus the personal qualities of an administrator have a great deal to do with the result achieved. George Berkley[2] says that a new organizational structure is emerging and that structure is moving from a pyramid to a circle — the management function is one of coordination and support rather than the exercise of authority. This new pattern is producing a new kind of leader, who is more tolerant of nonconformity; a new, humanistically oriented administrator is beginning to emerge in organizational life. Organizations are putting stress on ideas rather than resources, and they need administrators capable of coping with the trends, issues, and forces in society. Berkley sees the passing of the charismatic leader, which marks the beginning of a new era when people will look to themselves to supply their own human essence. The new administrator is the one who creates and maintains conditions that will enable people to do so. With the enlarged role of professionals and specialists in hospitals, the leadership role will become diffuse and almost invisible. Confucius once said that the right to govern is dependent on the leader's ability to make the governed happy; when the best leader's work is done, the people will say, ". . . we did it ourselves."

The nurse director who wishes to be effective must learn to get the right things done. Her work is governed by her concept of administering nursing service, her recognition of its potential, and her respect for the unique position of leadership. She will strive to remove every obstacle from the way of the nursing staff members who are actually rendering services. While nursing administration is involved in managing a myriad of activities within the hospital, the patient is not just one of many concerns of a nursing service department. The patient is the reason for the existence of the service, and the total effort of the service must be directed toward patient care.

[1] Marshal Dimock. *A Philosophy of Administration* (New York: Harper & Row, 1958), p. 5.
[2] George Berkley. *The Administrative Revolution* (Englewood Cliffs, N.J.: Prentice-Hall, 1971), p. 16.

Helen Weber, Professor of Nursing, Indiana University, says:

If whatever we know — even now — could be applied, we would be giving a quality of nursing care never before achieved. The universal problem is how present and future knowledge can be applied effectively. Applied effectively in spite of activity pressures; applied effectively where traditional ritualistic behavior and relationships exist; applied effectively within the economics of hospital care. . . . Leadership in the implementation of knowledge is essentially an administrative function.

M. D.

Acknowledgments

The first revision of this book would not have been possible without the assistance of the many persons who contributed to the original publication. Additional support, encouragement, and assistance have been given by: Dr. Peggy Ledbetter and Mrs. Jane Jenkins, College of Nursing, Northwestern State University of Louisiana, Shreveport; Mr. Earl Kephart and Mrs. Barbara Foss, Veterans Administration Hospital, Shreveport; Miss Ellen Lynch, Deaconess Hospital, Evansville, Indiana; Colonel Glennadee Nichols and Major Elizabeth Gortner, Academy of Health Sciences, United States Army, Fort Sam Houston, San Antonio, Texas; Miss Carol Buisson, School of Nursing, Louisiana State University, New Orleans; Mrs. Barbara Bilentnikoff, Southeastern Louisiana University, Hammond; Mr. John Watkins, Editor, *The Journal of Nursing Administration;* Mr. John Nelson, Schumpert Hospital, Shreveport; Mrs. Grace Peterson, De Paul University, Chicago, Illinois; Dr. Patricia Trussell, University of Central Arkansas, Conway, Arkansas; Miss Mary Roth and Mrs. Ivy Hill, Mercy Hospital, New Orleans; Mrs. Dorothy Hausman, University of Evansville, Evansville, Indiana; Mrs. Helen Roth, Mrs. Mary Mullin, and Mrs. Norma Madden, Evansville; and Mrs. Helena Karn, Mrs. Wanda Brooks, and Mrs. Janice Taylor, Veterans Administration Hospital, New Orleans. I am especially grateful to all those people who provided suggestions to build on the content of the original text.

I thank Little, Brown and Company — and especially Christopher Campbell, Nursing Editor; Mr. Robert Davis; and Mrs. Katharine Tsioulcas — for their guidance and counsel during the revision of this book.

M. D.

Nursing leaders need considerable knowledge and skill in politics, economics, social policy, normative values, and in management strategies and processes. They must be not only politically and intellectually astute, but they must be good risk-takers, fairly aggressive, active pursuers of issues, and alert to alternative strategies in pursuit of an objective. They must have strong egos, a positive sense of personal identity, and a determination to preserve desirable professional values.

Madeleine M. Leininger, The leadership crisis in nursing: A critical problem and challenge, *The Journal of Nursing Administration* 4(2):28, 1974

Part I. The Patient and His Needs

NURSE DIRECTOR ROLE

As administrative providers of health care, nurse directors must extend themselves beyond the walls of the hospital; they need to develop a social consciousness if they are going to provide the necessary leadership for nursing and health care. There must be a sensitivity to the many changes that are occurring in our social system and its health care. The progressive nurse director not only must be familiar with the best procedures and tools for the discharge of her daily responsibilities within the hospital but also must have extensive knowledge of the many environmental factors and trends that influence, or could influence, what she and the hospital can undertake. The nursing profession must be both informed and motivated toward understanding the rapidly changing scene in the delivery of health care as plans are made for patients and their needs.

TRENDS AND ISSUES

The necessity of designing an effective health care system is near the top of the priority list of our domestic problems. Health care has moved into the foreground of public policy debate. There is every indication that many difficult issues surrounding this complex field will remain at the center of public affairs for a long time. As is evident from the literature, a national debate continues to rage regarding the financial and organizational aspects of legislative proposals for health care delivery [10].

Social, political, and economic values are evolving in directions that will place the highest premium on upgrading the quality of life. Standards of what is important are changing. People at every level of life are seeking different goals, with which are associated higher values. Society is experiencing a change from competition to care, to a sophisticated concern for self-growth and self-actualization. The quality of life is as much a concern as life itself. All sectors of the population are seeking and demanding quality assurance health care [10].

The rising educational level of our population coupled with improved economic standards and federally supported programs for the geographically and economically disadvantaged has increased the expectations of people for health care services. The impact of third-

3

party insurance carriers and federal programs for prepaid health care contribute to public expectations of the services available for both preventive and acute care measures.

As a nurse director reflects on these changing times in health care delivery, she must explore what she believes about health; how health is defined serves as a base for action and a means for shaping the health care system. The meanings and perceptions of health vary, reflecting value judgments and the assumptions these judgments may hold regarding health. The perceptions of health are further determined by one's culture, historical period, and the role of the professionals. Aristotle said: "Health of mind and body is so fundamental to the good life that we believe if men have any personal rights at all as human beings, then they have an absolute moral right to such a measure of good health as society and society alone is able to give them."

It is part of our country's philosophy that:

1. Health care is a basic right of all people.
2. Everyone in our society should have access to health care.
3. Health care should be so organized that a person would know exactly where, when, and how to seek what is needed.
4. Health care means a focus on the quality of life in general and maintaining a healthy population.
5. The hallmark of health care is its comprehensiveness, with major emphasis on completeness and continuity.

With these forces in mind, health care trends point toward:

1. National health insurance.
2. Expanded role of consumers in health care delivery.
3. Health care as a right.
4. Focus of health care from illness to wellness.
5. Increasing role of government in the planning process of health care.
6. Involvement of health care professionals in meeting social needs.
7. Changing roles of health professionals.
8. Collective bargaining among health personnel.
9. Movement toward humanizing the delivery of health care.
10. Peer review among health professionals.

11. Development of quality assurance programs for health care delivery.
12. A more systematic approach to health care delivery.

With these trends are many issues that are of concern:

1. What can be done about the fragmentation and lack of continuity in health care services?
2. What can be done about the proliferation of new health workers?
3. What can be done about the rapid obsolescence of practice skills and knowledge among providers of health care?
4. How will health care be financed?
5. What can be done to cut health costs?
6. What is the proper role of power, authority, and leadership in health care?
7. How can physical facilities and manpower be redistributed for better utilization and accessibility?
8. How can the quality of care be controlled?
9. What can be done about obsolescence of the health care structure resulting from improved technology and automation?
10. What should be the role of the community hospital in the health care delivery system?
11. What should be the role of the federal government in the delivery of health care?
12. Should health-oriented facilities within a community consolidate services and facilities?
13. Should health care services be organized around the concept of profit?
14. How can consumers of health become informed and responsible participants in solving health care problems?

Leininger [9] says that there is growing public frustration concerning the dehumanization and depersonalization of health care. Some of the humanistic issues and questions she identifies are the following:

1. Are health care professionals becoming less compassionate and less sensitive to people's feelings, thoughts, and needs — and what factors appear to be contributing to dehumanizing services?

2. The most precise and scientific health treatment given without human warmth, interest, or compassion for another person will seldom be effective for most patients.
3. Helping consumers and health care professionals who are genuinely interested in ways to increase the quality and quantity of health care services based on a humanistic approach is undoubtedly one of the greatest challenges before us.
4. With the growing concern that health care is rapidly becoming machine-centered, machine-controlled, and highly impersonal, today's challenge for us is to reaffirm and reestablish the human dimensions of care. Philosophically, nursing has maintained a humanistic posture in the delivery of nursing care and is accorded that stature by the general public.

The humanistic point of view must become central, and human values must be restored to their proper order of precedence over impersonal forces and interests. A viable future will have to be humanistically rather than technologically oriented. The question is not whether we need technology, but rather how and in whose interest it is being used [9].

The responsibilities of nursing are evolving in response to the changing needs of society, as in health service; however, the *care* function remains constant. Nursing will continue to play a unique role in assuring health care delivery that is holistic, personalized, and humanized — to the individual, the family, and the community [9].

A nurse director needs considerable knowledge and ability to deal with the trends and issues in health care delivery; this knowledge is related to politics, economics, social policy, normative values, and management strategies and processes. The nurse director must also be a good risk-taker, fairly aggressive, and an active pursuer of issues [9]. The contemporary nurse director will be expected to serve as a political activist and to know what is happening legislatively; she must speak clearly and concisely to those areas affecting nursing and health care. She can assist political groups and candidates to define issues. By striving to know legislators — their interest and expertise — she can help to set the stage for issues related to health care.

An article by Agnes Flaherty in *The American Nurse*, April, 1975, stated: "The profession identifies nursing as a vital force in designing and implementing a viable health care delivery system." Nurses, recognizing the implications for political action, have established the Nurses' Coalition for Action in Politics (NCAP). Both the American Nurses' Association and the National League for Nursing are well committed to their role in becoming politically involved at a national level.

Nurse directors can participate in community, consumer, and other group activities to examine trends and issues in health care. Through political action, the community can be perceived as the basic building block in developing progressive health plans. It is obvious that the present health care system will change as a result of political action. Whether or not the changes under debate in the Congress today will provide more and better health care and whether or not revisions in the health care system will make it possible for nursing to maximize its contribution to health care should be a matter of concern to all nurse directors.

PROFESSIONALS, CONSUMERS, AND GOVERNMENTAL CONCERNS

Health care professionals, consumers of care, and the federal government recognize that the delivery of health care services is a major concern to all. Their efforts are being directed toward developing a more effectively, efficiently, and economically organized health care system. "As a nation we must provide better quality, more convenient health care for all the people, at reasonable cost, and in a manner in keeping with human dignity. This must be done because we accept one basic, irreducible principle: *Health care is an inherent right of each individual and of all the people of the United States*" [1].

Health Care Professionals

Health care professionals and providers are faced with the problem of meeting health care needs within a complex social setting of health care. The system is constrained, at least for now, by a shortage of qualified providers. The distribution and geographical location of providers limit the providing of health care to specific communities in our society. There is much talk about more interdisciplinary work among providers, and frequent recommendations are heard that they should collaborate more. Rarely is a clear analysis found of why such interdisciplinary, collaborative work is so infrequent or so difficult. Many of the pressing problems that face society today are so complex that no single health profession can ever hope to deal with them effectively. In this context, a basic criticism has been leveled at the health care professions — that they have failed to develop connections to other professions and have not prepared their practitioners in the skills of working collaboratively with other practitioners. Health providers have not been able to look at problems holistically, to use total systems concepts, or to identify the interconnections between areas they are traditionally responsible for, and they have not reduced the conceptual boundaries that exist among these areas. Health care providers are striving for autonomy when society's problems require more collaboration between professionals and consumers and among professionals themselves.

In developing an effective health care delivery system, the Hepners [5] say that beyond the physician, nurses, and other paraprofessionals who surround health care, the efforts of others are needed: (1) the architect, to build more effective facilities; (2) the anthropologist and the sociologist, to ensure that the facilities and procedures are in line with the prevailing cultural values; (3) the economist, to develop cost-effectiveness; (4) the lawyer and the politician, to make possible the location of health care centers in places ordinarily used for other purposes; (5) the engineer, to design better automated diagnostic procedures, prosthetic devices, and other mechanical aids; and (6) administrators, managers, behavioral scientists, clergy, educators, and many others, to help the community develop and effectively utilize the health-oriented facilities that are available.

Changing social values have caused providers of health care to call for rethinking of their roles; for example, they can (1) show concern with the poor, powerless, and those who cannot pay for services; (2) assume an advocacy role; (3) set out to improve society; (4) initiate change; and (5) challenge existing norms [5].

While much of the burden has been placed on the providers, there is another great source of untapped health manpower. Because of the responsibility of the individual citizen in the maintenance of his own health, and the increasing role of the patient and his family in the management of long-term illness, they, too, can share in providing health care.

Consumers

Consumers of health care are now much more sophisticated with regard to their health needs and rights (see Appendix 1) and expect to become involved in their care. Consumers' participation in health services has grown out of the efforts of the recipients of health care to influence the institutions providing this care to them. Consumers from diverse economic and social backgrounds want a greater voice in the delivery of health care for two reasons: (1) Increasing dissatisfaction with the current system has caused many people to believe that the health care system should be changed and that consumers of health care should participate in making the changes; and (2) the acceptance of consumer participation has been aided by the realization that many decisions involving health care delivery do not require highly technical medical knowledge, but, instead, knowledge of community wants and needs [14]. Consumers want: (1) the optimum available health care as a basic human right, rather than a privilege determined by ability to pay; (2) a more efficient system of health care that will preserve freedom of choice; (3) knowledge about health, disease, treatment, and rehabilitation; and (4) prepaid comprehensive insurance, even if this entails compulsory health insurance.

The docile patient who accepts treatment without questioning is rapidly disappearing. Patients are beginning to ask questions and to want understandable answers about their treatment in health-oriented settings. At the same time, the consumer must learn to accept responsibility for the maintenance of his own health and to respect other persons' health. Some people eat too much, while others may drink too much, work too long, exercise too little, or drive carelessly. The solution to many problems requires the active participation of the patient in the maintenance of health and the prevention of disease.

Communities are faced with a war against illness and poor health as well as poverty, social troubles, group conflict, individual greed, hunger, and hopelessness. These are the elements against which the health care system must fight to achieve the goal of adequate health care for all.

Role of the Federal Government

The federal government has designed health care programs in response to the needs of the American people. Through these programs, the government continuously seeks to bring closer the day when high-quality care will be equally available and equally utilized throughout the country. Major federal programs such as Medicare, Medicaid, regional medical programs, Partnership for Health, Hill-Burton, the Community Health Services and Facilities Act, and the Comprehensive Health Planning and Resources Development Act (see Appendix 2) have come into existence. The question in the minds of many people involved in the delivery of health care is what effects these programs will have on hospitals. Some experts in the field believe that the answer lies in an extremely constructive relationship and evolving interdependence between the hospital and its community. Solving the problems of health care cost and the quality and equality of medical care requires joint consideration by the hospital and the community [6].

The former Partnership for Health program has brought about state- and area-wide health planning groups. In order to bring comprehensive health services to the community, hospitals participated in planning activities and provided leadership. Consequently, a major impact of federal programs on hospitals during the next decade will be escalation of the hospital planning function, from the construction level to the full-scale, three-dimensional community service level. Comprehensive health planning, which includes all institutional, manpower personnel, and community health care needs, must be meshed with overall community planning if health care is to be effective [6]. The hospital is asked to support area-wide planning in cooperation with all other health care institutions in the community, because only through planning can the present and future health needs of the community be determined. Once this determination is made, each institution can identify its role, define its service area, and plan to meet its share of the community's health needs. Such action will prevent fragmentation, avoiding gaps as well as duplication of services. The planning aims at making a full range of services available for patient care [6].

COMPREHENSIVE HEALTH CARE NEEDS

Health services are being requested to meet the comprehensive health care needs of the community. Comprehensive care is a system of person- and family-centered service rendered by a well-balanced, well-organized group of professional, technical, and vocational personnel who, using facilities and equipment that are physically and functionally related, can deliver effective service at a cost that is compatible with individual, family, community, and national economic resources. The comprehensive approach may be perceived as including health care, medical care, and patient care [10]. DeGeyndt [3] recently delineated these terms.

Health Care

The primary focus of health care is on the quality of life in general and on maintaining a healthy population (see Figure 1). Health care encompasses preventive supervision, patient care, medical care, and rehabilitation or the maintenance of the individual at his maximum level of functioning. Health care includes social as well as physical health factors — adequacy of nutrition, housing, sanitation, the population's level of health knowledge, and the supply and distribution of

TYPES OF CARE SERVICES

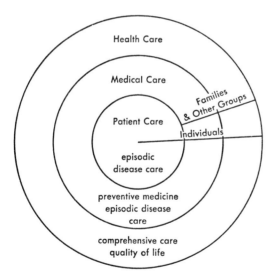

Figure 1. Types of care services. (Reproduced with permission from Hospital Administration — newly retitled Hospital & Health Services Administration — *the quarterly journal of the American College of Hospital Administration, Winter, 1970, p. 23.)*

health personnel and health facilities. The hallmark of health care is comprehensiveness, with major emphasis on completeness and continuity. Care need not be delivered solely by a physician; it may draw upon the whole spectrum of the health disciplines.

Medical Care

Medical care is concerned with the arrest of a pathological process and involves early diagnosis and physical rehabilitation when needed; the focus is on disease and the medical aspects of the care process. The terms *medical care* and *health care* include the concept of patient care but emphasize the appropriateness, availability, accessibility, and acceptability of a full range of services to prevent illness and disease and to maintain and restore health. Medical care and health care also include the social, economic, political, and organizational aspects of the delivery of care, not only to individuals but to families and other groups.

Patient Care

Patient care refers to the elements, procedures, and consequences of applying a number of inputs, including labor, capital and materials, knowledge, skills, and judgment, to the care of individual patients by physicians. The physician has a direct professional responsibility for each patient, and he may or may not be assisted by other medical, paramedical, or nonmedical persons. Patient care may be provided in a variety of settings: the home, the clinic, the office, the hospital, the extended-care facility, or the nursing home. Patterns of referral and consultation with other health professionals are taken into consideration.

HOSPITAL ROLE

A noticeable change can be seen in the role of hospitals. There is no such thing today as *the* hospital — there are hospitals. In programs, sizes, goals, resources, and histories, their differences are greater than their similarities. Hospital goals have gradually shifted over the years in response to changes in philosophy, scientific knowledge, and perceptions of the varied hospital services that are possible. In 1860 "the hospital" may have been described as an institution primarily concerned with charitable care of people in need. Today the word *hospital* must be modified in order to know what is meant, because shifts in goals have brought about specialization. There are general hospitals for care of the acutely ill, providing short-term care; chronic disease hospitals, providing long-term care; hospitals for specific illnesses; small community hospitals; large medical centers; government hospitals; and nonprofit voluntary hospitals. In its broadest modern meaning, the hospital is a social instrument whose purpose is to serve the whole community, the sick and the well. Service to the members of the community is not the hospital's only role, but one of a complex of services — education, research, and preventive and rehabilitative medicine as well [4].

A theme that seems to prevail in current health care literature is the concept of the hospital as the central core around which the community health center can develop. The hospital is beginning to act as the coordinating center for the community's total health care needs. Although experts recognize that the hospital as such does not have all the significant services necessary to provide comprehensive care, they believe that it is better equipped than any other institution to coordinate these services in a community setting.

In response to community needs, hospitals are broadening their vision and collaborating with one another in order to chart an effective course. The dimensions of the problem are so large that no one hospital has the physical or financial ability to carry the burden of comprehensive care alone. As social institutions functioning as health centers, hospitals are being asked to become the center of a configuration — a community pattern of health services. They will continue to command respect in their communities if they are genuine health centers rather than acute illness centers. Hospitals are no longer private, independent entities accountable to their own individual good intentions; they are publicly accountable.

The ultimate role of hospitals in relation to the delivery of health care is not yet clear. Will the hospital become a complex center of comprehensive and continuing health services? Health care responsibilities are not yet well defined; hence the need for study and research to identify a structural framework to coordinate the health needs of the people with resources, materials, and heterogeneous workers [7].

For the nurse director and her staff, this changing role of the hospital means greater participation with other health disciplines in contributing toward solutions for meeting health care needs. Together they must try to identify and understand the various and ever-changing systems of health care and determine how nursing is related to them. Thus sound nursing leadership at the service level is of paramount importance [7].

While hostpitals strive to accommodate and adjust to rapid changes, to complex care programs, and to outside pressure to expand their role, they must still furnish a proper environment in which the needs of patients can be met. The operation of a hospital must be directed toward providing for a patient's needs — physical, diagnostic, therapeutic, emotional, spiritual, and those connected with continuing care.

ADMINISTRATION

The hospital is held together systematically and holistically by a group of people — the board of directors, the hospital administrators, and the department heads responsible for major patient services. The administrators give cohesiveness, coherence, and order to the great mission of providing health care. Administration encourages effectiveness, efficiency, comprehensiveness, and economy in carrying forward the philosophy, purposes, and objectives of the hospital.

MEDICAL CARE

The patient needs to be assured of adequate medical care while in the hospital. The medical staff is the heart of the hospital, and the degree to which the physicians are organized determines the quality of patient care. The medical staff should be organized into essential committees that assume the responsibility of advising, disciplining, and evaluating performances of the members of the staff.

Emergency Care

As the medical center of the community, the hospital stands for service in any time of need. It has, for example, a moral obligation to provide a special unit for emergencies. The emergency service should furnish care and treatment for people requiring emergency measures. It should also be available as an information center for emergency questions from the community, especially concerning antidotes for poisons. The service may be used as a receiving area for the evaluation of acute-trauma accident cases, intoxication, and poisoning. Good medical coverage is necessary for good emergency service [13].

15

Outpatient Care

The recognition of health care as a right rather than a privilege implies the goal of a coordinated system of comprehensive health care. Adequate outpatient programs constitute an increasingly important part of that goal. They should include: multiphasic screening, preventive services, diagnostic and treatment services, home care programs, health-related social services, and a network of relationships with other health care programs. Providing such services may involve the hospital in operating satellite units of various types.

HOSPITAL ADMISSION

Patients need to be provided without delay with an effective and efficient admission process into the hospital. People entering the hospital are worried and apprehensive and would probably rather be any other place than there. Their first impression of the hospital depends upon members of the admitting staff and their performance. Patients in all stages of physical and emotional pain must be dealt with expeditiously and yet tactfully. Admission has many meanings for them and their families. Distraught relatives or friends are almost always present to "protect" and "comfort" those being admitted [13].

DIAGNOSTIC SERVICES

For the patient's diagnostic and therapeutic needs to be met, radiological and pathological services of adequate quality and quantity must be available to the attending physician. Radiological examination, properly employed, permits the recognition of many conditions not otherwise identifiable in a living patient and the planning of logical treatment. The pathology service is primarily concerned with investigations that reveal normalcy or degree of deviation from normal. Tissues, blood, bone marrow, cerebrospinal fluid and other body fluids, excretions, and other materials collected from the patient are examined. Postmortem examinations are conducted to determine causes of death and to study disease processes [13].

DRUG THERAPY

As a result of progress in the physical and medical sciences, numerous new drugs are available to treat the sick. These new drugs are extremely potent and widely used and have profound physiological and toxic effects upon patients. A wide variety of therapeutic agents are prescribed by physicians for patient care, and a knowledgeable pharmacist can be of inestimable help to hospital physicians in suggesting the best possible agents. Since the average inpatient of today receives large dosages of expensive drugs, the safety of the hospital and the patient demands that pharmacy personnel be acquainted with the stability, action, and toxicity of these agents [13].

PATIENT PROTECTION

The hospital assumes a heavy responsibility to the people who commit themselves to its care. It accepts the obligation to protect the patient's person, his property, and his reputation. His physical body must be guarded from injury, both physical and mental. He must be safe from exposure to known or suspected infectious disease and from known, suspected, or unforeseeable hazards [8].

Protection of property extends to the worldly goods that the patient may bring to the hospital. Protection of reputation extends to such confidential information as the patient may have revealed to his physician or members of the hospital staff for the purposes of obtaining treatment. This also includes his right of privacy [8].

The hospital must further shield the patient by ensuring accommodations that are safe and capable of providing the security and quality of care that his condition calls for. The administration must also be certain that the equipment used in the hospital is safe, adequate to the needs of the patient, and in accordance with up-to-date medical knowledge. Supplies have to be sufficient in quantity, modern, safe, and capable of meeting the needs of patient care, diagnosis, and treatment.

Careful consideration in the selection of physicians, hospital employees, volunteers, students, or others who will render services to patients is required. It is essential that personnel have the knowledge, the experience, and the general ability to carry out their respective tasks. The hospital has as great a responsibility to keep incompetent persons from caring for the patient as it does to guard against a short circuit in the electrical wiring. In addition, the hospital must protect the patient from doing injury to himself or from being injured by others.

NURSING SERVICES

The central focus of all nursing service activities is providing for the patient. This requires taking into account each patient's needs such as movement and exercise, spiritual well-being, hygiene, comfort, nutrition, safety, communication, and learning and then basing the plan of care on these needs. While nursing cannot furnish everything the patient requires, nurses have the coordinating responsibility of working with members of allied disciplines — medical staff, dietitians, social workers, pharmacists, and others — to supply a comprehensive program of hospital care. The nursing service department is maintained throughout the 24-hour period to implement that program [8].

SPIRITUAL CARE

The spiritual needs of patients are often apparent during illness, and the hospital should provide pastoral care. To offer a patient spiritual counsel is in keeping with treating the whole person. Many personal questions become urgent at a time of illness; the patient finds himself with time to think about himself and the world around him. The hospital chaplains and clergy of the community contribute significantly to meeting patients' spiritual concerns.

Nine groups of people who appear to be in need of pastoral care are: (1) patients who are lonely and seldom have visitors, (2) those who express fear and anxiety, (3) those whose illness is directly related to emotions or to religious attitudes, (4) those who are scheduled for surgery, (5) those who have to change their pattern of life as a result of illness or injury, (6) those who are concerned about the relationship between their religion and their health, (7) those who are unable to have their pastor visit or who would not normally receive pastoral care, (8) those whose illness has social implications, and (9) those who are dying [8].

DIETARY REQUIREMENTS

Goals of the hospital's service with regard to dietary needs of patients are: (1) optimum nutrition of the patient, (2) maintenance of morale, (3) dietetic education of patients, and (4) achievement of these goals with maximum efficiency and resulting economy. Proper nutrition requires knowledgeable purchasing of equipment and foods, professional planning of standard and therapeutic diets, scientific food production, and a well-planned system of food distribution from kitchen to patient. The morale function calls for consideration of the aesthetics of food service, including color, consistency, and temperature. The timing of meals is also important [13].

The dietary service staff has a significant contribution to make toward the education of patients and their families about their dietary requirements. Meals that are soundly planned, prepared, and served are in themselves an education to patients. This is especially true when patients and their families get together for an explanation and discussion about special diets [13].

SOCIAL SERVICE

The social factors that have helped to make the patient ill, the social problems that his illness creates for him, and the obstacles that may limit his capacity to make use of what medicine has to offer are of importance to his physicians and the health team.

The physician and the hospital personnel are concerned with understanding the patient's social setting, his relationship with the family group, and his socioeconomic as well as emotional resources. This type of understanding helps ensure integrated help for the patient.

To enhance the usefulness of medical care and to help the hospital achieve its purpose in medical treatment, a social service program should be provided. The social service department represents a logical and hopeful course of action, which the patient can understand, accept, and use to attain and maintain the fullest possible physical and social functioning. Achievement of this result, which involves treating each patient as a unique person, brings into focus a major responsibility of social work in the hospital. Increased knowledge of the close relationships among the physical, social, cultural, and emotional factors in health and disease has helped to bring about social work participation in collaborative responsibilities.

Each patient reacts in an individualized way to a given situation, according to his personality as well as his social and emotional needs. The social worker's knowledge and skill, therefore, are applied primarily through interviews with the patient and the family, in collaborative planning and sharing of information with the physician and other professional persons concerned and with community agencies with regard to the use of their services on behalf of the patient.

RECREATIONAL SERVICE

Recreation is generally recognized as a basic human need because it contributes to well-being and is therefore therapeutic. A recreational service for hospitalized patients does contribute to the therapeutic environment through refreshment and renewal of mind, body, and spirit. Programs must be adapted to the needs and interests of the patient, and they require approval of his physician. Recreational programs may include such activities as art, crafts, dancing, dramatics, hobbies, music, entertainment, nature and outing activities, and various kinds of social activities [13].

VOLUNTEERS

Hospital volunteers help meet the personal needs of patients, help them to accept their hospitalization better, help in their rehabilitation, help them retain or renew their contact with the community, and help break down their isolation from normal living [13].

THERAPEUTIC ENVIRONMENT

A therapeutic environment helps a patient grow, learn, and return to health. It is an atmosphere in which the patient is supported in his perception of himself as a person of worth. The therapeutic environment is oriented to the patient's needs and to his importance as a person capable of solving problems and making decisions. In such an environment patients are encouraged to participate as much as they are able. Psychological independence is promoted by: (1) encouraging the patient to participate in his own plan of care; (2) encouraging him to assume responsibility and make life decisions for himself, within his limitations; (3) helping him to develop patterns of response to stressful stimuli that are compatible with physical and psychological growth; (4) helping him to function in his sociologically defined roles within his family and the community; and (5) helping him to make realistic plans for the future [8].

MEDICAL RECORDS

The medical record is a written account of all significant clinical information pertaining to a patient; it is sufficiently detailed to enable the practitioner to give effective continuing care to the patient as well as to determine at a future date what the patient's condition was at a specific time and what procedures were carried out. It also enables a consultant to give an opinion after his examination of the patient. A written medical record is maintained on every patient admitted to the hospital as an inpatient, outpatient, or emergency patient [13].

The purposes of the medical record are to:

1. Provide a basis of communication between the physician and other professionals contributing to patient care.
2. Serve as a basis for planning individualized patient care.
3. Furnish documentary evidence of the course of the patient's illness and treatment during each hospital admission.
4. Serve as a basis for analysis, study, and evaluation of the quality of care rendered to the patient.
5. Assist in protecting the legal interest of the patient, hospital, and physician.
6. Provide clinical data for use in research and education.

Patients need to be assured that their care is being properly documented and that their medical record is treated as highly confidential. The fundamental reason for maintaining an adequate medical record is its contribution to high-quality individual care.

EDUCATION AND TEACHING

Both education and teaching are legitimate spheres of activity for hospitals. In order to meet the growing needs of patients and their families for information and knowledge regarding health and its deviations, the hospital can provide learning experiences for consumers. In addition, the hospital maintains a climate and an environment that are supportive of the continuing development of health care providers. By sharing its educational programs and resources (human and material) with the community, the hospital strengthens its ties between the providers and the public.

DISCHARGE SERVICE

Because hospitals provide a protective environment for their patients, the community outside sometimes becomes remote and threatening. At discharge, happiness at being united with one's family and being restored to a state of good health is often mixed with anxiety and fear about the future. A patient may be anxious about becoming a burden to his family or making an adjustment to life as a result of physical limitations. The psychological and physical needs of the patient at discharge can often be met by the patient and his family with support of the health team. Should the patient require the services of another agency, the referral is made prior to his discharge. If a patient is without a family or anyone nearby, members of the health team must assume the responsibility to plan with him, if he is able, for his discharge.

CONTINUITY OF CARE

Patients who are severely disabled or have long-term illnesses must be provided physical medicine and rehabilitation services. Special evaluation is concerned with the degree of disability and how it affects the patient, his family, his work, and his community. Such an evaluation is time-consuming, sometimes necessitates hospitalization, and utilizes the talents of many trained persons.

The basic elements of a department of physical medicine and rehabilitation are the medical section and physical therapy. Other elements are occupational therapy, speech therapy, social service, vocational counseling, prevocational laboratory, psychological services, and rehabilitation nursing.

PATIENT EXPECTATIONS

A majority of patients remain interested in personalized medical and hospital care, provided with competence and kindness and at a reasonable fee. There will continue to be a need for personal efficiency, promptness, and gentleness.

Health services cannot be effectively organized and provided without a clear understanding of the health needs of the people to be served, nor will the health services provided be properly utilized unless they are reasonably consistent with the expectations and demands of the users. Accordingly, there must be active and responsible participation in the decision-making process by the recipients served, including planning, financing, program implementation, and evaluation of health services. There must be a realistic accommodation between what people think their own needs are and what professional health personnel believe their needs to be, as well as an understanding of established needs and the available facilities, manpower, and financial resources [6].

Part I. References

1. American Hospital Association. *Report of the Special Committee on the Provision of Health Services.* American Perloff Committee, Chicago, 1970.
2. Bergen, S., and Schatzki, M. New directions for an urban hospital. *J.A.M.A.* 215:935, 1971.
3. DeGeyndt, W. Five approaches for assessing the quality of care. *Hosp. Admin.* 15:21, 1970.
4. French, R. *The Dynamics of Health Care.* New York: McGraw-Hill, 1968.
5. Hepner, J., and Hepner, D. *The Health Strategy Game.* St. Louis: Mosby, 1973.
6. Hospital Progress 50th Anniversary Symposium. *Hosp. Prog.* 50:61, 1969.
7. Illinois League for Nursing and Illinois Nurses' Association. *Nursing in Illinois.* Chicago, 1969.
8. Kozier, B., and DuGac, B. *Fundamentals of Patient Care — A Comprehensive Approach to Nursing.* Philadelphia: Saunders, 1968.
9. Leininger, M. *Health Care Issues.* Philadelphia: Mosby, 1974.
10. Mechanic, D. *Public Expectations and Health Care.* New York: Wiley, 1972.
11. Mote, J. Continuing Education: Enhancing the quality of patient care. *Hospitals* 50:175, 1976.
12. Novello, D. The National Health Planning and Resource Development Act. *Nurs. Outlook* 24:354, 1976.
13. Owen, J. *Modern Concepts of Hospital Administration.* Philadelphia: Saunders, 1962.
14. Somers, A. *Health Care in Transition.* Chicago: American Hospital Association, 1972.

Part II. The Nurse Director's Role and Management Functions

3. Hospital Organization and the Nursing Service

A hospital as a voluntary community organization is governed by a group of people who have full legal and moral authority and responsibility for the conduct of the hospital and the quality of care rendered to patients [16]. They are responsible for adoption of bylaws and for identification of the purposes of the hospital as well as the means of goal attainment. A competent administrator, appointed by the governing body, is continuously responsible for the management of the hospital, commensurate with the authority conferred on him by the governing body, and consonant with the hospital's expressed aims and policies.

The governing body further delegates to the physicians of the medical staff the right to assess the professional competence of its members and to get them involved in hospital affairs. The governing body requires the medical staff to establish controls that ensure proper standards of professional and ethical care.

The hospital administrator divides the work of the institution into major departments. He organizes functions of the hospital, delegates duties, and establishes formal means of accountability on the part of subordinates. Each department is under the direction of a competent director who is adequately prepared to assume a management role.

Each department director reassigns some of his duties to other managers, and the process continues until all hospital operations have been split into groups of tasks that individual persons can perform. When the hospital administrator places under the direction of one department head all activities relating to a single function, such as nursing services, the organization is said to be functionalized. In recent years, however, two other concepts have been introduced [25]. An administrator may divide and subdivide so that he can promote teamwork, thus narrowing the work assignments of each department. The coordination of activities through teamwork becomes more difficult when people concentrate on specialty areas alone. Another approach is to divide the work at the level of the workers. Those who can vary their work are sometimes greater in output than those who concentrate on a single activity. Even though certain types of activities differ, the hospital administrator may combine activities and put them under one department head because they need close coordination. A clearly recognized common objective is important in securing coordination among diverse activities and achieving success. While there is no magic formula for dividing the work, each administrator and

department director must look ahead and give thoughtful consideration to this task.

Each department is dependent to some degree on all the other
departments to provide patient care; none is functionally independent. The smooth working of the hospital depends upon each department's assuming its full responsibility and being willing to cooperate
and assist other departments.

Every organization or hospital of appreciable size has various levels
of executives: hospital executive directors, assistant executive directors, department directors, supervisors, and head nurses. Although
the titles may vary, all share in the management process. There is
little difference in meaning, except as defined in specific situations,
to denote differences in level of responsibility or prestige. The hospital administrator must therefore decide how much of the managerial function he will retain and how much will be assigned to lower
administrative levels. Should most of the management function be
passed along to the operational levels, or should a large portion be
kept at the highest levels?

NURSING DEPARTMENT

The nursing department must be maintained continuously for a 24-
hour period, 365 days a year, to provide nursing care and nursing services. A distinction is sometimes made between the terms *nursing
care* and *nursing service.* The implication is that *nursing care* refers to
the care of the patient with specific regard to nursing, while *nursing
service* refers to the coordinating responsibility of the nurse, who in
addition to giving nursing care also works with members of allied
disciplines in supplying a comprehensive program of hospital care [27].

This is the only department having daily contact with every patient
and every discipline involved in patient care. Other service departments are coordinated with nursing in order to present a unified effort to provide the best possible care to patients. It frequently happens that when others are absent from the hospital or at a distance
from the patient care unit, nursing administration assumes responsibility for contacting various members of the hospital staff to report
significant findings, and judging when these other staff members
should be called.

As manager of the largest department, the nurse director delegates responsibility to her assistants and supervisors for the actual operations of the nursing department. Supervisors are on the spot, observe what goes on, and are in frequent contact with workers. Supervisors may be assigned to manage two or more patient units within the department, and each unit in turn is managed by a head nurse.

The patient care unit is the area where things are done for and to individuals; it is where the action is and is considered the most costly segment. This is also the site of the most complex and difficult management situation. A myriad of diverse activities must be merged into a cohesive, individualized service for each patient located on the care unit.

TRENDS IN NURSING

In our rapidly changing society the traditional pattern of nursing organizational structure is undergoing experimentation and innovation. Trends indicate an increased decentralization of authority from the nurse director to the various elements in the nursing department. Authority has been confined as far as possible to the head nurse, increasing her responsibilities for administration of the unit and management of patient care planning.

Service Unit Management

Some hospitals are introducing an organizational concept for patient care known as service unit management (SUM) or ward management [32]. Under service unit management the responsibility for carrying out certain non-nursing tasks is given to a unit or ward manager, whose staff works separately from the nursing department.

Several service unit management approaches are in use and vary according to (1) the place of SUM in the hospital organization and (2) the responsibility of the unit manager. In the organizational structure there may be a difference in the person to whom the manager reports: the administrator, an assistant administrator, the director of nursing, or a nursing supervisor. The responsibilities of a unit manager may vary in terms of the number of nursing units, the number of patient beds, and the activities and tasks under his supervision [32].

The advantages generally cited for introducing SUM in hospitals include: (1) reduction in cost, (2) improvement in the quality of care,

(3) saving of professional nursing time and thus reduction of the nursing shortage, (4) increase in personnel satisfaction, and (5) setting the stage for further improvement [32].

Unit management is one approach bringing administration closer to the patient unit and to allocating tasks more appropriately to skill levels. Both nursing and hospital administration look at what is going on in the patient care function, bringing to the surface many of the real problems and issues. The unit management concept may set the stage for additional changes in hospitals such as reconceptualization of nursing, changes in the ancillary departments, decentralization of clerical and other administrative activities, and bringing policy making closer to the patient unit [32].

Clinical Nurse Specialist

The introduction of the clinical nurse specialist may well affect the delivery of nursing services in a hospital. Sims [30] defines her as a nurse with advanced knowledge and competence, capable of exercising highly discriminative judgment in planning, executing, and evaluating nursing care based upon assessed needs of patients having one or more common clinical manifestations. She is able to provide expert nursing care and treatment on the basis of scientific knowledge, clinical acumen, and professional judgment. She is not restricted by assignment to a work location or work period. She is free from a rigid time schedule, so that her skills are available at the most suitable period to meet patient needs. She is responsible for her patients 24 hours a day, seven days a week.

The role and functions of the clinical nurse specialist may include sharing with the physician responsibility for patient care. She makes a systematic assessment of the patient's needs, often with the help of members of the family; prepares a nursing care plan; discusses this plan with the physician in the light of the total medical-nursing regimen; attempts to see that the medical-nursing plan is carried out, with whatever teaching of personnel is required, herself providing any aspect of nursing care needed; continues visits to the patient for evaluation and psychological support, as indicated, even if he is transferred to another unit; provides assistance to the family when needed; coordinates aspects of the patient's care calling for the services of other departments; and makes certain that the patient and his family have received health counseling and assistance with the arrangements that are essential for leaving the hospital. The clinical nurse specialist may carry a case load of her own, is encouraged to undertake clinical investigations to increase her own competence and advance nursing knowledge, and is expected to view herself as a role model of expert clinical practice [30].

Because her position generally stands outside the organizational line on the chart, the clinical nurse specialist may have more freedom to move where and when she believes she is most needed. She serves as a consultant who also acts as practitioner, teacher, and supervisor. Her primary role, in cooperation with the physician, may be viewed as that of a representative of the patient's interests within the concept of comprehensive care [30].

This role raises a number of concerns within a hospital nursing service: The nurse would not be identified as a functionary in the organization, because no clearly defined title or pattern of activities has yet been devised for such a person; she might be resented by the head nurse or general duty nurse because of her apparent freedom of assignment and working time schedule; she would not fit the accepted title or activities pattern of supervisor because she would be more directly involved in patient care than supervision [30].

The role of the clinical nurse specialist has not, so far, made a great impact on hospital nursing services. There is still some question regarding the utilization of the clinical nurse specialist, and there are not yet enough prepared persons available. Each hospital department of nursing must determine for itself what it hopes to accomplish in employing the clinical nurse specialist and in making use of her services.

THE NURSE DIRECTOR'S MANAGERIAL SKILLS

The hospital derives its strength from capable leaders, equipped with superior management skill and a great capacity for hard work. As the hospital becomes larger, more complicated, and more business-oriented in its operation, the administrator will become more concerned that his nurse director fulfill her managerial responsibilities. The effectiveness or ineffectiveness of nursing services to patients can be ascribed to the effectiveness or ineffectiveness of the nurse director as administrator. For the objectives of the hospital to be realized, then, nursing service administration obviously must assure that the nursing service department achieve its purposes.

The nurse director and her nursing administrative staff in a hospital are engaged in two distinct and different professions, namely, nursing and management. Mastery of both is required to do a good job. Viewing the management of the job as a separate profession with a science and art largely independent of nursing has proved to be helpful in other fields of endeavor in developing good management practices [13].

As the task of administering a nursing department in a hospital becomes increasingly complex, the need for identifying and mastering the essentials of management becomes more apparent. Like managers in other kinds of industry, the nurse director has the responsibility for getting work done through others; she coordinates the services of a large number of people with differentiated but interrelated responsibilities so that patients will receive the best possible care. She must study and strive to understand the process of management. In so doing, she will establish a systematic view of management — a framework that helps her think in an orderly fashion about hospital and nursing service management. She will better understand how the essentials of management apply to her daily and long-range affairs. The strength and soundness of her personal convictions in activating management principles frequently are carried over into her management pattern for patient care. The effect of the pattern comes out in the hospital setting, for good or ill.

POSITION OF NURSE DIRECTOR

The American Hospital Association issued the following statement in May, 1971, on the position of the nurse administrator of the department of nursing services in hospitals:

1. The administrator of the department of nursing service should be a registered nurse because a nurse has the unique background to:
   A. Relate directly with the nursing staff.
   B. Represent and interpret nursing to other members of the administration.
   C. Work with the medical and other professional staffs to develop and recommend policies and procedures relative to patient care.
2. The administrator of the department of nursing service should be a member of the top management echelon.

A. Participation and cooperation of the administrator of the department of nursing in formulating policies and procedures is an essential element in accomplishing the administration's objective of coordinating functions among the various departments of the institution.
B. The department of nursing both affects and is affected by the functions of other departments to a significant degree.
C. The department of nursing has control of the single largest number of employees and thus has the greatest impact on payroll cost control.
3. The administrator of the department of nursing service should have sound educational and professional qualifications in administration. The effectiveness of the administrator of the department of nursing service depends largely on the knowledge and the application of management skills to establish and to accomplish goals relative to trends in nursing practice and health service.*

Functions of the Nurse Director

Statements about the recommended functions of nurse directors are available through professional associations and hospital accrediting associations [1, 3, 23]. A comparison of these statements reveals general agreement about responsibilities, duties, and activities. The nurse director is responsible for establishing an organizational framework through which patient care can be provided. She plans, organizes, leads, controls, and coordinates activities of nursing (see Figure 2). As part of her responsibilities she:

1. Develops and implements the philosophy, objectives, policies, and standards for nursing care of patients, which reflect the purpose of the hospital.
2. Provides a written plan of organization designed to implement and facilitate achievement of departmental objectives; indicates areas of responsibility, to whom and for whom each person is accountable, and the major channels for communication.
3. Develops, reviews, and approves departmental policies and participates in the establishment of hospital policies.
4. Determines a master staffing plan which will accomplish departmental objectives and standards of nursing care and promotes the maximum utilization of staff.
5. Prepares and recommends a departmental budget to implement nursing service objectives.

*Source: May 16, 1971, issue of *Hospitals, Journal of the American Hospital Association.*

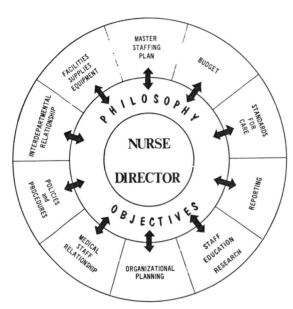

Figure 2. Nurse director responsibilities.

6. Participates in the formulation, implementation, and evaluation of a personnel program.
7. Establishes standards for measurement of the quality and quantity of nursing care to be rendered.
8. Provides and implements education programs and opportunities for staff development.
9. Estimates needs for facilities, supplies, and equipment and institutes a system for evaluation and control.
10. Provides for nursing personnel to plan with the medical staff and other disciplines for the total needs of patients.
11. Collaborates with the administrative staff, other department personnel, and representatives of allied groups in planning services for patients.
12. Establishes and maintains an effective system of records and reports.
13. Initiates and promotes studies and research on administrative, supervisory, and nursing care practices.
14. Plans with an educational institution for the use of hospital

facilities, which includes student learning experience and clinical practice.

15. Participates and promotes membership interest in the activities of a professional nursing association, in allied health organizations, and in community activities.

A s manager of the largest hospital department, the nurse director should recognize that management concepts and principles must become a part of her being. She is generally answerable for 40 percent or more of the hospital staff, and she is under obligation to get work done effectively through other people. She must improve the services of a large number of persons with varied but interrelated responsibilities so that patients may receive the best possible care.

WHAT IS MANAGEMENT?

Management is the process of getting things done through and with people operating in organized groups. It is a universal activity, practiced on one scale or another by almost everyone every day. Its principles extend from home to hospital, from school to the Army, and are fundamental to success in each enterprise. It is recognized, however, that the environment of management differs among these settings. The managing process can best be described by analyzing the functions of the manager, which include planning, organizing, leading, and controlling [17].

It is the task of management to carry out the policies of an organization with the fullest efficiency. It is also up to management to create conditions that will bring about the optimum use of all available resources, human and material. The scope of management is broad. At one end of the scale, management may be concerned with technical details such as the number and the order of movements needed to perform a given patient treatment or the test type of material for a particular nursing procedure. At the other end, it may be concerned with such intangibles as morale, the working climate, or the problems presented in the handling of others and the coordination of a network of human relationships and responsibilities. Management must build the whole into a team, with a working pattern, a rhythm, and a balance of its own [15].

NATURE OF MANAGEMENT

Management has been perceived as a blend of art and science. Scientific management is the result of applying scientific knowledge and methods to different aspects of management and the concerns that arise from them. Science needs to know, to ask why, and not to rest content until it has arrived at a testproof answer whose accuracy can be demonstrated. Scientific management depends very little on one's personality, given the possession of an adequate intelligence, an orderly habit of mind, and an ability to see a subject whole while observing the relationships of its parts. It is based on analysis and a theoretical approach; it can be taught, studied, and tested validly [15].

Some principal aspects of management to which science has contributed in study, in assembling and codifying data, and in developing principles founded on result relate to the selection of employees, training inexperienced workers, the physical background to work (fatigue, accidents, and safety), time and motion study, production planning, organization, administration, accountancy, statistics, and budgeting control [15].

Managers want employees to fit the job in two dimensions — skill and temperament. The potential employee must have an aptitude for the job and be equal (not only physically and mentally, but in the more complex matter of a certain balance of qualities in his or her makeup) to the assigned tasks and type of activities. Sometimes people are placed in a hit-and-miss fashion. Scientific management considers it a waste in human productivity and human satisfaction, as well as economically costly, to use such trial-and-error methods [15].

Scientific management has devised practical aptitude tests to show, in a reliable form, the degree of effectiveness in action to be expected from an employee in any particular job. The tests allow the selector to assess in a short time the kind of knowledge that normally would take months or even years of practical work to find out [15].

Management as an art starts where science leaves off. Science deals with the measurable, calculable, and predictable, but when management extends beyond these parameters, which it does in any busy day, art comes into play. Art is the ability to sense a situation, to respond to its nature and demands in terms of the inner or intuitive senses, which are capable of handling intangibles, rather than assessing by reason, analysis, and logic (with which the science of management must work) [15].

The art of management may be perceived as relating to one's personality. It requires certain qualities that can be learned, developed, and brought into balance by one's experience as his character matures, develops, and becomes rounded out and integrated. Education, training, and practice help. One valid test for management as an art is the production of successful results on a sufficient scale over an adequate period [15].

In certain management situations it matters less that a particular decision can be the right one than that a decision of some sort be given, right or wrong. However, to sense when to wait for the facts and when to render a decision whether the full facts are known or not is no small part of the art of management [15].

The necessity of reacting quickly and responding correctly to the unexpected is present in everyday management activities. Because managing is a social activity, people are faced with the unknown and the unpredictable and must act dynamically, producing change. The art of knowing "when" applies to management as to all other activities: knowing when to ask a question, to admit that one is wrong, to say "yes" or "no," to say nothing. The art of knowing "how" means realizing that, whatever the line of approach used in a specific situation, the outcome will depend not on what is said but on how it is said or put over to those affected [15].

The really progressive nurse director must strive constantly to lead her hospital to greater effectiveness and greater achievement in providing patient care. She recognizes that it is not sufficient, however, to apply sound management principles herself and neglect to instill them throughout the department. Skill in performing managerial functions can be acquired through assignment and through education and training. The nurse director should devote time and budget to supervisory training that goes beyond the needs of her administrative staff's immediate job; she should prepare these employees for advancement to higher nursing management positions.

MANAGERIAL FUNCTIONS*

The management process can be improved with practice and developed through the managerial functions of planning, organizing, leading, and controlling (see Figure 3). Examination of these functions soon reveals how closely they are related and how prevalent they are in every kind of organization.

*Some material in this section has been adapted from Newman, William H., and Summer, Charles E., Jr.: *The Process of Management: Concepts, Behavior, and Practice.* Englewood Cliffs, N.J., © 1971. Adapted by permission of Prentice-Hall, Inc.

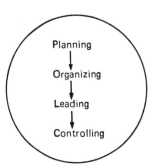

Figure 3. Administration moves into motion the management process.

These functions are present to a greater or lesser extent in all executive jobs — at different levels and in various fields. The job content will vary, but the underlying processes will be similar. In order to expose the full significance of each function, they will be considered individually.

PLANNING

The process of planning covers a wide range of activities, all the way from initially sensing that something needs to be done to firmly deciding who does what when. Planning is much broader than compiling and analyzing information or dreaming up ideas of what might be undertaken. It is more than logic or imagination or judgment. It is a combination of all these processes that culminates in a decision about what is to be done. A nurse director must draw many conclusions, such as determining what facts are important and whose word she can trust — and, broadly speaking, these are decisions [25].

Elements of Planning

A nurse director can improve her ability to plan — to make decisions — by asking herself two questions: (1) What are the elements of making a plan? (2) How are these elements actually carried out in an organization? The four essential elements are (1) diagnosing the problem, (2) finding the most promising solutions, (3) analyzing and comparing these alternatives, and (4) selecting the best plan (see Figure 4) [25].

In making a diagnosis, the first move is to identify and clarify a problem. For example, nurses in certain areas of the hospital were

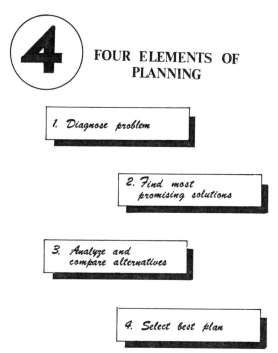

FOUR ELEMENTS OF PLANNING

1. *Diagnose problem*

2. *Find most promising solutions*

3. *Analyze and compare alternatives*

4. *Select best plan*

Figure 4. Four elements of planning.

being asked to obtain portable monitors, similar to those in the Coronary Care Unit, for use in the emergency unit, the delivery room, surgical intensive care, surgery, and the general nursing units. These nurses were apprehensive about using this specialized equipment. The nurse director recognized that additional equipment was needed to provide care to cardiovascular patients outside the Coronary Care Unit; she also realized that the nursing staff needed to receive additional instruction and orientation to their roles in the care of patients to be monitored.

Starting with a situation that needs improvement, the nurse director must locate the obstacles that stand in the way of achievement; she should spell out the essentials of a satisfactory solution. If there are critical restrictions on acceptable solutions, such as limits on money available or on personnel that may be used, she must also state them. A good diagnosis says what is wrong, identifies the causes, gives the requirements for a satisfactory solution, and indicates any significant limits within which the solution must be applicable [25].

In finding alternative solutions, the nurse director must be concerned with what could be done to overcome the obstacles identified by her diagnosis. This element requires imagination and originality. The alternatives can range from doing nothing to finding a means around the difficulty or removing it, to perhaps modifying the objectives [25].

The alternatives must be analyzed and compared. If a choice is to be made among the probable plans, the primary differences have to be recognized. All pertinent data, opinions or accepted facts, must be reviewed in the time available and related to the primary differences. Such an analysis will result not only in a list of advantages and disadvantages for each alternative solution but also in some evidence of the relative importance of particular pros and cons [25].

Finally, the nurse director selects the plan to be followed. Sometimes the one best alternative is not so clear that analysis alone provides the answer. Several factors may need to be balanced, such as morale, cost, acceptance, and patient reaction. Consideration must be given to the differences in probabilities of failure and the chances of partial success. Time and cost may prevent an exhaustive analysis, and the director will have to determine when decisiveness is worth more than increased accuracy. By blending these considerations with the results of objective analysis, she forms an authoritative decision on action to be taken. The course of action is then translated into a complete statement (objective) showing who, what, when, where, how, and why [25].

When dealing with problems, one may find that the elements for rational decision making vary in difficulty. Sometimes a solution is quite evident. Once in a while someone produces such a good solution to an unusual problem that analysis is unnecessary and the final selection is obvious. Few problems yield to an orderly, step-by-step procedure. New alternatives may appear at any time; a problem sometimes needs to be redefined as the analysis proceeds and values are formulated. The entire process is permeated with the gathering of facts and the need for judgment. The four elements comprise a mental framework for decision making rather than a procedural device; they serve as an aid in relating facts and thoughts in a rational pattern.

Purposes of Planning

The planning structure within an organization has several purposes: (1) to provide for consistency of action, which is necessary so that people both inside and outside the organization can anticipate its performance; (2) to provide for integration and coordination of organizational activities; and (3) to permit considerable economy of managerial effort [25]. Every organization has a set of basic plans, and these include objectives for the organization as a whole and subordinate objectives for its subunits. Objectives, policies, procedures, programs, schedules, and budget are all plans that provide a framework within which individual decisions are made [25].

Time Necessary for Planning

Sound planning takes time. It is desirable to consult with other members of the staff and to gather ideas and facts from many sources; this cannot be done on the spur of the moment. Deciding to make a major change in an organization's operations is often just the beginning of a wide range of planning necessary to implement the basic decision, and such planning is far from instantaneous.

The elapsed time involved in planning often serves good purposes. Expert help from different people is made available. The wisdom and consistency of a planning structure are incorporated into the operating decisions. The ramifications of a major decision are exposed, and opportunity for balanced, integrated action is provided.

Planning within an organization tends to become highly involved. The very effort poured into it sometimes complicates the decision-making process. A nurse director then needs to remind herself often of the basic steps in arriving at sound plans of action, and to determine how effectively the steps are being taken. Amid all the conferring, are problems being properly identified? Is creative effort being given to proposing good alternatives? Are the results of the various alternatives being projected with reasonable accuracy and completeness? Are final decisions being made on the basis of balance and objective judgment? Are the many potentialities of using an organization to plan being put to good use [25]?

Difficulties

Planning requires nurse directors to recognize that difficulties do arise. There is always some inertia when joint efforts of several individuals are needed, and someone must provide the enthusiasm and motivation to overcome it. Also important is managerial skill in organizing administrative work, in using planning instruments, and in coordinating the efforts of different personalities. Inept management may cause difficulty in planning.

One major concern is reducing organizational friction, which arises as people bring together their ideas to bear on a decision. A group undertaking inevitably creates problems in social relationships. It is essential that the nurse director be aware of such sources of friction as differences in perception of objectives, distortion and loss in communication, the persuasive ability of the impressive individual, the influence of informal groups, and personal needs. Despite some of these weaknesses, a well-designed organization of people is the best means of planning yet conceived.

The nurse director must then strive to obtain the greatest benefits from dispersion of planning and at the same time to lessen friction. Ways must be identified to reduce friction — for example, creating situations in which personal needs and organizational objectives are both met, building effective communication networks, controlling the influence of staff advisers, integrating informal groups and formal organization [25].

ORGANIZING

Organizing is the preparation for the action to come, with emphasis placed upon interrelating the required activities, practices, resources, and organization into a systematic and practicable pattern [29]. It is a configuration of people and resources put together in a manner apparently best suited to achieve particular objectives. Authority, responsibility, delegation, consultation, and decision making are part and parcel of organization.

Steps in Organizing

The task of organizing usually begins directly after the nurse director chooses the course of action that will best accomplish the desired nursing service objectives. As R. W. Ross [29] lists them, the four general steps of organizing include: (1) formulating departmental structure, (2) developing departmental procedures, (3) determining departmental requirements, and (4) allocating departmental resources (see Figure 5).

When the task of organization begins, one must be aware of certain

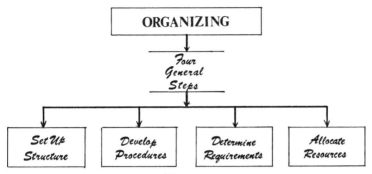

Figure 5. Steps in organizing. (*From Ross* [29].)

basics. Methods must be created for acquiring the necessary resources; structural aspects of the organization must be set up to indicate the activities to be performed and lines of responsibility and authority; policies, procedures, and controls must be worked out; a schedule for the details of performing the activities is needed; a timed plan for achieving certain goals should be devised. All these must be brought together into an operational system for providing nursing services. Then the resources are assembled and the department is brought into being [29].

It is helpful to understand the differences between an organization's *structural* and *procedural components.* The structural part deals with the interrelationships of functions and of people in doing a job; the procedural aspect is concerned with defining and bringing about the necessary conditions that make achievement of the predetermined objectives feasible. The purpose of organizational structure is to create a framework for effective operations, whereas the procedural part builds a system that will specify how to perform the various steps in a task. These components are not independent of each other, nor is it possible to complete one part of the process of organizing before moving to the other. Consideration must be given to the related factors in the entire action. Changes in procedural patterns generally affect the structure of an organization, and it is equally apparent that organizational structure influences the design of operating procedures [29].

The job of *ascertaining requirements for resources* and of *allocating and assembling them* generally follows the structural and procedural developments in organizing. It is assumed that the nature of the objectives, the plan, the structure, and the procedures determine the number and kind of resources necessary, their allocation, and their collection. This aspect of the job requires careful computation, judicious apportionment, and the assembly of resources into a sound pattern — no small task and a real test of managerial competence [29].

The *structural* aspects involve interrelating the different responsibilities. It must be determined which ones will be assigned to particular segments of an organization. The process requires identifying the scope and jurisdiction of the responsibilities growing out of the assigned job, showing the relationship that is decided upon, and developing a means through which orders may start or stop a management action [29].

Basic Structural Concepts

The basic concepts related to the structural element of organizing are unity of command, extent of command, homogeneous assignment, and assignment of responsibility with delegation of authority [29]. As these concepts are understood and practiced, a sound, strong, and workable organizational structure can develop.

Unity of Command. According to Ross [29], unity of command means that the final responsibility for and control of all actions directed toward the goals of an organization are vested in one person at each level of operation. This concept concerns itself with people and their interactions and with operating patterns and procedures. It establishes a definite chain of management echelons. At the same time it serves as a means of control by ensuring and protecting the unified system of procedural directives and orders. It becomes identical with managing a workable system, with making provision for it, and with being accountable for its smooth operation.

Span of Control. The extent of command concept involves the relationship that may exist between a nurse director and the staff she holds responsible for the performance of specific acts. It is based upon the restrictions that she imposes upon the span of her activities. These limits are divided into three parts: span of control of individuals, of distance, and of time. Span of control is sometimes defined as a set of abstract rules and generalizations regarding the number of people a given person may supervise and how much space he can cover [29].

The commonsense span-of-control approach prevents any hard-

and-fast conclusions, on a priority basis, of how many people one can supervise, what distance one can cover, and how to distribute one's time. The specific conditions in a given situation will decide the procedural setup, and the procedural setup will in turn determine the span of control [29].

How many individuals can one person effectively control? In the view of some writers, the optimum number of personnel reporting to one supervisor should be five or six. Modern writers, particularly behavioral scientists, have challenged the belief that a particular, rigid span of control must be adhered to. They contend that the span of control can vary, with wide limits, depending upon such factors as the personality of the manager, the complexity of the work, the level of competence of the subordinates, the geographical dispersion of the employees, and the closeness of control exercised [17].

A narrow span of control permits the manager to exert very close control over his staff. He can make most of their decisions for them. Those who favor rigid control tend to utilize a narrow span.

On the other hand, a wide span of control requires that the employees make their own decisions. They are given more freedom and latitude. A wide span of control encourages general supervision, and if it is to be effective, employees must be well prepared to perform on their own.

Homogeneous Assignment. Homogeneous assignments are those functions essential to the accomplishment of organizational objectives. They are grouped according to the closeness of their relationships to one another. Applying this concept calls for the use of a goodly amount of judgment, especially where the skills needed are not equal to those available. Consideration must be given to integrating related activities as opposed to the advantages of strict organization by function [29].

Delegation. From an organizational point of view, delegation means that when a job gets too big, part of it must be entrusted to someone else. The difficulty lies in identifying what part of the job can best be passed along. How can other people be encouraged to accept willingly the additional tasks, and how can one keep an efficient check on the delegated work being done?

Proper delegation involves three factors: responsibility for the work delegated; authority needed in order to fulfill that responsibility; and accountability, or the obligation to carry out the responsibility and authority.

By responsibility is meant, first, the obligation to do an assigned task and, second, the obligation to be answerable to someone for the assignment. Obligation implies a willingness to accept the burden of a given task for whatever rewards, as the result of success, or risks, as the result of failure, one may see in the situation.

The responsibility assigned to a subordinate implies commensurate authority conferred upon him. This relation is similar to the relation between action and reaction. There is no action without a corresponding reaction. In like manner, there is no assignment of responsibility without the delegation of corresponding authority.

Delegation of authority is preceded by the significant element of assigning a task. The right to action must automatically accompany the assignment of the task. While performance of an act may be assigned to a subordinate, the manager is ultimately always responsible for what the subordinate does. Every manager is responsible to a superior for the achievement of some portion of the organization's program, and his responsibility can never be delegated to anyone else; he can *share* his responsibility with a subordinate, but the fact that a manager has an assistant does not relieve him of the task of getting work accomplished [29].

A subordinate must be accountable for his actions. The superior expects the subordinate to carry out conscientiously the work assigned to him. Responsibility and authority can be delegated, but accountability cannot be delegated.

Effective delegation centers around a personal relationship between two people, the manager and his immediate subordinate. The manager, who is accountable for achieving certain results, looks to the subordinate for the performance part of the job and gives him permission to take certain action. Thus the relationship between these two people grows and shifts. The freedom and initiative that the subordinate is expected to exercise can rarely be spelled out in detail. Work habits and attitudes are shaped by the subtle interplay of the two individuals involved. Delegating a job requires considerable administrative skill. The assigned duties should be well defined and written out, indicating what is to be done. The person to whom work is to be delegated must be assisted to become self-sufficient; delegation will be ineffective if personnel have to keep checking back and asking advice unnecessarily. However, the person delegating the work must maintain contact with those doing the work and determine through some follow-up method whether the work is being done.

A common problem is that managers are reluctant to delegate adequately to their subordinates. A nurse director may fail to delegate to her subordinates if she believes she can do a better job herself. She may lack the ability to communicate to people what is to be done. She may be handicapped by a temperamental aversion to taking a chance for fear that the gains from delegation will not far offset the troubles that may arise [14].

Managers must also recognize that subordinates may not accept delegated tasks because it is easier to ask the manager than to decide for themselves how to deal with a problem. Fear of criticism for mistakes keeps people from accepting greater responsibilities. Lack of necessary information and resources creates an attitude that might make a person reject further assignments. Lack of self-confidence makes a person less inclined to take on more obligations [14].

The nurse director who understands and practices the art of delegation ensures prompt and effective performance of work under her supervision. She also creates the conditions necessary for cooperation and teamwork. Proper delegation is the first step in letting people make their own decisions and learn from their mistakes, and this is a basic ingredient in developing potential nursing managers.

Delegation means giving the employee freedom to exercise some initiative to get the job done. A director must place confidence in her subordinates and recognize that they will not carry out every assignment precisely as she, the director, would.

Delegation is one of the most difficult skills to acquire. It is important because a person's success may be measured largely in terms of work performed for him by other people. It has been found that the critical point in the career of many directors is reached at the stage when they must either learn to delegate or cease to grow. Delegation enables the director to multiply herself and to extend her knowledge, energy, and time through the efforts of others.

Line and Staff Responsibilities

Each individual has an immediate superior who issues orders and instructions. In any organization there are generally two types of positions — line and staff. Line responsibilities are action-producing. They stem from the chain of command that devolves from the top person of an organization down the line of assistants and supervisory personnel to the individual worker. Line positions are those without which the organization could not operate, even for a day.

Staff positions are advisory in nature. Individuals exercising staff responsibility have no line authority and no power to produce action. As a rule they are technical experts in their fields. For example, the personnel director of an enterprise may help a department head with developing safety programs, or in other areas in which his talents can provide assistance. At the top management level, staff persons may help formulate policy and advise and counsel line units. They usually exercise control over the line in their functional field.

The relationship between line and staff employees is often vexing. Confusion and conflict can arise when someone with staff responsibility attempts to assume line responsibility. Overeager staff persons may give orders to line employees, thus violating the principle of unity of command. If an organization has a host of functional people, each of whom has some contact with line personnel, it is obvious that direct order giving is unworkable. By background, staff personnel tend to be innovators, creators, cost reducers, and initiators of change. The constant pressure from staff is sometimes upsetting to the line people, who feel they must constantly defend their position. Line people may be perceived by staff people as being uncooperative. Staff specialists can generally reach the top executive officer more quickly with their proposals than can the line supervisor in many organizations. Usually staff persons are physically located close to the chief executive's office. They are charged with checking up on the performance of operating units. This is carried out by comparing results with standards that have been established, presumably with line participation. Harmonious and cooperative relations can be achieved by a better understanding of the other's role. Staff should look upon itself as a helper to line and not as an instrument demanding line obedience [25].

Organization also implies a group of people working together to achieve the goals of the enterprise. Anyone entering the hospital setting brings with him working habits, attitudes, command of skills, and a drive to accomplish something of value. Through the internal division of labor, an organization reflects the sum total of the interaction of many individuals. As organizational work and activities progress and the pattern of cooperation among the personnel changes through mutual adjustment, there develops what is considered an institutional structure, a way of operating and collaborating that is accepted by the people of the organization as the proper way. Some members of the institution will resist attempts to introduce changes in the setting [14].

Procedural Aspects

The procedural aspects of organizing are concerned with a prescribed way of doing things to achieve a predetermined objective. An operation does not move merely because resources are available; objectives are determined, an organizational structure is built, communication lines are established, and qualified personnel must be available. Procedures blend these elements. Procedures are the means for providing direction to effort and for coordinating it in place and time. Procedures will determine whether the operational system will perform in line with predetermined objectives [29].

LEADERSHIP

Assuming that adequate plans have been prepared and an effective management structure has been established, the third significant managerial function needed is leadership — the dynamic force that stimulates, motivates, and coordinates an organization. Leadership consists of interpersonal influence, exercised in a situation and directed by means of the communication process, toward the attainment of specific goals; it involves attempts by one person (the leader) to affect the behavior of others (the followers) in a situation [33].

The nurse director must deal directly with the use of personnel, material, money, facilities, and equipment, putting them in a definite relation to one another. In carrying out this function she is faced with the fact that one of her resources, personnel, is different from the other resources. Because of them, she cannot properly conduct an operation without some serious regard to the meaning and purpose of the work involved. While the different resources within an organizational system must be integrated, the peculiar characteristics of people require serious consideration because they are the generators of activities.

A director leads by personally and actively working with her subordinates in order (1) to guide and motivate their behavior to fit the plans and the job that have been established and (2) to understand the feelings of employees and the problems they face as they translate plans into actions [33]. The word *personally* in this definition implies that leading is a close, person-to-person relationship. Leading involves the reaction of individual personalities to each other, and it is rooted in the feelings and attitudes that have grown up between the employees over the entire time they have worked together. The word *actively* implies that leading is a dynamic, evolving relationship in which the nurse director must continuously communicate in a way she hopes will induce subordinates to support the hospital and nursing departmental plans and objectives.

The task of guiding and motivating the behavior of employees has many facets. Plans have to be communicated to people in a meaningful way, because some explanation of the purposes of, and reasons behind, a particular action aids a person to understand plans and helps develop his motivation. As plans are being executed, questions of interpretation arise, and adjustments are needed to overcome minor difficulties. Jobs well done should be recognized. Friction between staff members has to be resolved or minimized.

Personal relations and the reactions of individual personalities to one another play a major role. To improve one's ability to lead requires a high perceptiveness about the people involved in a specific situation. A nurse director must develop and understand the meaning of empathy, self-awareness, and objectivity toward others' personal behavior [29].

Qualities of Leadership

Empathy is the ability to look at things from another person's point of view. If the nurse director is to guide, motivate, and get information from a subordinate, she must be able to project herself into that subordinate's position. How does the subordinate feel about the nursing department and her job? How will she interpret the words and actions of her manager? What are her hopes and aspirations? What are her difficulties at present? Whom does she trust and whom does she fear? Empathy is not a matter of asking, "What would I do if I were in your position?" because anyone might bring to the position very different knowledge and feelings. A director is empathetic only when she can sense, almost intuitively, how another person reacts to a situation. A director may set up a new vacation policy or make some other change she intends as an aid to her subordinates, but if she thinks of the change in terms of how she would like it rather than how the people affected will like it, the move is likely to fail. To be empathetic one has to have respect for the other person as an individual [29].

Knowing oneself ranks with empathy as a requisite for leadership.

Each director must be aware of the particular impact she makes. She should know her own tendencies toward, say, taking action hastily, being curt with employees who do not understand directions the first time, or getting so involved in a specific problem that she bypasses supervisors in resolving it [29].

A leader must know how he appears to other people. Many people have images of themselves that differ from the way others see them. A nurse director may think of herself as fair and objective, for example, whereas some of her subordinates may consider her prejudiced in favor of young persons with college degrees. Regardless of what view is correct, she may have difficulty in motivating and communicating with a subordinate who is convinced that she is biased unless she knows the subordinate thinks so. With an awareness of her own preferences, habits, and weaknesses, and of what others think of her, the director should learn what impressions her actions make on others [29].

Another quality crucial to good leadership is objectivity in person-to-person relations. Something causes people to react as they do. If a director can identify the influences on a person's actions, she has taken an important step toward guiding her behavior. Instead of getting angry with someone for resisting a new policy or procedure, she will recognize the person's response and try to find out what caused it. Or if someone is unusually energetic, she will try to understand what motivates her, in the hope of finding a way to induce similar behavior in others [29].

Empathy fosters sympathy and personal identification with other people; yet a good leader must be both objective and empathetic. The viewpoint of a physician is similar to what a leader needs to reconcile these two attitudes. A good physician understands his patients' feelings and is highly empathetic. But his own emotional involvement with his patients must be restricted if he is to make an objective diagnosis. He is well aware of the problems of his patients as individuals, and at the same time he deals with such problems in a detached, scientific manner. An effective leader understands the feelings and problems of his subordinates yet keeps enough psychological distance to be fair, just, and constructively concerned with their performance [29].

A manager is endowed by his position with necessary authority to carry out his responsibilities. He can expect performance from others. Most employees see authority and orders as coming from above.

The power of a leader, and hence his effectiveness, is dependent upon the willingness of his subordinates to accept and support him.

It must be recognized that leadership is not the same as authority. The organizational manager has authority by virtue of the position he holds. He may or may not exert leadership. Authority involves the legitimated rights of a position that requires others to obey; leadership is an interpersonal relation in which others comply because they want to, not because they have to. Some people who occupy positions of authority are effective in their job, while others in such positions do poorly. The first type combines authority and leadership; the second has authority without leadership. In the first situation, the organization thrives. In the second, it deteriorates; sooner or later something must give — the people of authority are displaced or the organization becomes less and less effective.

In most organizations a person is a leader of his subordinates and a follower of his superior in the hierarchical structure. Stogdill [31], in a study of leadership characteristics, concluded that the pattern of leadership traits differs with the situation; no single personality typifies a leader. Evidence strongly suggests that leadership is a relationship existing among people in a social setting and that whoever becomes a leader in one situation may not do so in a different situation. A leader tends to have greater intelligence than his followers. A leader possesses social sensitivity and an awareness of individual values, feelings, goals, and problems. He is able to sense and judge human reactions accurately in order to influence people. A person is unlikely to move up to a role of leadership if he is inactive, apathetic, and aloof. Because a leader interacts with his subordinates as well as with others, he must be able to convey messages clearly and accurately, since fluency of speech promotes effective communication.

In a survey of literature relating to leadership, Wall and Hawkins [35] identify six principles of effective leadership:

1. The effective use of leadership contributes to the achievement of the goals of the group.
2. Effective leadership is a function of the characteristics of the leader, the group, the situation, and the interrelationship among these factors.
3. The effectiveness of a leader depends largely on how well he and his organization define his role and how completely they accept it.
4. To be effective, a leader must be able to analyze his group and determine what course of action will best help to achieve the group's goals and promote its morale.

5. It is important to the leader's success that his followers perceive him as effectively responding to group needs.
6. The effectiveness of the leader must ultimately be judged in terms of the group's survival and its progress toward its goals [35].

Leadership Styles

In classifying leadership styles, most authorities recognize three basic types: democratic, autocratic, and laissez-faire or free-rein (see Figure 6).

Democratic Leadership. A democratic leader assumes that employees are eager to perform their jobs and capable of doing so. They are willing to share decision making with their employees and believe that the latter have worthwhile contributions to offer. The group is perceived as having responsibility for goal determination and goal achievement, and self-expression is encouraged. Democratic leader-

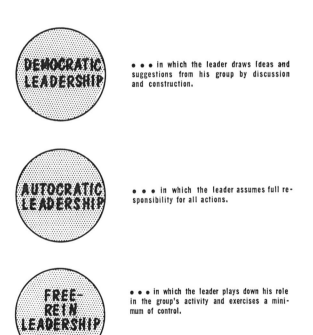

● ● ● in which the leader draws ideas and suggestions from his group by discussion and construction.

● ● ● in which the leader assumes full responsibility for all actions.

● ● ● in which the leader plays down his role in the group's activity and exercises a minimum of control.

Figure 6. Three types of leadership.

ship encourages enthusiasm, high morale, and satisfaction in employees, since basic human needs for recognition are being met.

The democratic leader uses rewards to create a positive motivation pattern. His study of human behavior has taught him that people in organizations today are more responsive to positive incentives — particularly psychological rewards, such as recognition, advancement, and responsibility.

Under democratic leadership an employee's orientation toward achievement and responsibility results in better performance. He shares in decision making and develops a feeling of participation in the overall accomplishments of his work group.

Under democratic leadership morale is measured in terms of the individual's motivation to contribute his talents to the achievement of organizational goals. Because he feels the support of the organization, his higher-order needs are aroused. He works toward recognition, the esteem of others, and self-fulfillment.

Performance of employees in a democratic leadership environment is characterized by awakened drives. Individuals are stimulated to participate in and contribute to the accomplishment of common goals. High achievement levels are attained because the resources of the whole group are utilized, rather than those of the manager only.

Autocratic Leadership. An autocratic leader gives direct, clear, and exact orders to his employees with detailed instruction as to what is to be done and how, leaving scant room for employee initiative. He delegates as little as possible and believes that in all probability he can do a better job than his followers. He does not necessarily distrust them but feels that an employee could not properly carry on without his direction. Such leadership tends to cause employees to lose interest and initiative, and to stop thinking for themselves because there is no need for independent thought. The autocrat believes he must direct the efforts of his employees toward organizational goals, and do it autocratically; he can do it benevolently or in an explosive manner, but *he* maintains control.

Although autocratic managers can be harsh or benevolent, they direct activities from a position of organizational power. The formal authority they possess gives them the right to command subordinates, and they depend upon and use this authority to get performance.

The autocratic boss uses a negative motivation pattern in the form of threatened loss of job, reprimand in the presence of others, and demotion. These penalties are employed as a means of frightening subordinates into productivity.

An employee finds it necessary to adopt an attitude of obedience to his autocratic boss. The constant reminder of his boss's power to hire and discharge forces him into a condition of personal dependency.

Under autocratic management the employee is expected to take his orders and follow them. Usually the level of morale attained is unenthusiastic compliance with rules and directions. As a result only his lower level or subsistence needs tend to be satisfied. He puts in his eight hours and makes enough to live on.

Because of the lack of motivation under autocratic management, the employee reluctantly gives only minimum performance and hopes for better things to come. The autocrat has centralized many functions in himself and thus usually works hard to keep ahead. Less than optimal goals are achieved, however, because the resources utilized are primarily those of the manager only.

Free-Rein Leadership. Free-rein or laissez-faire leadership is leadership in which each individual sets goals independently. It exists when a manager is too weak or too threatened to exercise the functions of leadership or when lack of trust within the group prevents unity. The manager who has great need of approval may practice laissez-faire leadership out of fear of offending his subordinates. He wants to please everyone and, in the attempt, fails to give strength and direction.

Such a free-rein leader may provide information to employees upon request but he gives little or no leadership. He tends to be preoccupied with his own work. Communication and directions to employees are lacking, and most do as they want. Very little teamwork occurs because there is no effective leadership.

The free-rein approach is the least efficient of the three types of leadership. It exists in "rebellion against autocratic leadership or because no leader is invested with responsibility and no one assumes the role . . . . Hostility generated by the autocratic leadership traditionally seen in [organizations] can result in a [leader] who is determined to be the opposite of all that was despised in the system. Because of lack of information, this [person] practices [free-rein] leadership in the mistaken belief that democratic rule is being practiced. Guidelines, rules and regulations, . . . and decisions are not seen as safeguards . . . but as infringements on the rights and dignity of the [staff]."* This "let alone" policy will repudiate any leadership that

*From Douglass, L. M., and Bevis, E.: *Team Leadership in Action*, St. Louis, The C. V. Mosby Co., 1970.

may have been present at the beginning, and the work situation will rapidly disintegrate into a disorganized hodgepodge in which no one knows or cares what he is supposed to do. A worker in this kind of atmosphere will lose all sense of initiative and desire for achievement [11].

Leadership studies indicate that the skill with which one applies the three basic styles determines an individual's personal success as a leader. Leadership styles continuously change, according to the leader, the environment, and the cultural climate in which the organization is operating. The effective leader strives to apply and shift his leadership style to fit the changing conditions, the problems, and the people. He perceives his role of leadership as a continuing process. His success in a leadership position depends on his own beliefs about his role and power, his value system, level of aspiration, confidence in others, feeling of security, and desire to lead. It further depends on his subordinates — their strength, needs, knowledge, job experience, and personal goals. The organization itself can be a contributing factor to a leader's success or failure — in its cultural values, size, effectiveness, and role within the community.

CONTROL

Control is the managerial function concerned with making sure that plans succeed; it means measuring and correcting the performance of employees to ensure that the planned objectives of an organization are achieved (see Figure 7). Planning and control are closely related. However, control means more than measuring, for in many instances it requires revised planning, additional organizing, and better methods of directing, thus closing the circle in the entire management process. Planning, organizing, and leading are the preparatory steps in getting the work done, while control is concerned that the execution be properly implemented [14].

The process of control has three elements: (1) standards that represent the desired performance, (2) comparison of actual results with the standards, and (3) corrective action. Standards may be tangible or intangible, vague or specific, but until the people concerned understand what results are desired, control will create confusion. Once a comparison is made between actual results and standards, it must be reported to the people who can do something about it. Control mea-

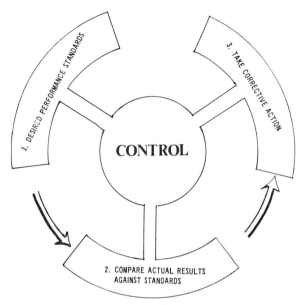

1. DESIRED PERFORMANCE STANDARDS

3. TAKE CORRECTIVE ACTION

CONTROL

2. COMPARE ACTUAL RESULTS
AGAINST STANDARDS

Figure 7. Elements of control.

surements and reports are of little value unless corrective action is taken when it is discovered that current activities are not leading to desired results [25].

Some basic guidelines relating to control are the following:

1. Control is a basic element in the structure of organization.
2. Action is the essence of control.
3. Plans and budget are important elements in implementing effective control because they outline what is intended and expected and the means by which the goals are to be achieved.
4. Control action can be taken only by the individuals who hold delegated responsibility and authority for the operation affected.
5. Control requires a system of information tailored to the specific management needs of key executives — information that is timely and adequate.
6. Management controls will not be of much value unless they cause people to alter their behavior.
7. The success of an organization and its parts depends on the degree of difference between what should be done and what is done.

8. When all members of the organization are aware of the major objectives being pursued and of the immediate objectives of their unit, control efforts are enhanced.
9. To be effective, a control system must be understandable and flexible and point out where corrective action should be taken.
10. Four activities can be controlled: quality, quantity, cost, and use of time.
11. Controlling is done so that performance can take place according to established plans.

A nurse director may be concerned with the overall activities of her department, but of course she is aware of more than broad concepts only. Many situations require facts, and, while she is not held down by operational details, a director must know where information is available. She should receive reports for the purpose of communication but does not necessarily examine every one she receives. The bulk of information, however, is at hand as needed to deal with problems or situations.

The response of people to standards, measures, reports, or other forms of control depends on the total situation. Controls may be rejected if there is no genuine interest in accomplishing organizational objectives or if standards of performance are considered too high. Controls may cause dispute among parts of an organization when the people involved lack confidence in the measurements. Controls that are enforced may serve as a guide to what must be done well and what can be done indifferently. People soon learn, for example, whether a "No Admission" rule means what it says or is merely a suggestion of desirable behavior. It is the action of the management in disregarding the standard or insisting it be maintained that gives meaning to control.

Control of operations in any organization is maintained by both its administrators and its managers. The administrator strives to create the setting in which the operations may proceed smoothly; he is responsible for the actual control of activities — for seeing that they are carried out within the limits determined by policy and that the end results correspond to the predetermined objectives.

The broad interpretation of the concept of control — evaluation of overall effectiveness — is a matter of answering two questions: Is the total job being done well? Is there any way of doing it better? A director who seeks and develops answers to these questions puts the crowning touch on her fulfillment of the managerial functions. An organization may have excellent plans and the instruments necessary for carrying them out, but without effective leadership to unify the actions of its members, chaos is likely.

The management functions of planning, organizing, leading, and controlling must be viewed as interrelated; they cannot stand alone. The successful nurse director develops each of these separate functions and simultaneously also develops their interrelationships. The integration of the management process and its functions into a well-balanced whole (system) is a major skill of an effective nurse director.

DECISION MAKING

Decision making is only one of the tasks of a nurse director. It usually takes only a small fraction of her time; however, making decisions is a specific administrative task, and decision making therefore deserves consideration in a discussion of the effective nurse administrator. The decision-making process in management is affected by the hospital environment of the nurse director, the role she assumes in the organization, and her mental processes developed in past experiences. The product of the process is called a decision — a course of mental action consciously chosen from available alternatives for the purpose of achieving a desired result. Wren [37] says that the choice of alternatives will depend on three social factors: (1) legitimacy, the decision maker's perception of what others expect of him in the situation; (2) sanctions, the rewards and penalties that accrue to the decision maker depending on the choice he makes; and (3) personal orientation, referring to the weight the decision maker places on the legitimacy and sanction dimensions of the decision.

Decision making is a common function in life and for those engaged in managing nursing care. All nursing personnel engaged in providing nursing care through the nursing process are involved in decision making. Opportunities should be provided for the nursing staff, through in-service programs, workshops, or self-analysis, to examine their decision-making skills.

Decision-Making Process

Ten steps that serve as a cyclic process for thinking about decision making are as follows:

1. Become aware of the problem.
2. Investigate the nature of the problem.
3. Determine the objective of the solution desired in light of total organizational objectives.
4. Determine alternative solutions which will solve the problem while being consistent with organizational objectives and without creating other problems through solving one.
5. Weigh the consequences and the relative efficiency of each alternative solution; if no solution seems acceptable, creatively seek other solutions.
6. Try out various alternatives — either in discussion with other people or possibly in trial-run experimental situations.
7. Select the best alternative solution.
8. Implement the decision by communicating it, training those who must carry it out, and seeing that it is being correctly carried out.
9. Check up on the solution at intervals to be certain that it is solving the problem and that it was the best solution.
10. Finally, change, correct, or even withdraw the solution, if the evaluation shows it is not working or was not the best answer [25].

Creative Process

The conscious mental activity of decision making involves a creative process. Five steps in the creative process identified by Newman and Summer [25] are the following:

1. Saturation: becoming thoroughly familiar with the problem and everything connected with it.
2. Deliberation: mulling over the problem, considering alternate solutions, and constantly rearranging all aspects of the situation in mind.
3. Incubation: relaxing, forgetting about the problem, letting the subconscious mind work on the problem.
4. Illumination: getting the new idea and sensing that it may work even though it does seem perhaps inappropriate.
5. Accommodation: refining and working out the new idea so that it is a practical solution to the problem.

Involving Others

There are times when the nurse director must make some decisions alone. At other times, to reflect and decide about a problem alone would be a sheer waste of the available talent and experience of the nursing staff or others. Listening to others can be of assistance to a nurse director. Listening to others will not hurt anyone, and it always opens the possibility that something useful may be said. There may be some decisions that will depend upon support and teamwork to be carried out. If listening to the suggestions of personnel adds impetus to the execution and gains acceptance for the final decision, it is worthwhile. One way of gaining allies is to ask these people for assistance and advice; they may say things that will make them part of the decision as it is finally made, and they will be identified with it. At many stages in the decision-making process, careful listening to the opinions of people who understand some special facet of the problem can improve the decision greatly. Listening to others and group decision making are probably less effective when rapid action is needed, when experts (on the subject) are not available, or when the results of a bad decision do not seem to be very great. There is probably no need to seek other views on a decision when the matter is covered by policy and seems clear-cut in terms of precedents under the policy. The decision has already been made, and the only problem is one of execution, which is more often a matter of individual action [37].

The effective decision maker does not start out with the assumption that one proposed course of action is right and that all others must be wrong. Nor does she start out with the assumption, "I am right and he is wrong." She starts out with the commitment to find out why people disagree [37].

No matter how high emotions run, and no matter how certain she is that the other side is completely wrong and has no case at all, the nurse director who wants to make the right decision must force herself to see opposition as her means to think through the alternatives. She uses conflict of opinion as her tool to make sure that all major aspects of an important matter are viewed carefully [37].

Delaying Decisions

Arriving at a point of decision, many nurse directors may vacillate, procrastinate, or in other ways refuse to decide. There is a myth that delay improves the quality of decisions. Flory, from the experience of many years as a consultant to executives, says that 15 percent of the problems coming to an executive need to mature, 5 percent should not be answered at all, and the remaining 80 percent should be decided right away. Those who insist on having all the facts before making a decision should remember the Pareto principle: If 20 percent of the facts are critical to 80 percent of the outcome, and a manager has those critical facts, then waiting until all the facts are in can be absurd; this practice has been dubbed "paralysis of analysis." Decisions that sometimes could be made faster with a minimum amount of information are delayed pending the availability of more data, most of which frequently reconfirm what the nurse director already knows. It is quite understandable that managers who are unsure of their authority are reluctant to make decisions. Organizational charts and job descriptions should be refined to clarify decision-making responsibility. This would prevent managers from avoiding or delaying decisions because others are involved [37].

Risks

There are some nurse directors who fear making mistakes; they wish something would happen so they would not have to make a decision. They may lack confidence in their ability no matter how many facts are available. However, few leaders have avoided making mistakes. The key issue is not that mistakes were made but that something worthwhile was learned, sometimes opening the door to larger successes.

Risk is implicit in all decisions; sometimes decision making is perceived as a problem rather than an opportunity. Fear of failure may so immobilize a nurse director that she is prevented not only from making decisions herself but also from delegating them, being afraid that mistakes by supervisors or head nurses will reflect on her. Thus the error — avoidance philosophy — dribbles down through the ranks, generating a pervasive caution that atrophies an entire nursing department. Gillerman [12] says that intelligent tolerance of mistakes is at the center of the problem of motivating people; if management is to motivate through challenge, it must insist on risk, which involves the distinct possibility of failure. He further says that an organization is either taking risks or dead.

Deadlines

It is common for managers to fail to set deadlines on decisions and to fail to stick to deadlines. The way a deadline is set may make a considerable difference in the attitude of the person responsible for meeting it. If the deadline is difficult to attain or unreasonable, or if it is imposed without discussion, resentment is almost sure to follow. Just as organizational objectives that are jointly determined will generate commitment on the part of those who achieve them, so with a deadline; a date that is set cooperatively will be more enthusiastically observed.

For the nurse director who gets things done, there are habits and patterns of behavior that make up the proper mix of fact gathering and decisions, in which her reflexes move surely from facts to action without undue haste, without any of the deliberation and delay that mark the indecisive person. Making effective decisions is a specific task of a nurse director; all the functions of management involve decisions. Decision making is based on communications, which clarify and improve decision making as incorrect decisions based on erroneous or incomplete facts are eliminated. The nurse director does provide feedback on the results of decisions, which is essential to the improvement of the decision-making process.

When a large number of people are involved in the decision-making process, it tends to appear democratic and improves the acceptance of the decision. Group decision making diffuses the responsibility for a decision and thus protects the individual from embarrassment from mistakes.

SYSTEMS APPROACH

To speak of health services as a system of care is now popular in the health field. The systems approach is being used increasingly in management, health, nursing, the social sciences, and other disciplines. Some believe that the systems approach is the only realistic way to manage health care institutions, which are now subject to complex and increasing pressure from all sectors of society. The systems approach provides a framework for analyzing an organization in relation to its environment. The pursuit of a systematic approach to achieving management effectiveness can make a significant impact on the problems facing today's nurse directors.

The complexity of modern organizational life is no stranger to nurse directors. The web of interrelationships and the intricate activities of an organization such as a hospital or a nursing service department require broad vision. A nurse director strives to grasp the "wholeness" of the situation and to view her own department in the same way. An understanding of the systems approach to managing the nursing department, as well as the hospital, allows the nurse director to look at the "big picture" — her total organization, the hospital, and its environment, the community. Systems is a total approach. Often much of organizational and personnel behavior is oriented toward a function, a department, or a person. The systems approach requires new patterns of thinking about organizations; it has its roots in general systems theory. The focus of this theory is a search for "an order of order, a law of laws in the universe" [19].

What Is a System?

A system has been defined as an organized or complex whole; an assemblage or combination of things or parts forming a complex or unitary whole; an array of parts designed to accomplish a particular objective according to plan [9]. Many definitions of a system exist; if sometimes a system is difficult to define and appears broad and vague, it is because the idea of systems is very broad in its conceptual framework — a true theoretical approach to management. Yet in spite of the difficulty of defining a system, examples of a system are familiar to everyone: the circulatory system; the legal system; the solar system; total man, a system; man, a biological system; an agency system, as a hospital; a neighborhood system; a community system. The key to each of them is its totalness. Each system is made up of individual functioning components, but the focus is on the total system and its end products, not on the parts or on the functions. The systems approach is a philosophy of treating the whole rather than bits and pieces; the concept of "wholeness" suggests that the system is greater than the sum of its components. Furthermore, to study the system one does not divide it into its components and then study each part in isolation. Instead, the system with all its interrelated and interdependent components must be studied as an entity [9]. This gathering interest in the systems approach replaces the previous notion that the whole can be manipulated piecemeal without affecting the other parts of its system. The systems approach to managing is total in its approach and concepts [9].

The systems approach provides a dynamic point of view that stresses changing relationships and interrelationships. In addition to its dynamic nature, systems theory provides a yardstick that can be used in (1) assuring a unified view of the interlocking components; (2) assessing the relationships within the systems and speculating as to how they will be affected by change within any one component of the whole; (3) pinpointing the crucial point where attack is most likely to bring about desired change; (4) determining the type and mode of intervention to be utilized; and (5) anticipating the probable results of intervention on each level [10].

A hospital may be viewed as a complex system made up of sets of interacting components (departments) that work together for the overall objective of the whole — providing high-quality care to the people of its community. Within a hospital there are patient care systems, information systems, financial systems, and other related systems. Generally a system can be broken down into less complex subsystems. This structuring of systems within systems is known as hierarchy [10]. A hierarchy of systems can thus be created, depending upon the nature, scope, and purpose of the systems study. This means that if a system (hospital) can be divided into subsystems (departments), then each subsystem can in turn be viewed as a system. However, the hierarchical concept cannot be applied in a haphazard way; it must result in a set of components and goals that conform to the definition of a system [10].

When thinking about a system, one should bear in mind that a system has a structure and a set of goals, properties, functions, input, output, and sometimes feedback mechanisms. A system connotes order, as opposed to chaos; the essence of a system is that its parts are supposed to work for the overall objectives of the whole [10].

In order to understand a system, Wren [37] says that we must be able to describe and represent it. A full description of any system will require specification of: (1) the objectives to which the system addresses itself; (2) the nature of the system (open or closed; static or dynamic); (3) the parts of the system; (4) the relationships among parts of the system; and (5) the procedures and mechanisms through which the system operates. Churchman [10] identifies five basic considerations as essential in thinking about the meaning of a system: (1) the total system objectives; (2) the system's environment; (3) the resources of the system; (4) the components of the system; and (5) the management of the system.

A set of systems goals represents some specific purpose that gives direction to the system and its components. The system and its components tend to be dynamic, in motion, reaching for an ultimate point — a purpose or goal that is perceived as desirable [20]. The interacting components of the system must be regulated to allow

movement toward goal attainment. Regulation includes planning —
determining required activities and control, determining deviations
from the plan, and making the necessary corrections. Feedback is a
required element of control [20].

The objectives of any system must be clear, precise, and specific
measures of the performance of the overall system. The measure of
performance tells how well the system is doing; thus, in the determination of a measure of performance, a nurse director will seek to
find as many relevant consequences of the system activities as she
can. The components of the system also address their objectives; if
the components of a system have diametrically conflicting objectives,
then such a system cannot long survive, even though each part may
be operating efficiently in advancing its own individual objective [20].

Environment. The environment of a system is made up of things and
people that are fixed from the system's point of view. For example,
if a hospital operates under a fixed budget that cannot be changed by
the system, then the budgetary constraints are in the environment of
the system. If the hospital can influence the budget, then some of the
budgetary process would belong inside the hospital system [20].

Resources. The resources of a system are the things the system can
change and use to its own advantage; the resources exist inside the
system. They are used to shape specific actions taken by the components of the system. Without some clear concept of the overall system and its priorities, it is difficult to specify the necessary resources
(manpower), the way in which different forms of resources (manpower) will interrelate, the kinds of physical facilities necessary, and
many other items of importance. Considerable resources must be
devoted to maintaining communication, the flow of information, and
clear goals [20].

Components. The systems approach is essentially comprehensive in
character. The various components are studied not in isolation but as
interacting parts of the system as a whole. The various components
that make up a system are not considered individually but in their
interactions with one another. Components belong together because
they interact, cooperate, and interrelate with each other. Components are recognizable, discrete, and dynamic, with their own individuality, objectives, and functions, yet each component is in some way
interconnected and interdependent. The components operate in such
a way as to produce a characteristic holistic and total effect. The
components may be looked upon as an entity rather than as a configuration of components [20]. The components exist in a state of

balance, and when change takes place within one, there are compensatory changes within the others. Systems become more complex and effective by constant exchange of both energy and information with their environment. When this exchange does not take place, they tend to become ineffectual. A system is not only made up of interrelated components; it is itself an interrelated component of a larger system.

As systems become more complex, their elements or subsystems will increase in specialization. These specialized components allow the system to cope with problems better and to move toward goal attainment [20].

There are components of a system that strive to maintain the status quo as well as those that are oriented toward activity and change. These different predispositions are related to the two basic functions of a system: (1) its internal job, to maintain the balanced relationship among the components of which it is composed; and (2) its external job, to perform the function for which it was devised and to relate to its environment. A system may move toward old age and death, particularly if it is closed and lacking the input of new energy. If too much energy is centered on maintaining relationships that have become rigid, the system can accommodate little input and expends its whole energy in maintaining itself; the system is unable to perform the task for which it was devised and becomes malfunctioning [20].

Management. The management of the system plays a major role in holding the system together. Management is concerned with the administrative organization and the management coverage of all the techniques related to the operation. Overlapping of functions with the other components is unavoidable. Management states the direction in terms of accomplishment of the objectives and strategy so as to avoid uncoordinated activities. Management plans, organizes, leads, and controls — supervising and regulating the activities that the system will operate [10].

Management by the systems approach forces planning, which is the most basic function of management and probably the most neglected. Systems cannot exist without planning, because for the system to exist and function it must be set up. Setting up the system is planning [10].

Open and Closed Systems

A system may be described as being open or closed. An open system allows for the exchange of information, materials, or energies with its environment. Within an open system a given final state or goal may be reached from different starting conditions; one set of initial conditions may lead to different final states. Equifinality, an essential characteristic of general systems theory, allows for reaching a purpose in a variety of ways for ultimate achievement of a desired goal.

A system is closed if there is no import or export of information, materials, or energies; therefore, no change can occur within a component or the system. Closed systems, with fixed and constrained resources, tend to run down. This tendency is termed *entropy*, and maximum entropy occurs when all energy differentials disappear. In a living system, entropy may be viewed as death.

Systems receive resources to perform their activities from other systems and likewise produce something of value to be used by other systems. For example, as new information about patient care is discovered, some hospital and nursing service administrators may close their minds to the new trends of care. They are willing to exist as they are: "We've done it this way all the time, and we plan to stay as we are." On the other side, if the hospital or the nursing department develops some new approach to patient care, they are not willing to share their new information with other agencies outside their system; they prefer isolation from their environment. An open system is well aware of trends, research, and new activities related to health care. Employees become involved in activities outside of the system; they attend workshops to improve themselves and share new information with others in their system [10].

At times it seems easier to look on a system and its components as a thing with certain specifications and to disavow human responsibility for its existence; nevertheless, any system is a vital composite of interrelating people whose attitudes, values, goals, and actions to accomplish those goals determine the character of that system [20].

Characteristics of Systems

Some property characteristics of a system are:

1. Every order of system except the smallest has subsystems.
2. All but the largest have a suprasystem, consisting of the system and its environment. There are factors in both the system and the environment which affect their structure and function. The factors in the system or subsystem are called variables; those in the environment are called parameters.
3. Every system has a boundary which distinguishes it from its environment. It

may be determined in various ways, but it is, in every case, an arbitrary distinction. The boundary is the region where greater energy is required for transmission across it than for transmission immediately outside that region or immediately inside it.
4. The environment of a system is everything external to its boundary. High order systems, therefore, are always part of the environment of lower order systems. For each system, moreover, there may be both a proximal environment, that of which the system is aware, and a distal environment, which affects the behavior of the system but is beyond the awareness of the system [22].

Concepts of the Systems

One of the most useful of recent developments is the utilization of concepts from systems theory. Some of these concepts are:

Systematic and Descriptive Factors
    Open System
    Closed System
    Subsystem (General purpose)
    Subsystem (Special purpose)
    Equifinality
    Boundaries
    Environment
    Field
    Order of Interaction
    Interdependence
    Independence
    Integration
    Differentiation
    Centralization
    Decentralization
Dynamics and Change
    Adaptation
    Learning
    Growth
    Change
    Teleology
    Goal
    Dynamism
    Dynamics
Regulation and Maintenance
    Stability
    Equilibrium
    Feedback
    Homeostasis
    Self-Regulation

    Steady State Maintenance
    Control
    Negative Entropy
    Repair
    Reproduction
    Communication
Decline and Breakdown
    Stress
    Disturbance
    Overload
    Positive Entropy
    Decay [20]

Implications of Systems for Nurse Directors

What implications does all this have for the nurse director whose task it is to improve the effectiveness of the nursing service department? How can she make practical use of the systems approach in her job? She may begin by asking such questions as:

1. What are the boundaries of the system or systems with which I am dealing?
2. What are the patterns and channels of communication, both within the individual system under consideration and among the external systems?
3. What are the explicit and implicit rules that govern the relationships among the components (internally and externally), particularly with respect to input (being open to new ideas, information, or material), processing (working with the new), and outgo (feedback or results of the work)?

When a nurse director thinks in systems terms she can see the whole picture, the relationship between the components involved, and the type of change that is necessary to achieve healthier balance; one hopes she can select the intervention that will be most effective. It must be recognized that systems change can be complicated, particularly as a nurse director deals with larger, diverse, older systems; the roles, relationships, and overall function of the system are rigid and sharply defined. A nurse director who wants to help change the hospital system or nursing service department system to make them function more effectively may find the job one that can be achieved only by pressure for policy and administrative change on a very high level.

The systems approach makes one keep in mind the totality of human experience as well as its erratic and balanced nature. Systems theory provides a set of rules regarding relationships that can be applied to the individual, group, institution, community, or society. Further, it gives specific indications for understanding and intervention, and increases a person's capacity to predict outcomes. It is a way of thinking, and it is only as effective as the nurse director who employs it.

1. American Hospital Association. *Management Review Program: Departmental Self-Evaluation, Nursing Service.* Chicago: The Association, 1971.
2. American Hospital Association. *Statement Position of Nurse Administrator.* Chicago: The Association, 1965.
3. American Nurses' Association. *Standard for Organized Nursing Services.* New York: The Association, 1965.
4. American Nurses' Association. *The Position, Role, and Qualifications of the Administrator of Nursing Services.* New York: The Association, 1969.
5. Bailey, J., and Claus, K. *Decision-Making in Nursing.* St. Louis: Mosby, 1975.
6. Bennett, A. New thinking required for development of management effectiveness. *Hospitals* 50:67, 1976.
7. Bertalanffy, L. *General System Theory.* New York: Braziller, 1968.
8. Brill, N. *Working with People.* New York: Lippincott, 1973.
9. Chapman, J., and Chapman, H. *Behavior and Health Care.* St. Louis: Mosby, 1975.
10. Churchman, C. *The Systems Approach.* New York: Delacorte, 1968.
11. Douglass, L., and Bevis, E. *Team Leadership in Action.* St. Louis: Mosby, 1970.
12. Gillerman, S. *Motivation and Productivity.* New York: American Management Association, 1963.
13. Gross, M. Should nurses be involved in management? *Hosp. Manage.* 107: 55, 1969.
14. Haimann, T. *Supervisory Management.* St. Louis: Catholic Hospital Association, 1965.
15. Hooper, F. *Management Survey.* London: Isaac Pitman, 1948.
16. Joint Commission for the Accreditation of Hospitals. *Accreditation Manual for Hospitals.* Chicago: The Commission, 1970.
17. Koontz, H., and O'Donnell, C. *Management: A Book of Readings.* New York: McGraw-Hill, 1964.
18. Kragel, J., et al. *Patient Care Systems.* Philadelphia: Lippincott, 1974.
19. Lill, D. *A Systems Approach to the Preservation of the Traditional Nuclear Family Unit.* Thibodeau, La.: Nicholls State University, 1975.
20. Levey, S., and Loomba, N. *Health Care Administration: A Managerial Perspective.* Philadelphia: Lippincott, 1973.
21. Massie, J., and Douglas, J. *Managing: A Contemporary Introduction.* Englewood Cliffs, N.J.: Prentice-Hall, 1973.
22. McKay, R. Theories, models, and systems for nursing. *Nurs. Res.* 18:393, 1969.
23. National League for Nursing, Department of Hospital Nursing. *Criteria for Evaluating a Hospital Department of Nursing Service.* New York: The League, 1963.
24. National League for Nursing, Department of Hospital Nursing. *In Pursuit of Quality Hospital Nursing Services.* New York: The League, 1964.
25. Newman, W. H., and Summer, C. E., Jr. *The Process of Management: Concepts, Behavior, and Practice.* Englewood Cliffs, N.J.: Prentice-Hall, 1969.
26. Odiorne, G. *How Managers Make Things Happen.* Englewood Cliffs, N.J.: Prentice-Hall, 1973.
27. Owen, J. *Modern Concepts of Hospital Administration.* Philadelphia: Saunders, 1962.

28. Reiter, F. The nurse-clinician. *Int. Nurs. Rev.* 13:62, 1966.
29. Ross, R. *Essentials of Management.* Washington, D.C.: R. W. Ross Associates, 1969.
30. Sims, L. The clinical nurse specialist — an approach to nursing practice in the hospital. *J.A.M.A.* 198:207, 1966.
31. Stogdill, R. Personal factors associated with leadership: A survey of the literature. *J. Psychol.* 8:35, 1948.
32. *SUM: An Organizational Approach to Improved Patient Care.* Battle Creek, Mich.: W. K. Kellogg Foundation, 1971.
33. Tannebaum, R., Wechsler, R., and Massarick, F. *Leadership and Organization: A Behavioral Science Approach.* New York: McGraw-Hill, 1961.
34. Walker, C. U. (Ed.). *Elements Involved in Academic Change.* Washington, D.C.: Association of American Colleges, 1972.
35. Wall, R. G., and Hawkins, H. Requisites of Effective Leadership. In Koontz, H., and O'Donnell, C. (Eds.), *Management: A Book of Readings.* New York: McGraw-Hill, 1964.
36. Weber, H. Nursing from Reality. In *Better Patient Care from the Organized Nursing Services Point of View.* New York: National League for Nursing, 1964.
37. Wren, C. *Modern Health Administration.* Athens, Ga.: University of Georgia Press, 1974.

Part III. Management Tools

5. Organizational Philosophy

Leaders in nursing have for many years attempted to identify the factors that make for a well-organized nursing service. They have succeeded in identifying certain managerial tools that contribute toward improving the quality of nursing care; one of them is organizational philosophy.

Any organization, in order to survive and achieve success, must have a sound set of beliefs on which it bases its policies and actions. Such a philosophy may be tacitly understood without ever being presented systematically or defined in a written document. It may be a reflection of an organization's traditions or of the character, experiences, and convictions of a single person. In some cases the collective character of the men and women who give the organization substance may transcend the personality of one person [90].

T. J. Watson [90] says that if an organization is to meet the challenges of a changing world it must be prepared to change everything about itself except its philosophical premises as it moves through corporate life:

> The basic philosophy, spirit, and drive of an organization have far more to do with its relative achievements than do technological or economic resources, organizational structure, innovation, timing. But they are, I think, transcended by how strongly the people in the organization believe in its basic precepts and how faithfully they carry them out [90].

The manner in which a nurse director performs is determined by her personal philosophy, which directs her activities. Her patterns of beliefs, attitudes, and values set the tone for a nursing department and for the hospital in all its relationships with patients, personnel, physicians, co-workers, and the community. Because philosophy can play a major role in shaping the character of a hospital nursing department, the director should strive to examine her own basic beliefs critically, shedding old and inadequate attitudes as necessary.

In order to develop an acceptable philosophy for administering nursing service, a director must have some comprehension of the concept of philosophy itself and its application to her area. She may ask: What is the meaning of philosophy? How conscious am I of my own personal beliefs? How well thought out are my beliefs? How do I translate my personal beliefs into everyday practices? What do I believe about providing care to patients?

The director has a set of ideals based on principles acceptable to her. Good, bad, or indifferent, these guides are derived from her belief about life. Aware of the world and human conduct, she has personal concern, involvement, and deep feelings about exploring the deepest questions in life. She knows that the wisest persons are not always those with the greatest amount of knowledge, for wisdom implies a mature outlook, a penetration and grasp that knowledge alone cannot supply [81].

The nurse director tends to be comprehensive in her thinking, viewing matters in a large perspective, seeing life steadily as a whole. One corner of experience does not satisfy her; she tries to discover relationships between diverse experiences as they relate to society. Her inquisitive and vigorous mind will generally go beyond the confines of any one setting. She may ask: Are we in nursing service operating in a vacuum? How do we view current issues and forces in our society that affect nursing? What means do we employ to bring our thinking together and produce a comprehensive plan of nursing action [81]?

When seeking a position, the director should determine in her interview with the hospital administrator, medical staff chief, and selected members of the nursing staff what their philosophy of patient care is. In identifying the basic prevailing beliefs, she must determine how compatible they are with her own thinking. Because her philosophical attitudes are significant, there must be considerable similarity, or conflict could develop.

HOSPITAL PHILOSOPHY

The hospital administrator recognizes the need for a set of principles that provide personnel with a common and consistent sense of direction. He applies a certain philosophy to achieve the purposes of the hospital. Even as conditions change, he strives to accommodate to them within the context of the hospital's beliefs.

Top management and all personnel must understand hospital philosophy and its application. If the basic beliefs appeal to the staff, the hospital's resiliency is increased, people are moved to desired action, and the result is improved patient services, satisfied personnel, and a productive setting. Each department director is responsible for establishing a departmental philosophy that is consistent with the credo of the hospital's governing body.

If a written hospital philosophy does not exist, the nurse director finds herself challenged to find a way to convince the hospital administrator of the need for one. Its absence should not deter her from getting started on a departmental philosophy.

NURSING SERVICE PHILOSOPHY

Departmental philosophies of nursing service (see Appendix 3) can and do vary because of the people, places, and time involved. It would be pretentious to think of one philosophical base so universal as to be called *the* philosophy of nursing service. Assuming that one purpose of any statement of beliefs is the establishment of a common point of reference, an integrated viewpoint toward certain ideas, attitudes, and practices, then what follows can be properly called a nursing service credo [15].

Developing a Nursing Service Philosophy

The task of developing a nursing service philosophy calls for understanding the significance of such a base of operation, knowing how to stimulate people to think about it, and getting them actively involved. It further requires a willingness to work with a process that is slow, demands mental action, and is very necessary to organizational life.

A nurse director must develop a plan for determining the nursing department's belief. Her approach will depend on her own attitude. Will she set it up alone? Will she let a nursing group be completely responsible? Will she mesh her thoughts with those of the nursing staff and create a credo that all are willing to support?

A common approach to development of philosophy uses the cooperative efforts of representatives of nursing service. The nurse director appoints a committee (or seeks volunteers) of the administrative staff — assistant directors, supervisors, head nurses, and the educational coordinator. In addition, there may be representatives of other nursing levels — staff nurses, practical nurses, nurse aides, or orderlies. This type of activity (1) provides a democratic atmosphere, (2) brings together different levels of nursing personnel, (3) provides an opportunity to bring out the talents and energies of personnel, (4) helps staff to find a common cause with one another, and (5) keeps people pointed in the right direction despite differences that may exist among them.

The nurse director's approach and presentation at the first meeting of the committee will have some bearing on their response to the task. She should provide an opportunity for the members of the group to get acquainted with one another. A simple and effective method is to allow members to interview each other in pairs, then let one member of the pair introduce the other to the group.

The purpose of the task group should be well defined and its members' roles and responsibilities clearly delineated. The nurse director should ascertain the group's present understanding of the concept of philosophy through discussion with the group, individual conferences, or a written questionnaire. In order to prepare the committee to function to the fullest, she may plan an in-service educational program to: (1) present guidelines for effective group participation; (2) expand knowledge and understanding of the concept of philosophy and the relationships between philosophy, principles, objectives, functions, and activities; and (3) allow time for the group members to clarify their understandings of the task, roles, and responsibilities.

In order to get the committee started, the nurse director or a few selected people may develop a tentative statement of beliefs to serve as a baseline from which the committee members can work. During their discussion the group may add, delete, combine, insert, or revise ideas. This process will continue over a period until the committee arrives at what it considers nursing service philosophy.

The committee submits the statements of belief to the nurse director and the administrative staff for consideration, review, and remarks. Supervisors and head nurses present the document to patient-unit personnel. As many people as possible should be allowed to participate in the review. A copy is given to the hospital administrator and chief of the medical staff to consider. The nurse director returns the proposed philosophy to the committee with any comments or remarks obtained during the review period. The committee makes any necessary revision of the philosophy and returns it to the nurse director for her approval.

Concepts

A review of eighty hospital nursing service philosophies indicated that the content ranged from a few sentences to three full pages in length. Among the more common concepts contained in the stated beliefs are the following:

1. Relationship of nursing service department to hospital, its philosophy and objectives.
2. Meaning of nursing, nursing care, comprehensive nursing, nursing services, patient care, administration.
3. Worth of the individual.
4. Christian concept of man.
5. Patient as a person.
6. Role of education in relation to the patient, his family, the employee, and the community at large.
7. Relationship to the other hospital departments, the medical staff, and other disciplines.
8. Democratic atmosphere.
9. Team nursing assignment.
10. Employee relationships.
11. Recruitment of personnel.
12. Survey, study, and research.
13. Significance of cooperation.
14. Coordination of patient care services.
15. Personal growth and development.
16. Utilization of qualified personnel.
17. Significance of interpersonal relationships.

No one philosophy epitomizes all the mentioned concepts. Each group identifies those closest to the people's beliefs, desires, and goals for nursing services. Members should be encouraged to develop concepts with the idea that they can be implemented in a superior fashion.

Statements of philosophy tend to be idealistic and to represent a state of perfection. Quality patient care presupposes superior performance from those providing services. An environment that calls for perfection is not likely to be easy to achieve, but aiming at it is always a goad to progress. A department is outstanding when it is willing not only to strive persistently for perfection, but also to take on seemingly impossible tasks. T. J. Watson said, "It is better to aim at perfection and miss than it is to aim at imperfection and hit it" [90].

Application of Philosophy

The real test of any statement of belief is its application to everyday activities and situations. A few selected examples are the following:

1. *We believe the patient has a right to expect that nursing personnel are qualified through education, experience, and personality to carry out the services for which they are responsible.*

This belief is maintained by careful screening of the qualifications and credentials of nursing personnel seeking employment. As new experienced personnel are employed, they are assigned to the nursing service educational unit and are temporarily under the direction of the staff education instructors. They attend hospital and nursing orientation programs for the purpose of becoming acquainted with their job responsibilities and new environment. They are made aware of the nursing department's policies, procedures, and nursing practices. Their specific needs are identified, and plans are made to meet them as much as possible. Only when the new employee is ready to take on her responsibilities is she assigned to a nursing unit. Supervisors and head nurses who receive new employees share in the duty of preparing staff for their nursing units, in conjunction with the staff education instructors. Employees are encouraged to attend educational programs provided by the hospital or other groups. Inexperienced personnel trained on the job (nursing assistants, orderlies, unit clerks) participate in a program of studies that prepares them to function in their respective roles. They too are encouraged to attend educational activities.

Individuals who consistently appear impatient, show lack of respect for the feelings of patients, or demonstrate other personal inadequacies are counseled and observed closely. Should such inadequacies persist, an individual is advised that the particular limitations revealed are undesirable in those charged with patient services.

Personnel are periodically evaluated by supervisors in order to assess their performance in relation to nursing care.

2. *We believe we have a responsibility to be creative and test new ideas that may improve the practice of nursing.*

An experimental unit has been established within the nursing department, the main objectives of which are: (1) to test new methods of providing nursing services; (2) to collaborate with other departments wishing to evaluate new approaches to patient care that will affect nursing; and (3) to do studies and research.

Staff members are encouraged to submit new ideas and to make suggestions that they believe may improve the practice of nursing.

3. *We believe the patient has a right to expect that he will receive the nursing care necessary to attain and maintain his maximum degree of health.*

A nursing practice committee has been established for the purpose of setting up and implementing standards that ensure safe and therapeutically effective nursing care of patients.

Staff members participate in the formulation of the nursing care standards.

Provision is made to acquaint all nursing personnel with the standards and their specific responsibilities in upholding them.

Each patient's medical and nursing care is planned, supervised, and evaluated by a physician and a registered nurse.

4. *We believe the patient has a right to expect that plans will be made with him and his family, so that nursing and other necessary services will be available to him throughout the period of his need.*

Nursing personnel are responsible for planning with physicians and other patient care disciplines for the total needs of patients. If, upon discharge from the hospital, patients should need continued nursing care, the physician, nurse, and social worker can plan and make arrangements for the service. The social worker assists by assessing the community health resources available for patient services and informing the physician, nurse, patient, and family.

5. *We believe the nursing department is a learning atmosphere for students of professional nursing and other allied personnel supportive to nursing.*

The hospital supports the belief that it has an obligation to contribute to the education of health personnel. A clinical setting is provided for students' learning experiences — e.g., nursing, laboratory work, x-ray examination, inhalation therapy, medical record keeping, or medical practice.

As students have an opportunity to become exposed to the clinical nursing units, for observation or practice, nursing personnel must be willing to cooperate and help make their experiences meaningful.

The few mentioned concepts and their applications and interpretations may vary from one setting to another. It is important, however, that the personnel learn from the nursing administrative staff how the basic tenets are translated into the daily work environment. If all employees are able to explain to others — patients and their families, visitors in the hospital, and people in the community — what the department believes, stands for, and strives to practice, it is hoped that the image of nursing service will be greatly enhanced.

Communicating the Nursing Service Philosophy

One opportunity to promote understanding of the nursing philosophy occurs during the introduction and orientation of new employees to the hospital environment and their duties. New employees can be given a written copy of the stated beliefs. A verbal explanation of the philosophy can be presented to the group by the director or her representative. As new staff are assigned to nursing units, the head nurse can further explain the implication of the beliefs within the patient care area. As a reminder to the nursing personnel of their commitments, a copy of the philosophy can be framed and placed on the bulletin board at the nurses' station.

If for some reason a departmental philosophy has not existed heretofore but is now available, in-service education programs should be held to acquaint all employees with the credo and its meaning. Practical situations should be discussed to show how they reflect concepts of nursing philosophy. Personnel must see that a philosophy can be realistic, workable, and practical, and still a means of striving for quality nursing services.

If the hospital administrator, physicians, and members of other departments have had a chance to share in philosophy development, it is likely their support will be gained. The hospital administrator has the responsibility of dovetailing all departmental credos with hospital philosophy. Once he understands what the nursing department is committed to, and approves it, he is able to look at operational activities, actions, practices, and services to determine how well the guiding principles are adhered to. When all personnel are optimistic and enthusiastic and give expression to those beliefs, their attitude will be felt by all, including the community.

As part of medical staff organization, the nurse director or her representatives or both meet with physicians. On these occasions both groups have a chance to understand and appreciate each other's philosophy and objectives for patient care, as well as the problems in which both must share. As an example of collaboration and sharing of philosophy, a group of physicians were interested in establishing a nursing unit specifically for the care of patients with neurological conditions. A physician and a nursing supervisor approached the nurse director. She encouraged them to develop a written justification and a plan of action to be presented to hospital administration. The plan was reviewed, approved, and programmed into the overall hospital objectives. Since the supervisor was aware of the significance of a philosophical base, she and the physician developed tentative guiding principles and objectives that they felt expressed their groups' thinking about the care of neurological patients. Once members of the nursing staff understood the significance of basic beliefs, they communicated this to others.

Because the nursing department relates to all other departments in the hospital, and its assistance is needed in order to accomplish the stated goals of nursing, it is imperative that the other departments understand what nursing strives for in relation to their services. An orientation session can be held in which representatives from various departments may hear an interpretation of the written nursing philosophy.

Revisions

Revision of a philosophy will depend on a group's desire to hold firmly to its guiding beliefs. If it appears to have achieved its objectives and has shown prosperity and growth, its basic philosophy is convincingly reaffirmed. Revision is not necessary when there is commitment to specific guiding statements; for example, "We believe in providing the best possible quality of service and nursing care to patients who come to us, adapting this care to his individual needs based on sound nursing practice." A reputation for quality service is one of a hospital's principal assets. If the personnel believe that quality service is a worthy goal, then means and ways are found and established to express this in everyday patient care. Such a belief will in all probability remain an aspiration ad infinitum.

Being a part of a dynamic and changing society may cause nursing staff members to review their commitments periodically and raise questions. They then identify what is worth preserving and what is not, and adhere to what they believe will sustain them in their everyday organizational life and service to patients.

NURSING UNIT PHILOSOPHY AND OBJECTIVES

The nurse director's responsibility for nursing care administration includes providing for the development of a philosophy and objectives for each patient nursing unit.

The management of care on a nursing unit will be based on what the staff believes about the care of patients. Nursing personnel must be accorded opportunities to formulate principles of nursing and patient care. The staff must be encouraged to look at their own activities and to develop a philosophy of nursing care. Each nursing care program, conceptually, has a philosophical origin arising from both staff and director. The nature of nursing care is dependent on the beliefs and intent of those who formulate objectives and stipulate procedures for the nursing unit.

The supervisory staff must be guided in writing out a statement of beliefs for patient care. The supervisors, in turn, will assist the personnel under their direction. For most groups, this task is not easy. It takes time to consolidate the thinking of people with varied educational backgrounds and work experiences. But slow as the process may be, a consensus eventually emerges.

As unit personnel strive to formulate their beliefs, they should be reminded to keep before them the hospital and nursing service philosophies and objectives; their statements must be in harmony with the total organization's precepts. The nurse director is able to multiply herself through others, and particularly her nursing philosophy, if by her words, actions, and demeanor she shows that she is concerned about quality patient care and about the staff's welfare and contribution to patient care. Once the unit philosophy and objectives are established, the supervisor and head nurse should plan for their implementation. The statement should be the guiding force in managing patient care and achieving nursing care objectives.

The nursing service department is more than an entity engaged in services to the people in the community; rather, it is a confirmation of the belief and principles of all the personnel who give it substance. The nursing service department is also a reflection of those who give it leadership in its development and in the conduct of its affairs. Having identified concepts that provide an impetus toward seeking quality patient care, the next task is to discover the proper objectives for attainment of the desired philosophy goals.

In current thinking and writing, the starting point for either a philosophy or the practice of management seems to be the predetermined objectives. The entire management process concerns itself with ways and means to realize predetermined aims and with the intelligent use of people whose efforts must be properly motivated and guided. Through its objectives, management attempts to create a climate conducive to achievement motivation, to goal-mindedness. In order for the concept of management by objectives to be effective, the use of participative management is essential. Participative management involves a relationship between superior and subordinate in which both share in goal setting and decision making.

Objectives are useful as they provide a course of action to follow in order to achieve desired goals. They determine what is to be done in the future. Deciding in advance what is to be done, how and by whom, where it is to be done and when, makes for purposeful, orderly activities. Objectives may be general or specific and may relate to a wide or narrow segment of an organization. They may concern the hospital as a whole, a department, a unit of a department, or an individual. General objectives are more manageable if translated into specific goals that are meaningful to people in their daily work. As they are divided into subobjectives, they are more tangible measures of progress. Assigning part of the hospital's objectives to a nursing department and then further subdividing them among the nursing units and staff creates a hierarchy of objectives [14]. Those of each nursing unit contribute to the purposes of the larger unit of which it is a part and at the same time promote cooperation and coordination among the staff. Objectives help set the tone for action by the staff members.

As a frame of reference for nursing service operational purposes, objectives may be classified as follows:

1. Ideals or permanent objectives are guiding statements that provide inspiration and values, with the hope of ultimate accomplishment, and that will continue as basic aims. The logical starting point for the development of these objectives is the nursing philosophy.
2. Long-range objectives flow from ideals; they advocate what is to be accomplished, but fulfillment may require an extended period of years.
3. Short-range objectives are steps toward long-range goals and make

the latter more tangible and meaningful. They exercise greater control over current performance. They are attainable within a 12-month period and can be further divided into intermediate objectives (for example, on a quarterly basis).

As objectives are being developed, the following principles are considered:

1. The overall objectives of the hospital are the core around which develop the nursing service department objectives.
2. Effective nursing objectives are evolved and refined through the cooperative efforts of administrator and nurse director.
3. Objectives that require work with another department in order to be accomplished should be submitted to and approved by those affected.
4. Objectives must be reasonable and attainable in the light of both existing and unforeseen conditions.
5. All staff members are to be involved in the process of accomplishing departmental objectives.
6. A systematic plan of action is necessary for the achievement of departmental objectives.
7. In writing objectives:
    a. Define specifically the results wanted; otherwise the objectives will be phrased in general or vague terms.
    b. Set realistic objectives that act as a stimulus, making the task challenging but reasonable.
    c. Develop objectives that are measurable. If results cannot be measured, they cannot be proved or denied. They should be measurable within a specified span of time.

A positive attitude on the part of the administrative nursing staff is essential to the fulfillment of the nursing service objectives. They are responsible for success or failure in achieving the hoped-for results. They use the abilities of the staff members, guiding them to: (1) understand the relationship between objectives and patient care; (2) recognize that valid, detailed planning depends on knowledge of where the departmental activities are going; (3) develop their own aims, which tie in with the immediate objectives and produce a sense of accomplishment; (4) provide adequate and suitable consultation as needed; and (5) recognize the need for teamwork and team outcomes.

If the nursing staff members have been sufficiently educated so that they understand and believe in the concept of objectives, there is less need for close control of their behavior. They understand the goals of the hospital, the nursing department, or a nursing unit, and where the personnel are expected to go. Such attitudes instill a sense of direction and responsibility for the success of an organization's purpose.

The administrative staff may be faced with what organization psychologists call a major stumbling block to achievement of organizational goals. Research has shown that in some settings the goals and needs of the staff are different from those of the organization, so that inescapable tension is built up between staff and administration. Such a situation challenges the administrative staff to maintain an environment that is supportive of the employee and at the same time is mindful of hospital goals. There are several possible ways to convey a feeling of support to the employee, such as: (1) trying to be sensitive to his feelings and needs; (2) helping him understand why his goals and those of the administration differ; and (3) planning future goals with the employee so that he can be actively involved. Providing a supportive environment assures a maximum probability that each staff member, in the light of his background, values, desires, and expectations, will view each experience and interaction as supportive — as something that builds and maintains his sense of personal worth and importance [69].

An effective, understandable procedure is necessary for identifying and setting objectives. Once established, the procedure should be communicated in writing and also verbally explained to the staff.

A suggested procedure is as follows:

1. During the first two weeks of the fiscal year all nursing personnel, under the leadership of supervisors and head nurses, share in identifying and listing those things they believe should be improved for patients and their families, physicians, personnel, hospital departments, and the community (see Figure 8).
2. At the end of the two-week period each nursing unit submits its list (see Appendix 4) to its supervisor, who, in turn, communicates the desired improvements to the nurse director.
3. The list of objectives is reviewed by the nurse director and her administrative staff to:
   a. Evaluate them in terms of their feasibility and contribution to hospital goals.

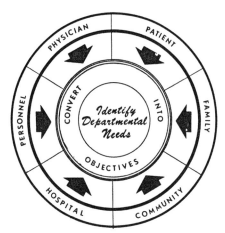

Figure 8. Setting objectives by identifying various departmental needs.

    b. Determine whether they relate to nursing service philosophy and the permanent objectives.

    c. Make some judgment as to which can be met through objective setting.

    d. Determine whether they should be converted into long-range or short-range objectives.

    e. Set priorities.

4. The approved needs are converted into tentative long-range or short-range objectives. If some objectives will require longer than a year to complete, they are broken down into short-range objectives, in which phases are attainable within a twelve-month period.

5. After discussing proposed objectives, the nurse director and her administrative staff finalize the list to submit to the hospital administrator.

6. The nurse director reviews the program of objectives with the hospital administrator and asks for his comments or suggestions. She revises the listing as needed.

7. Upon receiving his approval, she communicates the agreed-upon objectives to the nursing staff and others who are concerned.

    a. Supervisors and head nurses review and explain to their personnel the programmed goals for their unit and the department.

    b. Written copies of the departmental and individual unit objectives are placed on the bulletin board of each nursing station to serve as a reminder of departmental commitments.

c. A master plan of nursing service objectives is maintained in the nursing office. It provides an overall view of departmental, administrative staff, and nursing unit objectives. The manual is available to the staff.

d. The hospital administrator is given a copy of the master plan manual of nursing objectives.

e. As new persons are employed, they are introduced to the concept of objectives during their orientation period.

8. Subobjectives (arising from the nursing departmental objectives) are set at the beginning of each quarter of the fiscal year. Dividing the task over a twelve-month period makes it easier to measure and account for activity. Each head nurse formulates unit objectives and submits them to her supervisor. The administrative nursing staff does likewise, presenting unit objectives and their own goals to the nurse director. At this time, as subobjectives are being set, a progress review is made of prior quarterly commitments.

9. The nurse director then has an overview of activities within the department. She is able to report to the hospital administrator about activities taking place within the nursing department on a quarterly basis.

PROGRAMMING OBJECTIVES INTO ACTIVITIES

Once objectives are established, a plan of action must be initiated to ascertain the scope and complexity of the task and the range of activities required to accomplish goals. This will involve:

1. Identifying the specific steps needed to reach the objective.
2. Determining who will share responsibility for accomplishing specific objectives (nursing administration, nursing unit staff, or particular individuals).
3. Developing details.
4. Assessing resources needed, such as personnel, finances, equipment, supplies.
5. Assigning phases of the plan and setting target dates.
6. Reviewing and integrating plans.

PROGRESS REVIEW

In order for management by objectives to be effective, periodic evaluation is necessary to determine what is being accomplished.

1. Progress review sessions are held quarterly during the fiscal year. Additional meetings may be scheduled as needed.
2. Planned conferences take place between supervisor and head nurse, assistant director and supervisors, nurse director and assistants. As information is channeled upward through the hierarchical structure, the nurse director obtains a broad view of what is happening in relation to the predetermined objectives. All members of the staff are aware of the multiple reviews taking place at the various levels of organization.
3. During the session, consideration is given to the following:
   a. Are objectives being met? If so, how?
   b. If not, what are the obstacles?
   c. What action is necessary? Set new objectives or revise? Abandon objectives? Eliminate objectives because they have been accomplished?
   d. Promoting coaching and counseling as needed.
   e. Encouraging efforts to maximize contributions toward reaching objectives.
4. Toward the end of the fiscal year, fourth quarter, the nurse director and her administrative staff analyze the year's activities and accomplishments as well as problems that may have been encountered. A written annual progress report is submitted to the hospital administrator.

BEGINNING OF NEW CYCLE

At the beginning of the new fiscal year the cycle of goal setting is initiated again. Plans must be made to identify needs of the nursing department. The nurse director and her staff try to build future objectives on past experiences. As planning is considered she may ask:

1. What future hospital goals will affect nursing and its objectives?
2. What objectives are carried over from the past year?

3. What changes have taken place this year that will have a bearing on new objectives?
4. What areas of activity need further consideration?
5. Are all projects completed?
6. Are the proposed new objectives different from those of the last fiscal year?
7. What specific problems met this year can be helpful in preparing for next year's objectives?
8. What ideas in use outside the hospital may be considered for internal departmental use?
9. What ideas and suggestions do personnel have relating to the new objectives?
10. Are personnel encouraged to express their ideas and become involved?

Once the needs are identified, they are converted into objectives. An organized program of long-range and short-range objectives is established. The entire staff can work toward common purposes that are appropriately challenging and mutually consistent. Attainment of departmental objectives depends on the director's ability to provide leadership and to communicate the goals to others. Finally, control

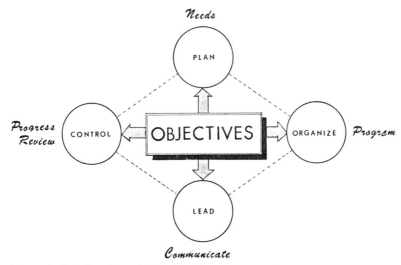

Figure 9. Relationship of objectives to management process.

is exerted by means of a progress review of objectives, to determine whether the goals are being achieved as planned (see Figure 9).

Objectives properly developed and applied can tell nursing staff in what paths, new and old, the department's total undertaking should be moving. They can guide both the day-to-day activities and the personal growth of the nursing staff. As objectives are accomplished with efficiency and effectiveness, they are powerful tools in serving the patient and others.

The usual expression of responsibility relationships among people and jobs is the organizational chart. An organizational chart is a management tool, a pattern to show how parts are put together to accomplish a particular purpose. It is effective only to the extent it is used, and it will be used only to the extent it carries out the aims and functions of the department. The purpose of the chart is not to change the established order but to enable it to operate smoothly. There should be no attempt to fit the department's functions into a new pattern just because it looks good on paper. Even something that has been shown to work well in one hospital may not be effective in another [3].

The chart indicates areas of responsibility, to whom and for whom each person is accountable, and the major channels of formal communication. It is interwoven with the organization plan of the hospital, indicating interdepartmental as well as intradepartmental relationships.

In drawing up an organizational chart a nurse director and the administrative nursing staff should:

1. Determine the purpose of the plan. There are at least three elements to be considered: (a) administrative control, (b) planning and policy making, and (c) relationships with other departments and related agencies.
2. Draw a chart of the present departmental plan — the actual working one, not the formal one. Sometimes there is a hidden organizational plan that differs from the formal plan and is quite effective. It is helpful to know what is happening in actual practice.
3. Review the departmental functions and determine what activities are needed in order to carry them out. It may be found that certain activities are duplicated; some may belong to other departments; important ones may have been left out of the pattern.
4. Classify the department's functions and activities, drawing up job specifications and finding out where the responsibility for decision making should be placed. With effective decentralization and delegation of responsibilities and duties, the nurse director will be relieved of details and allowed time to do long-range planning, evaluation, stimulation of new ideas.
5. Review relationship with other hospital departments. Determine what activities involve other areas, what working relationships are

necessary, and at what levels they are to be established in order to attain the objectives of the nursing department [3].

There is no one right way to organize a departmental chart. Organizational structure is not static and stationary. The personnel who are part of the organization change; the organization grows and adopts new technology; the social, political, and economic setting in which a hospital operates is continuously in flux. One task of a nurse director is to keep her part of the organization adjusted to these changes.

Careful and clear thinking about organization need not result in freezing duties and relationships. Organizational structure may require realignment as the necessary jobs change and the people who fit the jobs change. As nursing administration is able to predict changing conditions with reasonable accuracy, the chart or organization can be reviewed or revised. When changes do occur in the chart, all members of the department should be notified.

The pattern for administrative control should indicate an orderly chain of command, with lines of authority and responsibility clearly drawn. In that chain each person has an immediate superior and must not be expected to take directions from any other person. The number of levels of command varies [3].

ORGANIZATIONAL STRUCTURES

The traditional pyramidal concept has been a popular organizational structure. Some believe that the pyramid structure has outlived its usefulness; others believe pyramidal concepts are still valid. The need for accountability is still an inescapable fact of organizational life. As organizations experiment with new structural strategies in response to a swiftly moving scene, there is a need to find ways to modify and supplement the pyramid design. The results of empirical research on organizational structure offer convincing evidence that there is no single universally optimal organizational plan [45].

The reverse or downward pyramid goes in the other direction and gives greater scope for lateral relationships. Other variations of the pyramid structure are a beehive, a doughnut, a bell, a supergriddle, and a ladder. These structural variations aim primarily at toning down the strict autocratic nature of the pyramid structure, which is accentuated by its sharply pointed, defined apex. The bell structure depicts the idea of collegial management; the apex of the pyramid is broadened by a top management team of leaders. A beehive organizational structure attempts to soften the pinnacle of the pyramid by blunting it. The beehive is designed to do more than accommodate the trend away from autocracy; it also tackles the problem of trying to indicate the human relationships that do not show up in the pyramidal chain of command. The three-dimensional beehive consists of a series of concentric circles — the inner circle represents the apex of management, the surrounding bands constitute the supervisory echelons and correspond to the various levels of management, and the pie-shaped segments represent the organization's operating divisions. The doughnut structure is a circular chart that shows the close physical relationship of the staff with its manager; it represents a way to achieve a high degree of rapport with managers of every level by a freer flow of communications through the organization [45].

Some organizations see the ladder structure as the answer to the problem of where to locate the growing number of specialists being added to their staffs. Management services can be lifted out of the pyramid and placed in a neutral ladder apart from the hierarchy. This leaves executives free to call for the advice of any specialist without having to go through the hierarchy. It also releases the executive communication network from the obstruction of a specialists' department. The specialists should be able to pass up and down the ladder, temporarily entering the organization at various levels, wherever their services are required. Thus the specialists are left to their specialty, instead of being forced to climb to positions in the organization they may be incompetent to fill.

The supergriddle allows personnel to specialize in the type of skills they do best. For example, selling food to a hotel requires a different skill from selling it to a supermarket. The system is designed to ensure that salesmen are not promoted into jobs for which they are unsuited. There is no pressure on them to become sales managers. (In some instances, outstanding salesmen are earning more than sales managers.)

The pyramid structure for many years has been an ideal means for the person at the top to pass the orders to the subordinates under him. However, with the new knowledge that behavioral scientists have provided, people in organizations are now asking for some opportunity to share their voices and opinions about their place of work. The move toward participative management concepts offers, in theory, an opportunity for all levels of personnel to participate responsibly in the life of their place of employment. Associated with this person-centered concept of management is its tool, managing by objectives (MBO) — an approach that allows everyone to join in improving the life of a work setting — one hopes, to achieve hospital goals as well as the individual's goals.

The governing body of a hospital, on the basis of its philosophy and objectives, establishes principles that determine the institution's character and goals. It is on these principles that overall administrative policies and procedures are based. The nurse director may serve in an advisory capacity to formulate overall hospital administrative policies and procedures, or she may collaborate with other department heads to formulate interdepartmental policies. Her primary responsibility, however, is the establishment of departmental and interdepartmental administrative policies for the entire nursing department and the development of operational or specific policies to give direction at the nursing unit level. Written nursing care and administrative policies and procedures provide the nursing personnel with acceptable methods of meeting their responsibilities and achieving projected goals [13].*

A policy is a guide that clearly spells out responsibilities and prescribes actions to be taken under a given set of circumstances. Policies provide general direction for decision making so that action can be taken within the framework of the organization's beliefs and principles. A policy, however, does not supply the detailed procedure by which it is to be implemented; policy needs interpretation when applied to a specific situation. This is the point at which a written procedure frequently evolves. A procedure prescribes the steps that should be followed in order to conform to or carry out a policy. Policies and procedures seek to avoid the chaos of random activity by directing, coordinating, and articulating the operation of an organization [13].

USEFULNESS OF POLICIES

Written policies are useful, for the following reasons:

1. Uniformity of action is assured, so that each time a decision is made or a task performed, it follows a meaningful pattern. Policies do, however, leave room for individual judgment and extenuating circumstances.
2. It is easier to settle conflicts, issues, or concerns in terms of a

*Where indicated, sections of this chapter have been adapted from an article by Addison C. Bennett [13]. Reprinted with permission from *Hospital Topics*, November, 1967. Copyright 1967 by Hospital Topics, Inc.

written policy than in terms of personalities. The basis of conflict is the point for discussion rather than who is to blame for it.
3. A standard of performance is established. Actual results can be compared with the policy to determine how well the staff members are fulfilling their roles.
4. Personnel are generally assured of consistent treatment [13].

POLICY DEVELOPMENT

When planning for the development of policies, a nurse director and her staff must consider a number of basic principles:

1. Broad and durable policies provide a consistent course of action in handling matters that come up repeatedly.
2. Policies should fit the background and environment of the organization.
3. A policy is worthwhile only when it is carried out on a day-to-day basis.
4. Policies are interpreted when applied to a specific situation.
5. Policies are essential to smooth administration, providing continuity, uniformity, and consistency in the way things are done.
6. Deterioration of a policy is a reflection of management's failure to conduct its affairs effectively.
7. Policies should guide both internal and external operations.
8. Policy statements should be general enough to stand the test of time without the need of frequent revisions.
9. Policy changes should be thoughtfully considered, and changes should be promptly communicated to the staff [13].

The development of policies is not always premeditated. When a decision must be made three or four times in a row, a pattern that satisfactorily meets the need is identified. This may lead to a basic policy that not only solves the present problem but is likely to hold up well in future situations.

It must be determined how policies and procedures are to be initiated, reviewed, and revised. A policy committee, made up of nursing personnel, can be appointed to participate in policy development. For example:

Nursing Service Department
Policy Committee

Purpose
To develop policies and procedures for the Nursing Service Department that define responsibilities and prescribe the action to be taken under a given set of circumstances.

Objectives
1. To develop new policies to meet present and future needs.
2. To review policies submitted by clinical nursing units and other areas in the department.
3. To reappraise policies periodically and revise them if revision is indicated.
4. To submit recommendations to the nurse director regarding the development, revision, or modification of policies.

As a policy committee makes recommendations to the nurse director, she must ask: (1) Is this a recurring problem? (2) How often has it occurred? (3) Do others see this as a problem? (4) Is it temporary in nature? (5) Will a written policy help clarify thinking and promote efficiency of operation? (6) Does this problem require collaboration with other nursing personnel or hospital department heads? (7) Does this problem require a review by the hospital administrator? [13]

Once a policy or procedure is approved, the nurse director can delegate to subordinates the responsibility of applying the plan to specific cases. This delegation relieves her of the need to become personally familiar with each situation, while at the same time giving her confidence that work will proceed as desired.

COMMUNICATION OF POLICIES

The nurse director is responsible for establishing a method of communicating policies to nursing personnel. She must inform the administrative nursing staff of any policy changes. A written copy of the policy should be distributed to each member, eliminating breakdowns in communication that result when policy action is passed on by word of mouth. A verbal interpretation also should be presented to the administrative staff by the director. The administrative nursing staff members, in turn, verbally present the new policy to the nursing unit personnel. Copies of a new or revised policy are placed in the appropriate policy manual on the nursing unit.

The nurse director and her administrative staff have to assess how policies are holding up in day-to-day activities within the nursing department. Is the proper climate being created for making policy effective? The attitudes and opinions of the nursing staff who are being asked to comply with hospital and nursing policies are important. Supervisors and head nurses are in a position to feel and observe the staff's reactions to policies — favorable or otherwise. They can report reactions and offer suggestions for improving or modifying policy. As situations arise, the administrative staff will have the responsibility of interpreting policies. They must be able to make sensible exceptions to policies in the light of circumstances.

LEGAL IMPLICATIONS OF POLICIES

Because there are many practices in nursing that have legal implications, written policies serve as a safeguard for the nursing staff. An incident occurred in which the parents of a young child alleged that a staff nurse had negligently administered a hypodermic injection, causing a severe abscess on the child's right buttock. The child had undergone surgery, and his surgeon had prescribed injections of antibiotics for him every six hours. The plaintiff's legal adviser asked to talk with the nurse director. Among other things, he wanted to know whether the nursing department had any nursing policies and procedures. How often were they revised? How were employees informed of policies? What was the specific policy relating to the administration of medications and the giving of hypodermic injections? He requested a copy of the policies of the nursing department and was presented with the nursing service administrative manual, the nurse practice manual, and the pediatric policy and procedure manual. The nurse director discussed with him the written policies and procedures that had been established for safe, effective patient care and told him how often they were reviewed, revised, and disseminated to the staff. Liability suits sometimes require the nurse director to provide testimony on policies that guide the nursing personnel.

Licensing bodies, state health departments, boards of registration, and other agencies base many of their decisions on information found in hospital records. The presence of well-documented policies is indicative of the quality of care being supplied in an institution. The Joint Commission on Accreditation of Hospitals depends heavily on hospital records to assist it in reaching conclusions with regard to accreditation. Documented policies and procedures reflect the efficiency of hospital management and support other impressions gained through personal observation.

NURSING POLICY AND PROCEDURE MANUALS

A policy and procedure manual is a useful management tool that gathers together in writing the scope of departmental responsibilities and provides a comprehensive framework to implement nursing objectives. This manual is an instrument for orienting new staff, a reference when unexpected problems arise, a foundation on which to develop administrative procedures, and a firm basis for discussion when differences occur [5]. Policy and procedure manuals are important because they establish boundaries within which the hospital will operate and convey its beliefs. Without such manuals, management lacks direction and is vulnerable to inconsistent decision making.

A policy manual is meant to serve as an easy reference to policy. It provides guidelines and direction for nursing personnel who are accountable for the management of nursing care and staff. The use of written policies and procedures aids the hospital materially in its overall purpose — the delivery of quality care.

The general format of a manual depends on whether the hospital administration has issued specific directions or has left these to the nurse director and her staff. A "Nursing Service Administrative Manual" can be developed for overall departmental policies, procedures, and information related to nursing administration and the professional components of nursing care. It may (1) describe the structure and organization of the nursing department, (2) identify current departmental administrative and clinical nursing practice policies and procedures that are applicable to all nursing units, and (3) identify current hospital and medical staff policies and procedures related specifically to nursing.

Policies may be established within the nursing department that are applicable to all of its nursing units. Examples of topics that may be found in a nursing service administrative manual are: activities, departmental calendar, admission of patients, administrative nursing meetings, budget preparation, use of bulletin board, discharge of patients, emergency equipment, use of incident reports, master staffing plan, noting physician's orders, minutes of meetings, narcotics and sedative records, departmental objectives, time schedules, and visiting hours.

Internal departmental personnel policies relating to the nursing staff should be available in writing on each nursing unit. Policy topics may include: absence from duty, conditions of employment, employee safety, health services, leave of absence, leaving the nursing unit, orientation to nursing unit, overtime on duty, personal appearance, and scheduling of time.

Policy topics related to patient care may include: administration of medications, assignment of nursing care, appraisal of nursing care, chapel services, use of dangerous materials, leave of absence, patient teaching programs, private duty nursing care, safety, precautions to prevent suicide, and orientation to nursing unit. Policies not necessarily initiated by nursing but related to it can be placed in a miscellaneous section.

An adjunct to the nursing service administrative manual is the "Nursing Unit Policy and Procedure Manual" for each nursing section or related area of the nursing department. This manual can (1) describe the structure and organization of each specific clinical nursing unit or related area of nursing services, (2) identify administrative and clinical nursing practice policies and procedures related to nursing units, and (3) describe hospital and medical staff policies and procedures related specifically to a particular unit of the department. Either a departmental or a clinical unit nursing manual may be organized into the following sections:

1. Cover sheet
2. Foreword
3. Table of contents
4. Introduction
5. Statement of philosophy
6. Objectives
7. Organization

8. Administrative policies and procedures relating to:
   Department or unit
   Personnel
   Patients
   Other (e.g., hospital)
   Medical staff
9. Index

The nursing manuals can be prepared by the nurse director and the policy committee, in cooperation with the nursing practice committee, administrative nursing staff, department heads, hospital administration, and medical staff.

One of the problems encountered in developing policy manuals is the insertion of new policies or deletion of outmoded policies. A system should be devised by which policies can be removed or inserted with ease and facility so as to keep the manuals current.

A manual can be organized so that various sections are typed on colored paper to indicate a particular area. Once a policy is initiated or revised, it can be placed in its proper section. Each section has its own numbering system (Roman numerals) and each policy is given a specific identification number (Arabic) based on page location. In the case of a new policy, a page number is assigned following the last number in the section. If a policy is deleted from a section, its page number remains unused, and another policy may be placed on that page as the occasion arises. If a new or revised policy has a subpolicy condition, it will be identified with a small letter.

For example:

Policy	Section	Page	Addendum
Staffing	II	1	1-a
Employment	IV	2	
Overtime	IV	3	

With the many changes that occur daily in a hospital and a nursing department, policy development requires a clear-cut procedure on maintenance of the manual. To ensure accuracy of contents and to provide a check that the procedures described in the manual are followed in practice, some sort of control mechanism must be available.

The major responsibility in these areas rests with supervisors and head nurses. The size of the department and the ability of individual managers can substantially affect the success of such efforts. An auditing process could be used to pinpoint areas of weakness, so that necessary changes can be made to ensure adherence to nursing policy.

A good audit consists of (1) review of all manual contents at least once a year; (2) continuous random sampling of operating practice within the nursing department; (3) regular reports of audit findings to supervisors and head nurses; and (4) report by supervisors to the nurse director, indicating any actions taken on the basis of audit results [21].

All nursing personnel must understand how and to what extent the manual is to be used. Each employee must know all the policies and procedures described therein and must recognize the fact of being accountable for failure to comply with them. Dependence on the manual should help employees to do a better job.

One of the most complex problems facing the health care industry is that of spiraling hospital costs. Because hospital management is charged with delivering efficient, high-quality health care, it must accurately define all cost factors in order to maximize the effects of necessary expenditures. The budgeting process, carefully thought out, properly developed, and wisely administered, is a tremendous management tool to satisfy this responsibility. When understood, the budget provides a department director with the ability to define in detail the many cost factors involved in delivering the best possible patient care at the lowest possible price.

The financial operation of the nursing department represents the greatest percentage of the hospital's total expenses. While a nurse director's ultimate goal is to provide good nursing care, she must recognize that this objective can be strongly affected by her own concept and practice of financial management. She cannot relinquish this responsibility or feel unconcerned about financial matters; they require her special interest. Improper management of fiscal affairs can be detrimental to patients and the services they receive. The nurse director and administrative staff must strive to learn as much as possible about the process and overall aspects of budgeting. Concentrated study and effort should be given to planning, preparing, analyzing, and reviewing the nursing budget and expenditures. Once a systematic financial plan is established and brought to the attention of nursing personnel, a substantial step toward adequate cost control will have been achieved.

DEFINITION

A budget is a plan that states anticipated results in dollars and cents; it is the financial translation of that part of the goal of the hospital that applies to nursing. The budget serves as a guide for the fiscal year for which it is prepared, specifying a framework within which the nursing department can function, appraise results, and modify organizational tasks. Its prime purpose is the prevention of expenditures in excess of reasonable needs of an organization's operation. The budget is a means of checking the progress made in keeping expense and cost in compliance with an organization's financial plans and allowances.

ADVANTAGES

The establishment of a budget offers the following advantages:

1. A complete and detailed program of activities is planned in advance.
2. The analysis of operations required in setting up a detailed budget helps to clarify the assignment of responsibility and authority, facilitating the task of supervision and administration.
3. The cooperation and support of all department heads can be obtained toward the accomplishment of a common objective.
4. The orderly handling of financial matters is assured — a necessity for sound operation of an activity.
5. The budget has a balancing effect on the total organization; the quality and quantity of service that can be given the patient should closely equal the expected revenue. If monthly trends are defined, advantage can be taken of peaks and valleys in activity. Because hospital departments are interrelated, future plans of one department must complement those of other affected departments.
6. Budgeting encourages the exchange of information; ideas are traded, and cross-stimulation in budget interest and understanding occurs.
7. The process stimulates team approach. By enabling each team member to contribute to organizational planning as well as to see the results of good team play, the budget becomes a stimulant to employee commitment and efficiency and an effective guide to proper utilization of resources.
8. The budgeting process gives the hospital administration a chance to evaluate the thinking of department directors. Is the budget planning realistic? Are the standards too high or too low? The budget can aid in evaluating quality and initiative in performance.
9. Once the budget standards are set, actual expenditures and budgeted standards can be compared with little effort.

PREREQUISITES

In order for a budget to be meaningful, the following prerequisites should be met:

1. The hospital must have a clearly defined organizational structure with responsibilities defined and assigned.
2. Responsible personnel at all levels of management must participate in budget development.
3. The personnel involved must have an understanding of the service ideals and financial goals of the hospital.
4. There must be an adequate system that provides reliable financial and statistical information to the person responsible for the budget.
5. Budgets must allow enough freedom to accomplish departmental objectives.
6. Budgets must be flexible enough to allow for unpredictable expenditures.

TYPES OF BUDGETS

Operating Budget

Financial programs usually consist of three types of budgets: operating (expense), capital expenditure, and cash. These may be supplemented by other financial plans, estimates, and forecasts. The nursing department is directly concerned with the operating budget and capital expenditures. The operating budget includes the accumulated estimates of operating revenues and expenses for a specific period of time. It predicts future requirements and expenses for personnel, supplies, and other items, whether the activities are devoted to direct or indirect patient care or are income- or nonincome-producing.

The expenses in the nursing budget as prepared by the nurse director are ordinarily only those under her control, and they are related, for the most part, to estimation of direct expenses. These operating expenses are charged directly to nursing on the hospital's general records.

Some of the items that may be included in the operating budget are the following (see Appendix 5):

Personnel salaries and wages
   Administrative (salaried)
   Staff (hourly employees)
Education
   In-service education

On-the-job training
Travel to professional meetings
Educational leaves
Scholarships
Uniforms for personnel
Books, periodicals, and subscriptions
Dues and membership fees
Medical and surgical supplies
Laundry service
Provision for depreciation
Repairs and maintenance
Drugs and pharmaceuticals
Legal and professional fees
Recreation

Institutions vary as to whether medical and surgical supplies and equipment are included in the nursing department budget. These items, however, are requisitioned by nursing personnel and will appear on the breakdown of budget to the individual nursing units.

Heat, light, power, and housekeeping, for example, are considered indirect expenses. The portion of the total of these expenses applicable to the nursing department is determined by extensive and technical cost studies. Since the nurse director has no control over these expenses and is in no position to make a determination of the portion applicable to her department, the amount must be furnished to her if the hospital policy requires that such expenses be included in her budget. Even though the nursing department may not be charged with the control of these items, personnel should cooperate in eliminating waste and unnecessary cost.

Capital Expenditure Budget

The capital expenditure budget outlines the need for major equipment or physical changes in the plant requiring large sums of money. Adequate cash must be available for these expenditures. The meaning of capital expenditures may vary from one hospital to another. For example, a nurse director and her staff may identify those items of equipment (see Appendix 6) or supplies necessary for patient services — among them, perhaps, a CircOlectric bed. If such an item exceeds some arbitrary amount — say, $100 — it is classified as a capital expenditure. The ceiling is established by hospital administration. Capital items are usually requested on a special form accompanied by a written justification for the item. If the number of requests for capital expenditures is unusually great, a priority list should be set. Where possible, the time when items are needed should be specified.

Included in the capital expenditure requests are cost estimates of installation, delivery, and maintenance as well as trade-in credits and, when available, names of manufacturers and suppliers. Where physical improvements are necessary within a department, reasonable cost estimates and completion dates should be obtained from the maintenance department. The purchasing department generally provides the department directors with estimates of equipment costs. Because the plant and equipment budget is dependent upon working capital, payment plans for larger expenditures should be investigated.

It is a joint responsibility of hospital administration and its department directors to develop a meaningful capital budget. Because of the high cost of major equipment, no organization can afford all the equipment that it wants. Each department director should thoroughly review capital needs, so that capital expenditures are handled as efficiently and effectively as possible.

The hospital administration usually provides guidelines. What equipment is to be considered for capital budgets? What type of items should receive priority? How should items being requested be listed? One hospital utilizes a simple system in which the department director states the desired new equipment needed, approximates the cost, notes the date it will be requested, and includes a brief narrative justification for the equipment.

Cash Budget

The cash budget forecasts an estimate of the amount of money being received — cash flow. It consists of the beginning cash balance, estimates of receipts and disbursements, and the estimated balance for a given period corresponding to that of the operating and capital expenditure budgets. The cash budget is prepared by estimating the amount of money collected from patients and from other sources of income and allocating it to cash disbursements required to meet obligations promptly as they come due. It is desirable that the money needed for operations, fixed assets, and long-term indebtedness be treated separately and combined in summary to reflect the overall requirements.

BUDGETARY FACTORS

Nursing service needs are determined by many factors, which the staff should be aware of as budget planning proceeds:

1. The type of patient (medical, surgical, maternity, pediatric, communicable disease, chronically ill), the length of stay, and the acuteness of the illness.
2. The size of the hospital and its bed occupancy. It takes more total personnel in the *large* hospital than it does in the smaller hospital to care for the same number of patients.
3. The physical layout of the hospital, the size and plan of the ward — open ward, small units, private ward.
4. Personnel policies:
   a. Salaries paid to various types of nursing personnel, including pay for overtime;
   b. The length of the work week and work period as well as flexibility of hours;
   c. The extent of vacation, statutory holidays and sick leave;
   d. Provision for in-service education programs including instructional staff as well as relief staff;
   e. Provision for development of staff through university preparation, refresher courses, etc.
5. The grouping of patients: for example, segregation demands more standardization of equipment; specialized units, such as neurological services, intensive care units, will have differing needs.
6. Standards of nursing care: The kind and amount of care to be given as it affects the number of hours of bedside care, for example, frequency of giving baths, changing beds, turning patients; assisting the patient to be dependent when necessary, for example, patients with coronary attacks; assisting the patient to adjust to the degree of independence of which he is capable, for example, the patient with a fracture; health teaching including methods of adjusting to normal living in the community.
7. The method of performing nursing procedures, simple or complex; the method of record-keeping and charting, for example, whether or not: all routine procedures such as baths and back rubs must be charted; all medications must be recorded in the nurses' notes; a work sheet and checking system are in use. In the nursing analysis project of 1953, directed by the University of Pittsburgh School of Nursing and Method of Engineering Council, it was determined that if the methods of nursing procedures and

routines in the medical center were improved, the services of 38.9 people working 40 hours per week, 50 weeks per year could be saved.

8. The proportion of nursing care provided by professional nurses as compared to that provided by auxiliary personnel.
9. The availability of graduate and allied personnel and the utilization of both groups according to competencies and preparation.
10. The amount and quality of supervision available and provided; the efficiency of job descriptions and job classifications.
11. Method of patient assignment, for example, team nursing.
12. The amount and kinds of labor-saving equipment and devices; flash autoclaves; intercommunication systems; telautograph; carrier and pneumatic tube systems; electronic monitor for determining vital signs, etc.
13. The amount of centralized service provided: sterile supply; central oxygen service; postoperative recovery room; messenger and porter service; linen service including distribution of linen.
14. Whether or not non-nursing functions such as clerical, dietary, housekeeping, messenger, and porter service are the responsibility of the nursing department.
15. The nursing service requirements of ancillary departments; clinics; admitting office; health service; emergency department, etc. These activities may be included in the responsibilities of the nursing department but should not be charged to nursing.
16. Reports required by administration, whether simple or complex.
17. Method of appointment of medical staff; size of staff; activities of medical staff; kind and frequency of treatments and orders.
18. Affiliation with a medical school: Inexperienced medical students need more equipment and supplies.
19. The presence, or not, of a school of nursing [96].

NURSING BUDGET COMMITTEE

The nurse director and her administrative staff are responsible for preparing an estimated departmental budget based on their understanding of the job to be done. A budget committee should be formed within the nursing department. It might be composed of assistant directors (day, evening, and night), supervisors, head nurses, and an administrative assistant (not a nurse — if one is assigned to the nursing office).

The committee is charged with setting overall budgeting policies of the hospital. It should also establish broad outlines of the operational plans before the budget is prepared. The committee ultimately will review each nursing unit budget separately and then look at the total

departmental plan. It can assist and advise the nurse director before
the final departmental budget is completed.

PREPARATION OF THE BUDGET

The director must be aware of any special instructions available from
hospital administration about preparation of data and the annual procedure for budgeting — and so inform the committee and unit personnel responsible for budget preparation. She must also obtain a copy
of the hospital calendar budget (see Appendix 7), which will provide
sufficient information for internal budget planning and a timetable
of proposed activities. The nursing budget committee initiates a
calendar (see Appendix 8), based on the hospital calendar, which will
also serve as a schedule to outline activities leading to the preparation
and completion of the nursing budget.

Past operations records need to be analyzed, and the overall master
staffing plan must be reviewed. Each supervisor should work with
her head nurses to determine the staff requirements for each unit.
They should consider such factors as: (1) assurance of standards according to the philosophy and objectives of the hospital and the department of nursing, (2) past experiences of the unit, (3) anticipated
needs for the unit, and (4) percentage of unit occupancy.

The estimation of staff for each unit should also include, for example, provision for vacation, sick leave, holidays, average amount of
illness per staff member, and on-call pay. The number of hours of
nursing care and nursing service hours per patient should be estimated
from the total.

As these figures are identified for each unit within the nursing department, there emerges a visible method of interpreting nursing care
needs to the nursing budget committee and later to hospital administration.

Consideration should next be given to any new activities that will
occur within a unit or have some bearing on the overall department,
such as new services for patient care, changes in in-service educational
programs, or changes in other hospital departments that affect the
nursing services required.

A review of the number of nursing hours per patient per day should
be done to determine whether the amount of care provided was com-

parable to what is considered minimal for safe nursing care. The hours may be maintained by the nursing office or data-processing office and available to nursing administration. Each supervisor and head nurse should receive a monthly report of nursing hours and should have a cumulative record from the previous fiscal year to review. These figures must be scrutinized, moreover, to find out whether the quality of nursing care met the predetermined standards of care and whether it could be maintained by using other levels of personnel, with fewer professional personnel, by a prearrangement of duties and responsibilities — for example, the addition of unit clerks to the evening tour of duty.

The next step in the preparation of the budget is to ascertain the amount and kind of supplies needed for the operation of each nursing unit, or those which are for total departmental use. A review of the last fiscal year's expenses provides data for planning. For budgetary purposes, the year's expected expenses can be divided by 12 or, where possible, calculated month by month. Generally, a 5 to 10 percent increase in cost of supplies is figured because of rising prices. Each unit should identify its needs in writing. Each nursing unit also submits a list of its own capital expenditure needs, and they are compiled into the total departmental requests.

As each supervisor or head nurse completes the preparation of the proposed budget, she meets with the nursing budget committee to make a formal presentation of her unit financial request. The purpose of the session is to review the operating and capital expenditures and allow for an explanation and justification of unit requests. To be discussed are: (1) personnel staffing requirements, with a justification if additional persons are needed; (2) general impact of supplies needed for use; (3) capital equipment to be replaced or requested, with documented justification, and other items requiring financial assistance; and (4), in some situations, specific recommendations for equipment and supplies prepared by the nursing unit staff with the chief of staff.

The unit budgets are approved as recommended, or revisions may be requested by the committee. Once the unit budgets are reviewed, classified, and summarized, the next step is to examine the departmental nursing budget appropriation and the actual expenditures for the current year, using information furnished by the accounting department in conjunction with the statistical data, such as average daily census per unit per service for the past year, and anticipated census for the fiscal budget year; percentage of bed occupancy by months; average length of patient stay for the past year; total patient days and outpatient visits; nursing service hours per patient per day; number of employees divided into their various classifications; and expenses for supplies.

BUDGET PRESENTATION

The nurse director compiles and completes the final draft of the nursing service budget. She should carefully reflect on how she will present the budget to the controller, budget officer, or hospital administrator. Presentation of the proposed budget affords her an opportunity to outline future nursing service plans for the department and the hospital, to define goals, and to set forth her ideas for achieving the desired results. It also allows her to review her department's past achievements and appraise them with some degree of perspective. A carefully planned budget presentation will reflect favorably upon the administration; a haphazard presentation may place the director in a less than favorable position.

Because the nursing department employs about 40 percent or more of the hospital staff and is the prime user of supplies and equipment, the hospital administrator is especially interested in the nurse director's presentation. She may choose to offer the budget alone or to capitalize upon the special knowledge of members of her staff by skillfully fitting their part of the budget presentation into the total picture.

A fundamental principle to keep in mind when selecting statistical data to include in the proposed budget is that the presentation should enlighten, not confuse. Data that are meaningful and depict the nursing functions should be chosen. After the nurse director selects the statistics she believes most pertinent, she must decide on the method of putting them forward. She must be able to highlight important information with a minimum of detail. Simplicity is essential, and times does not permit the study of many details. The details should be available, in case a question is asked that calls for further enlightenment, but they are not necessarily a part of the submitted budget [79].

BUDGET REVIEW

After the departmental budget has been reviewed and revised as needed, it becomes a part of the overall hospital-prepared plan. The hospital board of directors reviews the hospital budget and either approves it or suggests areas for revision. If any major changes are made in a departmental budget by either the hospital administrator or the budget controlling group, the director should be informed before the budget is finally acted upon. Once the hospital budget has been approved, it becomes the formal tool for measuring the progress of each department director toward her goals during the fiscal year.

BUDGET CONTROL

Once the department director receives her approved budget, a plan of action is necessary for review and control during the fiscal year. Effective implementation requires that she get timely and meaningful operating reports. These reports should contain sufficient detail and explanation of budget variances so that they can be used to evaluate the action required to correct the variances. Accurate monthly budget reports should make the department director cost- and budget-conscious and give her a sense of responsibility for the financial success of her department.

Budget development is only one of the major steps toward effective financial management in the nursing department. The nurse director has the obligation to organize the department so that she can operate efficiently and effectively within the budget throughout the year. The ultimate test is the evaluation of budgetary performance.

The nursing staff also has a responsibility to the patient and to the community to manage funds and resources well. Good budget administration is achieved only when the staff members feel that whatever can be done without a budget can be done much better with one.

Staffing is one of the most persistent and critical concerns facing nursing service administrative staff; yet there appears to be no definitive evidence on whether the problem is one of quantity, quality, or utilization of personnel. The numbers of graduates entering the labor force, the turnover of staff, the expansion of health care facilities, the changing role of delivering health care, the knowledge explosion, and the resultant changes in medical treatment — all affect the staffing process [77].

Staffing activities include such areas as: recruiting nursing staff; interviewing and screening personnel; employing all categories of nursing personnel; assigning staff to a clinical nursing unit and to specific work hours; preparing time schedules for the various groups of personnel; long-range planning for scheduling; short-range planning for supplementary staff (floaters or temporary staff); maintaining the daily and weekly work schedule; adjusting to meet needs of patients when the needs change or some staff members are absent; adjusting time schedules daily among the three tours of duty, as well as providing for transfer of staff within the nursing department among its units; keeping records significant to staffing such as budget, turnover, and hours; and developing and maintaining policies [77].

DETERMINING PERSONNEL REQUIREMENTS

Personnel requirements for any nursing department depend on such factors as the size of the hospital, its physical design, its patient population, the type of personnel available, the medical staff, and hospital policies and procedures. Because each setting is unique by virtue of these and other factors, there is no guide that can stipulate the correct number of personnel needed to provide high-quality care to patients. As a nurse director and her administrative staff study their own department, they can evaluate current nursing and staffing practices, identify areas that need improvement, and determine how they can best supply service based on available nursing resources.

Several methods may be used for predicting personnel requirements of a nursing department. The first approach is a subjective determination of personnel needs based on empirical evidence. The supervisor and head nurse will request a certain number of personnel according to how many people they think are necessary to perform the work on their specific nursing unit. This method gives little consideration to the ratio of professional to nonprofessional personnel. There is a tendency to adjust the staffing plan to the reality of the existing situation and availability of personnel rather than to develop a plan based on the number actually required. There is no way to explain or justify the actual personnel requirements. Very little research has been done in the area of staffing, and empirical evidence is still the best guide. The number of variables involved in hospitals of differing size, control, and services necessitates an individual rather than a general approach to developing a staffing pattern.

A second method is to adopt the commonly used rule that each patient is to be provided approximately so many nursing hours each day. The nursing care hours per patient are based on the nursing unit bed capacity or average daily census. It is difficult to determine the level of care needed and to establish a proper ratio of professional to nonprofessional personnel. The personnel requirements for care may vary widely from patient to patient; even the same patient may not have to have the same amount of care throughout his hospital stay. The amount of nursing care called for on a nursing unit is determined not merely by the nursing unit census but by the needs of each patient. Unfortunately, no available standards as to how many hours of nursing care patients require have been based upon adequate research.

A third method for developing a staffing plan is the use of scientific management techniques. This approach consists of conducting activity studies for all levels of personnel on a nursing unit, determining what each person does and how long it takes. Activities are then combined into tasks. At the nursing unit level, meetings are held with all personnel, and tasks are discussed — those currently being performed and those that should be performed to improve the quality of patient care. The unit group identifies all tasks as being related to nursing or not related to nursing. The nonrelated tasks are referred to hospital administration to be redistributed to other hospital departments. Tasks are redistributed either to reduce cost or to improve nursing services through better utilization of all levels of personnel. Tasks that properly belong to a nursing unit are analyzed to be sure that the appropriate employee is performing them. On the basis of the amount of time needed to carry out a specific task and the determination of the worker who will be performing the task, the proposed plan is calculated.

Another method that may be used for developing a staffing plan involves assessing patient needs by means of a numerical figure or index that predicts the nursing load. This is based on a realistic evaluation of patient care requirements. The approach provides a guide for classifying patients according to their nursing needs. An informal classification is done when the nurse in charge determines what category of personnel should care for each patient. The progressive patient care system is one application. It places each patient in the hospital area most suited to his needs — intensive, intermediate, and self-care.

As greater emphasis is placed on staffing according to the needs of patients, the scientific method will dictate what proportion of the staff giving direct patient care should be professional nurses. It can then be determined how the various levels of nursing personnel are to be utilized. The usual criterion for deciding whether a task shall be performed by a professional nurse, a nursing assistant, or a practical nurse is the simplicity or complexity of the task. Recognition of the difference in tasks performed for patients and the nursing judgment required is paramount in providing quality nursing care.

STAFFING OBJECTIVES

In accordance with nursing philosophy, staffing requirements and patterns can be designed to achieve objectives such as the following:

1. To provide continuous quality nursing care to patients with the available staff.
2. To evaluate staffing practices periodically in order to determine the scope of staffing problems.
3. To recruit qualified nursing staff.
4. To utilize the talents and skills of each level of nursing to their fullest through the team nursing concept.
5. To provide new employees with an adequate orientation period.
6. To establish personnel conditions of employment and adjust as needed to current practices.
7. To utilize centralized (or decentralized) staffing as a means of scheduling.
8. To develop personnel policies that attract and provide effective staff members.

9. To establish a master staffing plan for allocating personnel based on an assessment of patients' needs.
10. To maintain records pertinent to staffing data.

FACTORS AFFECTING STAFFING

Nursing staffing is complicated by such concerns as:

1. The need to provide hospital and nursing services 24 hours a day.
2. Unpredictability of the patient census.
3. Differentiating between nursing care and patient care.
4. Budget limitations that do not provide for realistic personnel requirements.
5. Time spent by nursing personnel performing non-nursing duties.
6. Employee satisfaction or dissatisfaction.
7. Improper utilization of personnel.
8. Unpredictable turnover of nursing personnel.
9. Instability and inflexibility of staff.
10. Decreased continuity of patient care due to high ratio of part-time personnel.
11. Staffing for weekends, holidays, and vacations.
12. Span of supervision.
13. Lack of qualified professional nurses for leadership positions.
14. Communications among different levels of personnel.
15. Staff development programs.
16. Absenteeism among staff.
17. Physical facilities, supplies, and equipment.
18. Extent of knowledge by the board of directors about patient care and nursing services.
19. Ability of the hospital to understand nursing needs of patients.
20. Meeting changing needs of patients.

As the nurse director identifies staffing problems, she should involve the nursing staff in collecting the necessary data to support a change of direction. For example, much has been written about freeing nurses of non-nursing duties. As nurses are released from those activities, the quality of care to patients should increase, and nursing personnel should concentrate on those tasks related to nursing services. A plan of action should be developed to identify non-nursing areas and also to indicate how the additional nursing time will be used. The plan can be presented and interpreted to the hospital administrator, showing the need for other hospital departments to become self-contained. The director will be able to suggest a study of those departments to see how they can be organized in order to release nursing man-hours.

FUTURE DIRECTION

The administrative staff must live and work with the current situation while planning for the future. If sufficient numbers of graduate nurses are not available to provide all the nursing care people expect, the strengthening of the educational programs for registered nurses, practical nurses, nurse assistants, and technicians is imperative. Personnel appointed to the nursing department should be judiciously selected, and any assignment should be preceded by a carefully planned orientation program.

The supply of nursing services to patients in hospitals or any other health care agency depends on two factors. The first is the number of persons employed, and the second is the effectiveness with which these persons undertake their responsibilities. The question should be raised within every health care setting: Is there really a shortage of nursing personnel, or is there a misuse of nursing personnel? Great effort and concern must be directed toward making the work situation and condition of employment attractive, so that the supply of personnel is likely to be adequate and the effectiveness of their work performance is likely to be high. A nursing recruitment committee should be developed with the assistance of the personnel department or any individual or group interested in attracting people to nursing or to entering a nursing educational program. It must be made clear that the quality of care to be attained will be in proportion to the available personnel and how effectively they can function in nursing tasks [77].

MASTER STAFFING PLAN

A master staffing plan is an administrative tool that increases organizational efficiency. It is an estimate of the total number of nursing

personnel, professional and supportive, required by the nursing
department to provide nursing services for the fiscal year. This plan
is based on a study of the needs of patients and the availability of
personnel. It is a practical and efficient device for the control of positions allocated to each nursing unit, as well as the total department.
The plan further offers a visible means of identifying vacant positions. It virtually becomes the personnel budget, establishing the
number and kind of positions for each unit and the salary scale for
each position [34].

Development of a master staffing plan requires effective projection
and cooperative effort by the nursing service administrative staff.
Each supervisor or head nurse submits an estimate of personnel requirements for her unit. If additional positions are needed, a written
justification must also be presented. Each unit plan is discussed by
the supervisor and head nurse with the nurse director. Together they
are able to adjust, add, or delete positions. Once all unit plans are
reviewed in this manner, the director prepares the departmental
master staffing plan. She must be sure it is simple to interpret and
easy to understand. She must be able to explain and justify it and
prepare the necessary written information to substantiate her
requests.

The master staffing plan is then submitted to the hospital administration for approval. The nurse director has a responsibility to make
known the degree of care patients may generally receive on the basis
of the proposed plan. If staffing problems exist, she must use this opportunity to express her growing concern and make recommendations.

The hospital administrator may endorse the plan or suggest changes.
When the plan is approved, it becomes the official administrative
tool for personnel budget control. It must be recognized that the
plan is subject to change in the event of changing circumstances or
emergencies, when the necessary personnel adjustments can be made.

The master plan, as well as each unit plan, should be available to
all who are interested. It will keep everyone aware of what is happening in terms of staffing. The nursing personnel will be able to identify
filled and vacant positions, so that they can apply for the latter if
they are perceived as opportunities for advancement. The plan also
serves as a means of control — identifying as it does the actual number and kind of positions approved for the fiscal year.

A master copy of the plan can be maintained in the nursing service office. Commercial staffing boards are available to show, at a

glance, all positions, filled or vacant. Kardex card files may be used for the same purpose, as it is possible to view each unit plan or segment thereof separately; large bulletin boards may hold individual copies of unit staffing plans and present an instantaneous visible picture of the total plan (Figure 10).

Each nursing unit, as illustrated, has its own plan, which indicates the various levels of nursing positions, names of persons in the positions, assigned tours of duty, and the authorized hours per person per pay period. The plan also reflects the total number of hours allotted for each nursing unit's operation within a two-week pay period. This latter figure is used to determine the number of nursing hours allotted per patient based on the individual unit plan.

SCHEDULING

Scheduling personnel is a complex task, time-consuming and frequently perplexing; but it must be done. Actual scheduling may be performed centrally by the nursing office, or the smaller units may make up their own schedules.

If it is believed that centralized staffing is best for departmental scheduling, whether done by a supervisor, an assistant director, or a centralized staffing secretary, this approach provides a central control of staff. It means that personnel can be distributed in a more balanced manner among the nursing units, and understaffing or overstaffing is eliminated to some degree. Since full responsibility for staffing is delegated to one person at the departmental level, the head nurse is relieved of a time-consuming task. Centralized staffing provides an overall picture of the staffing situation. As schedules for the department are reviewed, it is easier to make adjustments in case of illness, emergencies, or changes in patient care needs among nursing units. Under this system, specific time requests by personnel tend to decrease. Centralized staffing is likely to eliminate the personal contact that develops between a head nurse and her personnel as it relates to employee work schedules. The person in charge of centralized staffing finds that she knows very little about the person she schedules on time sheets.

Even if scheduling is established by a computer, someone must check to see that the schedule is truly equitable and that it is compatible with actual needs. Data processing does not completely do

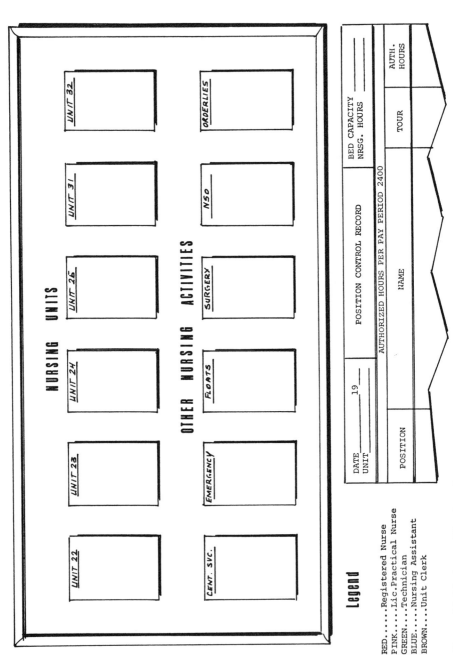

Figure 10. Master staffing board.

away with the need for a person or persons to be responsible for staffing; the validity and feasibility of the suggested programmed schedules and reassignments must be evaluated and approved by someone in the nursing office.

Circumstances in some instances may support the decentralization of scheduling, which means that the head nurse or a unit manager plans work time schedules for personnel. The decentralized system presumably allows the head nurse to base her scheduling plan on her knowledge of the personnel assigned to her unit. She feels "more in control" of the activities on her unit. However, the system does limit the ability of a nursing unit to be self-sufficient in relation to staffing. In cases of illness or emergency the head nurse has little recourse among her own unit personnel for additional coverage. Decentralized staffing can work as long as the nursing office maintains some reserve personnel for use where needed. The nursing office should not (in fact cannot) ever relinquish authority to move staff from place to place according to patient needs.

Decentralized scheduling sometimes makes it difficult for a head nurse to be completely objective; she may be prone either to under-staff or to overstaff when she herself is on duty, depending on how she views her role and the capabilities of her staff. Staff members may feel that the head nurse is not objective, and they may miscon-strue undesirable scheduling as punishment for poor performance or as evidence of dislike on the part of the head nurse. Each head nurse under decentralized staffing tends to develop and utilize her own staffing patterns, and, as workers on various units compare schedules, dissatisfaction may arise.

Cyclical scheduling is another method of staffing. It involves central-ized planning and development of schedule patterns that are repeated at regular intervals with decentralized responsibility for imple-mentation. Schedule patterns are set for a certain number of weeks and are repeated (every two, four, six, or more weeks, as desired) within the given cycling period. This approach divides responsibility for the staffing process and its implementation between the nursing office representative and the nursing unit supervisor or head nurse [42].

The actual work schedules are management tools accompanying the master staffing pattern. In planning these schedules, the sched-uler is faced with developing work time sheets that balance the needs of patients and personnel. There is also a concern for increasing the ability of the staff to respond to fluctuations in patient care needs and staff changes such as those caused by illness, holidays, and vacations. There must be an equitable distribution of the desirable as well as the undesirable tours of duty. An employee must be assured that her assigned time on duty will not fluctuate unless an extreme emergency arises, and only with her permission. Scheduling practices should reflect fair and just treatment of all employees in regard to scheduling of hours [77].

Scheduling policies must be identified that will promote effective staffing. At the time of employment, conditions relating to hours on duty need to be clarified. The new staff member is entitled to know what is meant by the work week, rotation of hours (if used), floating and part-time employees, and similar terms [77].

Standards of performance are established by each department of the hospital to guide the actions of the personnel into purposeful, safe, and effective patient care. The nurse director and her staff have to be aware of those standards that have any relationship to the care of patients. For example, the hospital has fire safety standards for the general welfare of patients and others within the hospital: "If fire or smoke is detected, remove all patients in immediate danger from the area; notify the Fire Department by using the nearest alarm; fight the fire until relieved by the Fire Department."

Standards for nursing — nursing practice and nursing service — are the responsibility of the nurse director and the administrative nursing staff. Nursing care concerns itself with (1) the provision of care through nursing practice and (2) the provision of care through nursing services. The first involves the actual use of nursing skills of all kinds in direct contact with the patient and his family; the second has to do with the facilitation of this practice through the use of administrative, supervisory, and teaching skills. Each of these parts of nursing requires a set of standards. Central to the determination of nursing care standards are working definitions of what nursing is [33].

Each nursing group, for example, must define nursing as it relates to its own operation. In practice there is no universal definition. The basic meanings found in the nursing literature and promoted by various professional organizations form sound guides and, if desired, may be used profitably without change; other definitions developed and formulated by a particular group may be helpful. It is questionable, however, whether progress can be made toward quality nursing care without some idea of what it is.

DEFINITION OF NURSING

In formulating a definition of nursing care (see Appendix 9) one must recognize that each individual's concept of nursing is influenced by his or her own perspective, experience, and background. Each nurse's value systems and beliefs will serve as a basis for giving care to patients. The nurse director must strive to mesh the thinking of the staff in order to arrive at some operational meaning of nursing care that the staff will support and implement. Once established, the meaning of nursing care must be interpreted to the members of the nursing department and others who are interested.

It is also necessary to define the practice of nursing legally, so that the boundaries of that practice will be clearly understood by all personnel giving nursing care. A legal definition may be more mundane and less inspirational than some of the definitions found in the nursing literature; it is nevertheless very important that such a definition exist, to protect both the nurse and the public [78]. The nurse director and her staff must be aware of the definition of nursing practice that allows individuals to practice nursing in a given state.

Standards are criteria against which performance can be measured. Standards of nursing practice should be clear, concise, specific sentences worded in terms of action and behavior that describe intended outcomes that can be seen, measured, and judged. The standards are derived from a definition of broad roles the nurse practitioners fill in relation to the patient. Activities the practitioner will carry out to reach a goal must be selected. Nursing administration is responsible for determining who is to author the statements and who can make the standards useful for producing quality nursing practice. People who are innovators in the realm of ideas and practices and thoroughly experienced practitioners who have developed expertise in giving care to clients need to collaborate in the development of standards.

Methods should be formulated for maintaining standards, and ways identified to inform the staff and others whom they may affect. The standards of practice are usually minimal standards, describing the safety measures and expertise necessary for performance of a job.

Nursing practice procedures should be established to assist personnel to make correct decisions in the performance of nursing care. Written procedures should be available as evidence that standards have been set up for safe, effective care, taking into consideration the best use of available resources and personnel [78].

A committee of nursing personnel can be appointed to develop, review, and revise performance standards. Members of the medical staff and other health professionals should be invited to participate on the committee as needed for direction and guidance. Standards of performance can be compiled into a nursing practice manual or a quality assurance program manual, which can serve as a tool for the management, as well as accountability, of nursing care.

The nursing department should have a specific, written policy in its administrative manual indicating that the nursing practice manual is the department's official guide. A copy of the nursing practice manual should be placed on each nursing unit. Copies should also be available to the hospital administration, the medical staff, and other departments that may need to be aware of these standards.

A general medical and surgical nursing practice manual can serve as a basic guide for nursing care but is to be accompanied by procedures relating to such specialized areas of nursing practice as pediatrics, maternity, psychiatry, and surgery.

Standards for organized nursing service have been developed by the Joint Commission for the Accreditation of Nursing Services, the National League for Nursing, the American Hospital Association, the American Nurses' Association, and others. These generalized statements can be studied and tailored to an individual hospital nursing service and related to standards for practice. For example, if a standard states: "The nursing department promotes safe and therapeutically effective nursing care through the implementation of established standards of nursing practice," it can be assumed that it is the function of service to provide the numbers and levels of personnel needed, the physical facilities, the supplementary educational programs, the motivating atmosphere, the necessary administrative hierarchy, and the administrative channels for the nursing staff to practice. How all this is provided will differ in every hospital. The hospital's philosophy, budget, types of programs, and many other factors will influence its specific standards.

In setting both types of standards, nursing administration should consult everyone who is directly affected, and those who know the most about a subject should have the most to say in making decisions about it. If the effort is to be effective, it must be collaborative. Knowledgeable, talented, and experienced people should be sought to provide a foundation on which to build nursing standards.

QUALITY ASSURANCE PROGRAM

The concept of quality assurance refers to the accountability of health personnel for the quality of care they provide to patients. The accountability involves provision of evidence as compared to an agreed-upon standard [74].

It is evident in the literature as well as in practice that nurse directors and their staffs are reviewing and planning programs to ensure the provision of quality care. Society grants to nursing (as well as to other health professions) authority over functions vital to them and allows considerable autonomy in the control of their own affairs. In return, the nursing profession is expected to act responsibly, always mindful of its public trust and accountability for its own practice. Self-regulation and self-discipline are recognized as hallmarks of professionalism [74].

No longer is quality assurance a purely professional need in the pursuit of excellence; rather, it is a public need in defense of the entire health care system to ensure its creditability. Quality assurance of service is necessary because the consumers who receive care have high expectations; it is also necessary for those who provide the setting with high liability; and, finally, it is necessary for those with fiscal responsibility, who have high costs. Third-party payers want legitimate assurance that the costs of care are justified. Medical staffs as well as hospital professionals have a legal responsibility to the governing boards of hospitals, and the governing bodies in turn are accountable to the communities from which they draw their patients [76].

The enactment of the Social Security Amendments of 1972 (Public Law 92–603) has brought into focus the urgent need for effective quality assurance programs in patient care and management by the providers within the health care system. Auditing at a state or regional level for effectiveness and cost efficiency has been made the responsibility of the Professional Standards Review Organizations (PSROs). The purpose of this auditing program is to ensure that services are medically necessary and that they are provided in accordance with professional standards [75].

In 1971 the American Hospital Association began development of its Quality Assurance Program for Medical Care in Hospitals, a program that includes the best elements of proved traditional review mechanisms and incorporates the measurement of performance with cost effectiveness. The Quality Assurance Program guidelines accommodate evaluation procedures that lead to the identification of a need for corrective action if care does not meet established criteria of quality. Through this inherent control factor, review becomes primarily an educational process and also a management tool [7]. One of the new standards of the Joint Commission on the Accreditation of Hospitals requires that quality assurance and corrective action mechanisms be built into hospitals' provision of care.

Providing Quality Nursing Care

The nurse director and her staff must continuously evaluate the quality of care patients are receiving. A question to be raised is: What is quality care? The definitions can range from general to specific. For example, here is a general statement: "Quality nursing care is the wise use of knowledge, skill, and compassion to meet the needs of the patient" [98]. *Knowledge* includes not only formal nursing education and experience but other formal education, as well as life experiences and understanding. The social, biological, and physical sciences are applied; clinical knowledge can be used; and an understanding of administration, teaching, and other supportive aspects can be applied to nursing. *Skill* must be demonstrated in the light of knowledge, which becomes operational in the giving of care. Skills range from manual to communicative and include evaluation, judgmental, and coordinating skills. Skill encompasses the ability to apply the many facets of knowledge. *Compassion* reflects the concern and interest of those who give the patient care. Knowledge and skill applied without compassion will not fulfill the needs of patients, and the element of practical compassion is vital to quality care [98].

Quality nursing care, defined more specifically, consists of:

1. Careful development of the physician's therapeutic plan for the patient as delegated to the nurse — including treatments, administering medications, pertinent observations, and coordinating of nursing with the activities of the medical team in therapeutic approaches to the patient. This aspect of quality care invokes the nurse's whole knowledge and skill in the area of medical science and technology. It calls for her participation as a senior member of the medical team — informed, responsible, and accountable.
2. Basic physical care of the patient for his comfort and welfare. This aspect of quality care falls to nursing service; it includes simple areas of personal care — care of the hair, shaving, oral hygiene, baths, skin conditioning, body alignment, assistance with meals and elimination, regulating room temperatures and ventilation.
3. Recognition of individual needs, and use of nursing, hospital, and community resources to meet them. The third part of the definition of quality care touches recognition of the patient's individual needs — social, economic, emotional, psychological, religious, and rehabilitative. This requires sensitivity to patient reactions that go beyond the medical treatment and physical needs, and it extends into the family and the community. The extensive and wise use of referrals is one indication of sensitivity, interest, and concern for the patient's welfare as well as the alertness and effectiveness of the staff [91].

The nurse director and her staff must encourage their group to define quality nursing, appraise current practice in terms of the definition, and then plan for every activity to close the gaps and reinforce the strengths. They must clarify what they believe should happen to the patient before they plot a way to achieve it.

A nurse director and her staff should be concerned with two questions: (1) How can we develop quality nursing care? (2) How can we appraise the effectiveness of what we develop?

In response to the first question, consideration should be given to identifying written materials, which might include:

1. Statements or articles on quality nursing care and quality assurance programs.
2. Self-evaluation guides from professional organizations.
3. Performance evaluation methods and forms for staff providing care to patients.
4. Evaluation guides provided by accrediting, professional, and local licensing groups.
5. Study and research identifying patient needs.
6. Models for internal surveys to identify reactions to care by the patient, family, physician, and nurse [91].

In response to the second question, the nurse director and her staff must identify the tools within the nursing department that are available to judge the quality of care being rendered. These may include:

1. Standards set by professional and accrediting bodies: American Nurses' Association, National League for Nursing, American Hospital Association, Joint Commission on Accreditation of Hospitals, state licensing board.
2. Nursing audit of the patient's record.
3. Results of patient questionnaires following discharge.
4. Review of infection records.
5. Analysis of accident reports.
6. Patient and family comments or complaints.
7. Study of medication errors.
8. Analysis of employee critical incidents.
9. Rounds on the nursing units.
10. Quality of patient written nursing care plans.
11. Adherence to nursing departmental and nursing unit philosophy and objectives.
12. Effectiveness of team conferences and reports.
13. Effectiveness of patient teaching programs.

14. Peer review program.
15. Review of staffing patterns for each nursing unit.
16. Interviews with terminating personnel.
17. Use of nursing care plans.
18. Observation of nursing activities.
    a. To what extent have the nursing care objectives of the patient been achieved?
    b. To what extent and with what degree of skill have nurses carried out the nursing process?
    c. To what extent are the conditions under which nursing care is given judged to be conducive to the delivery of good nursing care?

As the nurse director and her staff examine what is actually happening to the patient in all these areas, they should have some idea of how effective their nursing services are. Areas in need of improvement and corrective action can be located.

Role of the Nurse Director and Nursing Staff

As the hospital system strives to achieve quality care for its consumers, nursing participates and collaborates with other health care providers to (1) develop criteria for the outcome of patient care and (2) monitor the overall program of quality assurance. A multidisciplinary team approach within the hospital can design patient care criteria that reflect actual conditions and can ensure that decisions appropriate to hospital patient populations are made. Health team members must strive to demonstrate that they can develop quality assurance mechanisms that are available, sound, and economically feasible for the delivery of health care. While nursing is concerned with promoting positive nursing care results and outcomes, it is the outcome of a patient's total care that matters.

The nurse director provides the leadership both within her department and as a member of a multidisciplinary hospital team to contribute toward the development of a quality assurance program (QAP). A QAP estimates the degree of excellence in nursing care outcomes and in the cost outcomes of activity and other resources; its major concern is evaluation and improvement of care. A QAP has two functions: (1) to assess the results of an ongoing program, and (2) to estimate the value, rank, or degree of excellence of care. A

QAP requires a method that will allow the nursing staff to move from findings to actions that will result in improvement, and to report the results of care to successively higher levels in the hospital [98].

Leadership in the implementation of knowledge about quality assurance care is essentially an administrative function. The nurse director's concept of quality assurance care, her recognition of its potential, and her respect for its contribution to patient care will reflect the leadership she provides.

The nurse director is responsible for the development and implementation of a quality assurance program as a management tool for nursing. She provides the organizational and administrative structure for accomplishing the goals of a QAP through the commitments and cooperation of the nursing personnel, hospital administration and its departments, medical staff, and consumer. The nurse director is directly concerned with obtaining what is needed to provide high-quality care. High standards of nursing care must be established and maintained, and the nurse director then delegates to the nursing staff the primary responsibility for review and development of quality control.

An effective nursing review plan must have approval from the nursing administration, hospital administration, and committees related to quality assurance. The plan must involve frequent meetings, patient population selections, methodology of reviews, records, reports, and forms, recommendations, follow-up, and assistance from the nursing administrative staff. Quality assurance requires much time and effort, but high-quality care is a right — not a privilege — and cannot be compromised.

A quality assurance program committee can be organized within the nursing service departmental structure and, preferably, it should have representation from various clinical nursing departments. The working committees may include a nursing care committee, a nursing audit committee, and others that contribute to the goals of quality assurance. The committees may establish advisory committees to provide input from other segments of the hospital or community. Recommendations from the nursing QAP committees are referred to the nurse director, and she in turn refers them to the hospital administrator or to other persons who share administrative responsibility for quality assurance patient care. This delegated responsibility renders the nursing staff accountable to the hospital's administration, which shares the nursing department's responsibility for the quality of care provided in the hospital.

Objectives of a Quality Assurance Program

The objectives of a QAP in nursing may include:

1. Providing quantitative measures that will indicate the level of quality of nursing care.
2. Measuring the existing quality of level of care in nursing.
3. Providing feedback about deficiencies of nursing care that call for corrective action.
4. Monitoring the work effectiveness of nursing personnel upon the quality of nursing in nursing services and functions to patients.
5. Collaborating with other health care programs to achieve quality health care.

Quality Assurance Program as a System

QAP in nursing may be viewed as a system composed of three components — structure, process, and outcome; the ultimate goals of the system are directed toward the achievement of high standards of care. The structural component focuses on the organization of patient care in which nursing is given; the process component emphasizes the actual performance of care through the nursing process; the outcome component concentrates on patient welfare, the end results of nursing care, and professional measurement using criterion measures.

Development of Criteria. Basic to any evaluation is the need to develop criteria against which actual care is judged. Criteria are categories of nursing actions or patient outcomes that are representative of quality nursing care. Criteria are classified in various ways: medical diagnostic categories, nursing diagnostic categories, degree of illness, and nursing problems. The categories facilitate the development of specific criteria. Watson and Mayers [89] suggest that criteria be established by nurses who are providing direct patient care. The criteria are written in two forms: (1) desired nursing actions (process criteria), which the nursing staff members believe are important for achieving satisfactory patient outcomes, and (2) desired patient outcomes (outcome criteria) or clinical manifestations, or both, which represent the desired patient responses to nursing care activities. A criterion must be achievable, specific, concise, and understandable; it serves as a guide to nurses for professional performance, is functional for auditing patients' charts, and is representative of the values of the hospital [98].

In developing criteria, one should look at what is being said and done in the literature as well as in practice. Criteria should be written in specific, measurable terms, and their applicability to patient care areas in the nursing department should be determined. The criteria must be relevant to nursing practice; they should yield a range of scores and values that are written for a population of patients with common pathological conditions that can be identified. A criterion is a predetermined measure established to determine the highest achievable level of care; it consists of elements of care of major consequence to the nursing outcome of patient care, standards for that element, and any clinically recognized exceptions to that standard. Criteria should produce reliable and valid data, from which proper generalizations about the quality of care can be made and used for improvement. The development of criteria provides a method for abstracting data, allowing comparisons of actual results with desired results and judgment of the results of comparison, in order to make decisions about implementing improvement actions, reassessments to determine patterns as they develop, and needed accountings for results.

Consumers must be allowed to communicate to professionals what is important in nursing outcomes.

Some nursing staff members look upon criteria development as a peer responsibility, belonging to nursing; however, it must be recognized that the care of patients is a team responsibility, and that collaborative development of criteria reinforces the team concept of the hospital system.

Developing a Quality Assurance Program

Characteristics. The characteristics of a QAP are the following:

1. The model for quality assurance in nursing should be especially designed for evaluating nursing practice in terms of the contemporary model of such practice and should be developed and applied by nurses.

2. The program should be primarily directed toward evaluating quality of care rather than any other characteristics of care.
3. The program should be designed in such a way that the resulting data can be used for accountability and improvement purposes.
4. The evaluation instruments should measure nurse performance rather than the outcomes of care.
5. The evaluations should yield both quantitative and descriptive data.
6. The criteria and instruments of evaluation should be widely applicable both geographically and with respect to the nursing problems of patients [75].

Steps. The steps necessary to fulfill the requirements of the QAP in nursing are the following:

1. Develop measurable outcome criteria.
2. Examine and evaluate the care rendered to patients.
3. Compare the results of care with anticipated outcomes based on criteria; identify discrepancies.
4. Take corrective action (if indicated) to remedy shortcomings.
5. Reassess the outcomes after corrective action has been taken to determine whether outcomes equal expectations after action taken.
6. Share evaluation of nursing care with the nursing staff and the larger system of which nursing is a part.

Development of Model QAP. The nurse director responsible for developing a QAP should:

1. Develop written standards of nursing care for patients.
2. Identify the desired nursing outcomes for a definitive population of patients with specific health problems.
3. Determine the nursing activities as well as the cost of the resources required to reach the desired outcomes.
4. Establish criteria designed for use as a comparison against the findings or results of care.
5. Develop tools (forms and directions) to be used during the process of assessing the quality of care received by patients and to measure nursing competence.
6. Develop a rating scale for each measurement tool.
7. Develop an evaluation form to record results of measurement assessment findings against the established criteria.
8. Establish procedures for assessing the nursing care given to patients.

9. Establish methods to document evaluations and criteria changes as well as what facilitated the change.

Corrective Action

When it is observed that nursing outcomes do not conform to established criteria (and are less than satisfactory), the nurse director and her staff can have recourse to meaningful, planned change and corrective action through:

1. Peer review — nurses scrutinize their own process data for deviations from accepted practices, with resultant clues for improvement, and, conversely, for care outcomes that are more than satisfactory. When the goal is to improve nursing care, it is not the outcome that can be manipulated; rather, it is the professional nursing practice that must be changed, with the expectation that outcomes will also change as a result.
2. Educational programs, for individuals or for the entire nursing staff based on demonstrated needs identified through QAP.
3. Administrative or organizational changes that will correct observed shortcomings of nursing care.
4. Individual or group changes through counseling and guidance.

The board of directors, the hospital administration, the medical staff, and the nursing staff, through summary performance reports and information concerning correction of shortcomings, will be constantly and adequately advised about the nurses' performance so that they can fulfill their obligation to the community for assuring high-quality care.

Benefits of a Quality Assurance Program

The benefits of a QAP in nursing are the following:

1. It provides a well-developed and widely communicated method for quality assurance in nursing.
2. It provides an appropriate mechanism for the nursing staff to fulfill its mission.
3. It provides nursing staff members with information as to where they are going.

4. It identifies where nursing stands and what must be done to improve nursing care for the consumers.
5. It upgrades the quality of nursing care and the skills of nursing personnel.
6. It points toward greater assurance that the nursing objectives of patient care will be met.
7. It identifies weak areas in the structure, process, and outcomes of nursing that must be changed to strengths.
8. It promotes cost containment.
9. It provides valuable documentation in case of any litigation.
10. It provides interdisciplinary opportunities to achieve broad health care goals of quality assurance.
11. It generates self-satisfaction to all those delivering nursing care and can ensure the consumer optimal service and satisfaction.

PEER REVIEW

Peer review is an ongoing process in which professional nursing can demonstrate accountability and responsibility for nursing actions. Peer review is oriented toward the manageability of the nursing role. The major focus of peer review is the use of peer judgments to implement standards of nursing practice. As the nursing director and her professional staff begin to think about the development of such a program, this author recommends as a starting point the Peer Review Guidelines developed by the American Nurses' Association, Ad Hoc Committee on Implementation of Standards of Nursing Practice of the Congress for Nursing Practice, November, 1973 (see Appendix 10).

In the publication *Quality Assessment: Program and Process*, National League for Nursing, Western Regional Assembly of Constituent League, March, 1974, and March, 1975, Forums for Nursing Service Administrators in the West, Joan King raised the question: Who is really qualified and able to help in reviewing the performance of the nursing service director? A Peer Review Tool for the nursing service director was presented at that Forum (see Appendix 11).

12. Methods of Assignment

The philosophy of the nursing department generally determines the method of assigning staff to care for patients. There are five methods of assignment that may be used, individually or in combination with other methods.

The case method involves assignment of complete care of one or more patients to one member of the staff. Individualized care is possible; patient-nurse rapport is heightened; and the satisfaction of both patient and nurse is ensured. The case method facilitates a close relationship of the nurse to family and friends.

The functional method involves assignment of selected functions to all personnel, with no one person being responsible for any total nursing activities. Emphasis is on the task, and the jobs are grouped in the interest of time and expediency of service, such as having a medication nurse or a treatment nurse.

The case-functional method of assignment involves a combination of both of the foregoing: case for morning care, functional at mealtime, in the afternoon, or at night. This approach may be used when certain staff members are not prepared to provide for the total needs of patients.

The team method of assignment has the staff working together as a team to provide care to patients. A professional nurse serves as leader of the team. This approach incorporates all personnel in group processes, recognizing interdependent values and challenging the best individual and combined efforts. It allows the head nurse to share responsibility with her staff and to extend her own ability. It promotes and builds a sense of belonging on the part of all, an esprit de corps.

There are situations in which the case method is desirable, but exclusive use of a one-to-one ratio is unrealistic in terms of staffing and economics. The functional method provides for smooth division of labor according to tasks but prevents use of personnel to their fullest potential. The case-functional method utilizes one approach today and another next week and may render the learning of values and acceptability of either method questionable. Under the team nursing method, all personnel have contact with patients and share in planning and providing nursing care. However, team nursing is difficult to manipulate with relatively unstable staff members; it is impossible if the head nurse does not delegate authority to leaders of teams. The method of assignment becomes a nursing administrative decision based on nursing staff resources, physical facilities, nursing service standards, and budget.

ASSIGNING STAFF TO PATIENT CARE

Primary nursing is an organizational pattern for nursing units in hospitals that calls for nurses to assume a new role. Primary nursing may be defined as distribution of nursing care in such a way that the total care of an individual patient is the responsibility of one nurse, not many; it can be differentiated from team and functional nursing, which require that the total care of any one patient be shared by several nurses during a single shift [59]. Primary nursing, like case method care, assigns one nurse to each patient. Whereas the case method nurse may be responsible for her shift only, the primary nurse is responsible for the patient 24 hours a day for the duration of that patient's hospital stay. The primary nurse assesses the patient's nursing care needs, collaborates with the physician and other hospital personnel, and formulates a nursing care plan that the nurse is responsible for carrying out around the clock every day. The primary nurse may delegate to a secondary nurse the responsibility for carrying out the care plan on other shifts; delegation is accomplished by means of nursing care plans, recordings, or notes and never proceeds through a supervisory third person [59].

ASSIGNMENT SHEET

In order to plan and direct nursing care, assignment sheets are used to indicate the total work program for a 24-hour period or for seven days a week (see Appendix 12). Written assignments for nursing staff are generally made by the professional nurse based on the data found in the written nursing care plans and on the abilities of the staff.

The nurse director is responsible for reviewing periodically how assignments are being made:

1. Are assignments written clearly, concisely, and legibly?
2. Are assignment sheets posted in an area where they are easily accessible for the team members to use as a reference?

3. Are assignments related to previous assignments, so as to provide a progressive type of learning experience?
4. Are duties overlapping?
5. Are assignments made out on a weekly basis and adjusted to meet the needs of patients? [57]

Individual assignment work sheets may be developed to serve as a guide and reminder for nursing personnel (see Appendix 13).

THE NURSING PROCESS

One way of thinking about the management, practice, and delivery of nursing care to patients in the hospital is through use of the nursing process. The idea of the nursing process has generally been accepted as the very core of nursing. In order to promote the nursing process effectively to the nursing staff, hospital administrators, and other hospital departments, the nurse director must be able to assist others in developing an awareness of the ultimate benefits derived from utilization of the process in meeting hospital goals.

Goal of Nursing

The main goal of nursing is to assist individuals in progressing toward the highest achievable level of wellness. To reach this goal, a process must be set in motion. The process must have coordination of its parts without interruption or cessation until the goals are achieved. Since the process is centered upon people — adaptive organisms influenced by social, psychological, cultural, and physical factors — the process becomes complex. Because of its nature and the context in which it takes place, this could be called more accurately the nursing process [49].

The nursing process itself is a cycle of action that includes multidimensional components: assessment, planning, implementation, and evaluation. A dynamic, interdependent relationship exists among the components, with each one giving direction and impetus to the other. Research is perceived as permeating all components of the process, whether it be in the form of applied research or formal research. The nursing process encompasses all the activities that are implemented in the care of people; wherever the nurse cares for individuals, this same process could and should be performed. Both theory and clinical expertise are necessary for adequate application of the nursing process.

Properties

General properties of the nursing process, as identified by Little and Carnevelli [57], include a pattern of thinking and behaving that: (1) is cyclic and recurring; (2) may be carried on either with awareness or almost automatically; (3) can be learned in terms of skill and speed; (4) may be carried out with varying speed, ranging from almost instantaneous thinking to protracted deliberation; (5) integrates priority setting and feedback mechanisms into every step; (6) is dependent upon the effective use of a body of knowledge; and (7) involves verbal symbols (words). These general properties are an integral part of each step of the nursing process as well as of the totality of the concept.

The nursing process seems to have evolved as a result of several factors:

1. The need to describe what nurses do in some type of scientific measurable terms.
2. The need for nursing to upgrade the quality of nursing care as a result of several issues (accountability, consumer demand).
3. The need for nursing to defend itself as a profession in an attempt to upgrade the status of nursing.
4. The need to apply scientific terms to the process of nursing; this results in an emphasis on an intellectual, behavioral, and functional role of the nurse, rather than on the technical "doing" aspects alone [86].

Meaning and Definitions

The basic meaning of the nursing process — assessing, planning, implementing, and evaluating nursing care — is not new; systematizing the process makes the difference. If the nurse director can assist the nursing staff to restudy the basic steps of a systematic approach to nursing care, to apply the nursing process to their work situation, and to utilize the nursing process fully, a better quality of care will be provided. The nurse director can encourage nurse practitioners to reappraise their own delivery of nursing care. It is easy to begin to take one's abilities for granted and to act intuitively or become hurried to the point of overlooking important aspects of care. The nursing process is a refreshing, effective, and challenging way to analyze what nursing is, and the functions of nurses. As a framework on which to base and improve the quality of nursing care, the nursing process can be adapted and evaluated in a variety of situations. Nurses strive to meet the needs of patients; this may well be overwhelming at times. One method of coping with this sometimes frustrating situation is to say, "There are only so many hours in the day or at work to accomplish this number of things." The other alternative of coping is to become more efficient and systematic (assessing, planning, implementing, and evaluating care). By using the nursing process as a framework and a guide, it is possible for nurses to remove the randomness from their efforts and to proceed with a planned, deliberative method of nursing care [86].

The evolution of the definitions of the nursing process proves that nurses have been assessing, planning, implementing, and evaluating all along, but now it can be defined systematically:

Nursing process is viewed as the vehicle through which nursing is practiced. The nursing process is defined as a dynamic, on-going interpersonal process in which the nurse and the patient are viewed as a system with each affecting the behavior of the other and both being affected by factors within the situation [22].

The nursing process is an orderly, systematic manner of determining the client's problems, making plans to solve them, initiating the plan or assigning others to implement it, and evaluating the extent to which the plan was effective in resolving the problems identified [97].

The phrase *nursing process* [is used] to refer to the sum total of nursing care activities performed to attain and maintain high-level wellness for the patient [30].

The term *nursing process* has been used interchangeably with the terms *problem-solving approach* and *problem-solving method*. Some writers elaborate on the characteristics of the nursing process by referring to its interpersonal nature, a framework, or a system of relationships. Others disagree and say that it is not a problem-solving process, but, rather, a communicative interaction process [22]. The rationale for this concept is explained as follows: The nurse does not identify the problem for solution or select the alternative for decision as if they existed passively "out there" in the real world awaiting discovery [22].

The nursing process may be viewed as a problem-solving process, since it is an ongoing, systematic process of assessing, planning, implementing, and evaluating nursing care. These four components are accomplished by and through communication and interaction [86]. The nursing process is further referred to as *goal-directed nursing*, a *problem-oriented system*, and a *systems approach*. The terminology is not uppermost, since even if the name *nursing process* were used concurrently by all, some variations would still persist in individual meaning and interpretation of the concept [86].

The nursing process describes the activities that nurses perform — activities in the broad sense, including intellectual and physical functions. It is a rational, ongoing, dynamic, systematic process based on relevant theories, concepts, and principles from the physical and social sciences; it is a process by which nurses manage through assessing, planning, implementing, and evaluating nursing care to meet the needs of a patient or group of patients [86].

Components of the Nursing Process

Assessment. Assessment consists of collecting subjective and objective data from sources such as records, observations, interactions, interviews, self-reactions, appraisal of the pertinent literature, and physical, physiological, or psychological measurement. Organized information is gathered, classified, analyzed, and summarized to determine an individual patient's nursing problems or needs. Assessment involves astute observation, purposeful listening, and a broad knowledge of human behavior. Assessing is the first step of the nursing process, but it must be continued throughout the process in order to update patient care. The end result of assessment is the nursing diagnosis — a comprehensive statement of the problem or the identification of specific nursing problems. Tools and techniques that may accompany the nursing process during the assessment phase include: physical assessment skills; admission interview; health (or nursing) history; data collecting sheets; contact with the patient and his family; contact with the nursing staff, the health team, and patient records; and the nursing care plan.

Planning. Planning is a systematic approach toward meeting the patient's needs and consists of developing a written plan of action. The nursing care plan is formulated with specific measures designed to assist the patient in achieving both immediate and long-term goals. The planning phase involves the use of sound nursing and management knowledge, scientific principles, and team conferences.

Implementation. Implementation is an action-oriented activity and requires the active involvement of the nurse, the patient, and members of the health care team to carry out the nursing care plan. It is a shared responsibility, but the nurse is needed to provide its leadership. Tools and techniques that may be used are direct care, counseling, guidance, teaching, and referral activities. Indirect care involves supervising, directing, and guiding team conferences.

Evaluation. Evaluation is a comparison of the patient's response with the expected outcomes identified in the nursing goals to measure goal achievement; it involves reflecting about the actions taken to determine their effectiveness in reaching desired changes. Tools and techniques that may be applied to this phase are physical assessment skills, team conferences, individual reports (from the patient, family, health care team, and others), physicians' orders and progress notes, nurses' notes, consultation, rounds, nursing audit, and peer review.

Sense of Accomplishment

Modern management is being challenged by forces developing out of a changing environment. Important among these forces are the generation of tremendous amounts of knowledge, the development of almost unbelievable technology, the wide alterations in the general environment in which management operates, and the deluge of changing human values.

Health-related work, when well done, is socially approved and rewarding. When the sense of accomplishment is lacking, it is common to find the individual or group involved in health care frustrated and easily fatigued. Important elements of the combination of factors leading to a sense of accomplishment are having sufficient autonomy to make decisions and having authority commensurate with responsibilities. In too many instances, autonomy and authority are not granted in the degree appropriate to the functions of health professionals and, as a result, levels of productivity are minimal, to the detriment of comprehensive health care. It is hoped that this situation will change as the nursing process concept gains ascendancy; this should satisfy the need for a sense of importance of the job as well.

Change

Toffler suggests that future shock "may well be the most important disease of tomorrow." He defines future shock as " . . . a time phenomenon, a product of the greatly accelerated change in society. . . . It is culture shock in one's society" [84]. It is his belief that man handles technological innovation by going through three phases: idea creation, idea application, and idea diffusion [84]. To paraphrase Toffler and apply the phrases to nursing, use of the nursing process would involve the same three phases. First, there must be a creative, feasible idea and the suggestion that the situation is one in which nursing can be of help; this is an area in which nursing offers some expertise to resolve a problem or to prevent a problem from developing. Second, the process must have a practical application. Having identified the area of need, assessed the problem or potential problem areas, and arrived at a plan for coping, one must be ready for action. This action includes implementing as well as evaluating aspects of the process. Constant recycling through phases is an inherent part of the nursing process. The third phase in the utilization of the process involves "diffusion through society." Translated into the language of nursing, this concept involves convincing those who do nursing that orderly movement through the process ensures the "how" of nursing. The process ensures a systematic and orderly movement through the necessary phases of nursing so that the problems of patients can be thoroughly assessed and action for coping can be planned and implemented. A final and continual evaluation of the process is as essential as each of the other three phases. Challenges for the future of society, of health care, and of nursing care are coming into focus; the nursing process is the significant process for meeting some of these challenges [21].

Future of the Nursing Process

The future of the nursing process can be seen from four points of view: (1) continuing development and refinement of the process itself; (2) contribution toward the growth and development of the profession of nursing through its use; (3) influences on the personal and professional growth and development of users of the nursing process; and (4) improvement of the health status of recipients of the process [21].

As disenchantment with the health care delivery system grows, the pressure for change and new perspectives will increase substantially. It is estimated that by 1980 the financial outlay for medical care will reach $200 billion [21]. Being aware of "an orderly, systematic manner of determining a client's problems, making plans to solve them, initiating the plan or assigning others to implement it, and evaluating the extent to which the plan was effective in resolving the problems identified" should be a major step forward in assisting both the hospital and nursing administration in accomplishing the goals of the institution [21].

NURSING CARE PLANS

The nurse director delegates the direct management of nursing care to others on her staff — supervisors, head nurses, and staff nurses. She gives them the tools, the support, and the overall direction they need to perform their jobs successfully. The nursing care plan is one tool of the management of nursing care (see Appendix 14). It is a proposed method of action, indicating the results to be achieved, the steps to be taken in achieving them, and the means to be used. The nurse director is responsible for seeing that the plan is made and the groundwork is laid for its effective use [4].

In order for nursing care plans to be effective, nursing care objectives need to be clearly defined. Some objectives will apply to the care given all patients, reflecting what the nursing department believes is quality care. With the overall objectives as a guide, a basis is provided for determining specific objectives for the individual patient — objectives unique to him and his individualized nursing care needs [4].

To facilitate the implementation of nursing care plans, appropriate supportive policies and procedures need to be developed to answer questions such as:

1. Who is responsible for initiating a nursing care plan?
2. How is the plan initiated?
3. How are new staff members oriented to the use of the plan?
4. How do the physician and nurse use the plan together?
5. Do nurses make rounds with physicians?
6. What are the responsibilities and functions of the various levels of nursing personnel for the plan?
7. Who can safely carry out nursing actions and to whom can they be assigned?
8. How is the plan coordinated over the 24-hour period?
9. What disposition is to be made of the plan after discharge of the patient?
10. What provision is made for periodic evaluation and review of the methods for preparation and use of nursing care plans?

Because the successful development and carrying out of the plan depend upon knowledge of the patient and his illness, the nursing staff must know the physician's plan for care. Therefore, the relationship between the nursing staff and the physicians and their ability to communicate are very important. What policies and procedures facilitate this two-way communication? What are the reporting methods? How does the nursing staff communicate with other departments involved in patient care or community agencies?

In order for the nursing care plan to be a successful tool in the management of nursing care, the support of the hospital administration and the medical staff is important. It is up to the nurse director, as a representative of top management and a representative of nursing, to interpret to the administrator and physicians the goals of the nursing service and the means selected to achieve them. She is in an influential position to bring about the development of hospital policies and administrative procedure that will promote the carrying out of nursing care plans.

NURSING ROUNDS

Nursing rounds are a means of providing contact between the nurse director and each individual in nursing service. Seeing the personnel in their work situations provides the nurse director with personal insight into the working conditions and morale of the staff, which reports fail to convey. Being seen in the various nursing areas gives her an identity, a personal image to the staff. It also indicates that a channel of communication exists from top to bottom levels within the nursing department. Nursing rounds supply firsthand knowledge of the general situation in the hospital and provide a means of coordinating activities and improving interdepartmental communication and understanding.

Nursing rounds also yield firsthand information concerning the quality of care being rendered to patients. The nurse director and her administrative staff should make rounds periodically within the nursing department. Each person's objectives in making rounds will depend to a degree on her specific responsibilities. The following outline may serve as a guide:

MAKING ROUNDS WITH A PURPOSE*

Every Activity Should Have a Definite Purpose

A. Purpose of periodic supervisory rounds:
  Supervisory rounds should be used as a continuous survey and evaluation of the nursing service given.

*Reprinted by courtesy of Helen Weber, Professor of Nursing, Indiana University.

B. Procedure:

Continuous survey and evaluating requires a definite planned schedule of observation and reporting with provision for follow-through based upon the facts observed.

C. *Questions to be answered* in establishing a pattern for systematic productive rounds:
1. What should be observed? How frequently?
2. How to compile, record, and report observations.
3. How to coordinate and pool 24-hour observation.
4. How to identify patterns of performance.
5. How to determine area limits to be covered by rounds.
6. How much time should be allotted to each scheduled round? When should these be made?
7. Whom to make rounds with?
8. How to avoid rounds becoming a social visit or glorified messenger service.

D. *Survey and evaluation of:*
1. Quality of patient care
2. Work performance
3. Assignment and utilization of personnel
4. Services provided by other departments
5. Physical facilities
6. Safety and security measures
7. Recording and reporting
8. Equipment
9. Supplies
10. Inter- and intradepartmental relationships
11. Admission and discharge of patients
12. Effectiveness of communication system
13. Public relations: visitors, press, community

Each of the above lends itself to observation. A systematically planned schedule should provide for concentration on *one specific* area during each scheduled round.

E. Planned observation:
1. Area to be surveyed
2. Recommendations based upon facts observed
3. Follow-through on recommendations

F. Observation schedule:
1. Schedule should be mapped out in advance so as to assure that areas requiring frequent or continuous observation are not overlooked.
2. System set up for permanent record of observation, recommendations and actions taken.
3. System set up for periodic review of #1 and #2.

G. Joint planning regarding development of continuous survey:
1. Involve Nurse Director and departmental supervisors, head nurses (rotate assignment on committee), and other departments as needed.
2. Method of approach to the problems as they arise:
   a. Original personal planning should be tentative.
   b. Before implementation involve others in: (1) more detailed planning of areas, (2) timing of visits, and (3) recording.

c. Share results:
By reports to various individuals and groups
By carrying out commitments
By commendations and recommendations on good work done

H. Periodic evaluation of the result of *continuous survey:*
Suggested procedure for planned observation (Section E)
Area to be surveyed: *public relations as it touches visitors*

1. Rounds deliberately made during visiting hours
2. Specific observations of hospital routines affecting visitors:
   a. Control exercises by information desk
   b. How questions are answered
   c. Availability of physician to answer questions
   d. Time and length of visiting hours
   e. Waiting room facilities
   f. Facilities for relatives of seriously ill patients
   g. Number of visitors per patient
   h. Sensitivity of nursing staff to the unvisited patient, the worried visitor, the over-tired patient
3. Recommendations based upon facts observed by the day, evening and night administrative nursing staff during the rounds:
   a. Need for orientation of new personnel regarding hospital's visiting policies
   b. Need for clarification with physician on what information can be given to visitors
   c. Need for additional waiting room facilities
   d. Need for more explicit directions and markings for routing visitors to nursing units
   e. Need for food dispensing machines
4. Follow-through recommendations:
   a. Revision of visiting rules
   b. Brochure on visiting rules prepared for patient and visitors
   c. Coffee and sandwich machines installed
   d. Identification markers installed
   e. Other

ADMINISTRATIVE MEETINGS

I t is important to involve personnel in the planning and evaluation
of nursing activities and services. Opportunities must be provided for
free communication between the administrative nursing staff and
other levels of nursing personnel. Ways must be discovered in which
the energies and talents of personnel can be utilized not only for self-
expression and development but also for the welfare of patients.

A democratic atmosphere in which people share and participate to
some degree in the decision-making process will succeed only if various levels of nursing personnel can work together to achieve departmental objectives and employee needs. Interaction of administrative
staff and nursing personnel can be brought about by periodic meetings between the two groups that:

1. Provide a free flow of communication between the nurse director
   and her staff.
2. Present information to the staff and help them to understand how
   the information can be used effectively in relation to their jobs or
   the hospital.
3. Obtain staff's advice needed to solve a problem or to initiate a
   course of action. Information, facts, and opinions can be elicited
   from a diverse group. Certain individuals may have specialized
   knowledge that is needed. Personnel will be more receptive toward
   accepting decisions as they have a chance to recommend solutions
   to problems.
4. Discuss any problems that staff members want to express and
   strive to develop a workable solution.

Assuming that work time schedules are planned four weeks in advance, administrative meetings are scheduled at a fixed time and day
of the week during the four-week placement. A calendar of meetings
and events is prepared and posted on the nursing unit to serve as a
reminder for the nursing staff.

All personnel should be made aware of the date, time, place, and
agenda of the meeting in advance. They should be encouraged by
the administrative staff to be present. Special consideration must be
given to arranging meetings for the evening and night duty personnel,
as well as part-time employees.

The taking of minutes is an important part of the process. In order

163

to provide consistency and uniformity in record keeping, the committee secretary should receive guidelines and directions concerning the task. Someone should be appointed to take minutes routinely; if it is possible to release a nursing office secretary or unit clerk to keep records, there will be a greater opportunity for all staff members to participate. The minutes should include a record of the actions taken — problems, reports, discussion, or recommendations — which can be reviewed and referred for administrative deliberation.

All minutes should be typed and signed by the chairman and secretary. A copy can be maintained in the nursing office that is available to the nursing staff upon request. Copies of the minutes may become a part of the nursing service monthly report. At the end of the fiscal year, minutes can be bound and stored for future reference.

It is desirable for the nurse director to be present at all the administrative meetings; in this way she can get to know and understand the personnel better. Since there may be several levels of managers between her and the staff, these meetings afford her a chance to communicate with the staff members personally.

If for some reason the nurse director is unable to be present at the meetings, she delegates this responsibility to a member of her administrative staff. She must, however, keep in touch through the minutes of the meetings, which should reflect areas of concern or interest to the staff. If the meetings can provide a place in which the employees can be heard, and if the employees view them as occasions on which nursing administration will hear them out, they should be meaningful and productive. Failure to notice employee suggestions, recommendations, or concerns may lessen the employees' confidence in those who set up objectives to get them involved.

It is no small task to keep aware of all the problems or concerns that may occur in the largest department of a hospital. A method must be developed that will assist the administrative staff to plan systematically for the identification of areas that need attention and action. It is then possible to parcel out to others the situations that need study or follow-up. Several study committees can be working to arrive at conclusions and recommendations.

COMMITTEES

The committee technique offers a number of advantages: A committee is formally organized; it has an assigned job to do; it has a leader; it keeps written records of its proceedings for future reference; and it knows results are expected.

As a nurse director plans for the achievement of nursing objectives, her use of committees can be one of the most important forces in the department. This is particularly true if committee members are selected for the contribution they can make and are made to feel that it is an honor and privilege to serve. The wise use of committee members capitalizes on the experience of a variety of personnel, generating many ideas and, with more ideas, perhaps more creative solutions to problems and more meaningful ways to accomplish nursing goals and to improve nursing organization.

Standing committees (see Appendix 15) can be responsible for a specific part of the regular, ongoing work of the department. Special committees can be chosen to do particular jobs. When a special committee's goal has been accomplished, it is dissolved. If the job is of long duration, it is often wise to plan for a rotation of members in order to provide the group with fresh ideas.

The selection of nursing staff for committee activity is not left to chance; one must guard against inviting inefficiency and low productivity. Consideration should be given to the following factors:

1. Which of the nursing personnel have an interest in the kind of activity in which the committee will be engaged? Participation should be voluntary.
2. Who in the nursing department has the knowledge and skill or access to information needed by a committee? Personnel with specialized training or experience, or aptitude for the task, should be given special consideration.
3. Who of the nursing staff can benefit most by serving on a committee with experienced members? The opportunity to learn by doing is helpful in developing committee members.
4. Are there members of the nursing staff who might develop a greater sense of belonging or commitment to the nursing department by working on a committee?
5. What staff representation is needed on a committee? There are three kinds of representation to weigh: (1) representation of different opinions or points of view; (2) representation of different levels of nursing personnel; and (3) representation of persons outside of nursing. The nature of the committee's goal will determine whether any or all are needed.
6. Does the chairman of a committee have any preference as to the

committee members? Because the chairman does have much responsibility, it is well to consider her suggestion for committee appointments [52].

The selection of a committee chairman deserves careful attention. The chairman must be willing to give leadership to the committee and to stimulate it toward the accomplishment of committee goals. She should be capable of organizing the members into a productive working group. She is chosen for her ability to lead the group.

The size of the committee depends on its purpose. If the purpose of the committee is such as to require wide representation of nursing staff, the group will be somewhat larger than one whose task calls for the effort of four or five people. It should be remembered that the major reason for appointing a committee in the first place is the greater efficiency and flexibility offered by a small group. Size will be determined by the optimum number of people needed to accomplish the purpose of a committee.

Once the decision is made to appoint a committee, the nature and composition of the group, along with its duties and responsibilities, should be clearly defined. In order that the members have an accurate idea of what they are to do, it is helpful to put the assignment in writing and give a copy to each member. Personnel who are to serve on the committee should be informed at the time of their appointment whether it is a standing committee or a special committee.

The standing and special committees are advisory to the nurse director. After weighing the advice of the committee, the nurse director makes the final decision about matters within her area of responsibility and becomes accountable for their implementation. Matters outside her jurisdiction are referred to the hospital administrator. Minutes are maintained similar to the administrative meeting records.

RECORDS AND REPORTS

Every nurse director should give some attention to whether the records and reports in her department provide the right kind of information, to the right people, at the right time to enable her controls to work effectively. As she reviews reports, she needs to know departmental achievements, exceptional problems, operating conditions, labor morale, and patient attitudes.

The nurse director may be expected to issue reports monthly, quarterly, semiannually, and often at a moment's notice. To be able to do so efficiently, she needs to know the value of records, to set up forms to make meaningful data available, and to analyze and use data for the betterment of nursing service. Recognizing the significance of records and reports, she interprets them and makes the findings accessible to all who in turn can use them to further the cause of quality nursing care. She shares accomplishments indicated by records with her staff and encourages all concerned to meet the challenges inherent in the weaknesses that present themselves.

Administrative Records and Reports

In order to maintain a viable administrative and organizational structure, the nursing department needs to have ready access to information that:

1. Provides a scope of activities within the department.
2. Ascertains whether the volume of work is increasing, decreasing, or remaining the same.
3. Allows for an evaluation of programs.
4. Provides for the coordination of activities.
5. Contributes toward budget preparation.
6. Furnishes content for educational experiences.
7. Serves as basis for preserving information of historical significance.
8. Draws attention to how well performance matches acknowledged standards so that corrective adjustments can be made.
9. Serves as a source for legal purposes.

The kind of administrative records and reports, the design of the forms, how and where they are filed, and methods for obtaining the information depend upon each hospital's particular requirements for information, ease of collection, and the way the information is to be used. The responsibility of the nurse director for maintaining certain records and reports differs according to the size and type of hospital, the size and complexity of the nursing department, the functions of other departments, the extent of computer facilities, and the requests of hospital administration.

Statistical Information

The management of an organization requires statistical summaries of the work for any given period. The purposes of collecting data should be well defined at the time of their compilation. For example, data obtained from a patient census may serve as a basis for revising the personnel staffing assignments; they may help to establish new patient care services; or they may point up the need for additional facilities for the next five or ten years.

Data collected should be relevant to their purposes; they should be analyzed and presented in a meaningful manner. Finally, consideration needs to be given to how statistical data will be used in making decisions leading to action. It cannot be overemphasized that the value of such summaries lies not in the report per se but in its intelligent interpretation and utilization.

In the case of statistics, management is as always well advised to ask six basic questions:

1. Whom are the statistics for?
2. Are they in a format that will be understood by the people who receive them?
3. Are they, or can they be, circulated in time to influence the action to which they relate?
4. What actual action (if any) is taken at both the preparing and the receiving end?
5. What do they cost, in time spent at both the preparing and the receiving end?
6. How do the costs compare with the gains in more effective management? [38]

The six questions are proper to scientific management; they will be found to cover the principal avenues for the use (and abuse) of statistics in their practical application [38].

The types of data that may be received from another department or maintained in the nursing office are, for example: bed occupancy, analysis of departmental operational indicators, professional activity study, hospital administrative service reports, expense sheets and account analysis, personnel productive hours, labor (personnel) transfer account charge, staffing statistical report, overtime hours, ratio of professional personnel to allied personnel, and summary of nursing unit hours per patient.

Annual Report

The annual report of the department of nursing is an important management tool. It serves as a progress report on patients and nursing activities and accomplishments to the hospital administration. The organization of content and format is an individual matter. The nurse director should discuss with the hospital administrator those areas of content that he believes would be helpful. Most administrators, limited in time by having to read many reports, appreciate brevity.

The report may include areas such as: (1) significant projects undertaken, completed, or discontinued; (2) major changes in departmental policies and procedures; (3) effects on nursing service of changes in interdepartmental policies and procedures; (4) activities of the in-service education program; (5) nursing issues; and (6) plans for the forthcoming year [3].

Other topics that may be included are: progress report on yearly objectives (if management by objectives approach is used); recommendations to implement the plans (objectives) for the new fiscal year; recommendations for the solution of identified problems; annual summaries of statistical data, such as nursing hours per patient, ratio of professional nurses to allied groups, turnover rates; annual summary report of nursing committee activities and accomplishments; and acknowledgments, which offer the nurse director an opportunity to give credit to the departments, community agencies, and individuals who made substantial contributions to the progress of the department of nursing during the year.

Another approach to developing the annual report is to use the criteria established by various groups as a guideline. For example, the National League for Nursing's *Self-Evaluation Guide for Nursing Service in Hospitals and Related Institutions* (1967) lists ten criteria that may serve as content for annual reports: (1) philosophy and objectives, (2) organization plan, (3) written administrative policies, (4) personnel policies, (5) budget, (6) control of equipment and supplies, (7) reports and records, (8) program for nursing care, (9) in-service education, and (10) evaluation [68].

How the report will be prepared depends on the nurse director. Does she see this tool as her complete responsibility, or is it one in which she will involve her administrative staff? Does she require supervisors and head nurses to submit annual reports in order to build this annual report? Does she provide structured guidelines to assist them in the development of their annual report or leave it to the staff's ingenuity to approach the task creatively?

The annual report should correspond to the hospital's fiscal year. A copy of the report is sent to hospital administration, and other copies should be accessible to the medical staff, the nursing staff, and other interested groups. A copy should be retained in the nursing service office as a reference source as well as for organizing, planning, and evaluating nursing activities.

The Patient's Medical Record

A patient's medical record provides a written record of data about the patient; thus it serves as a means of communication among the professionals sharing in his care. The patient's chart is the basis for planning his care and carrying out the plan, and it is evidence of the course of his illness and his treatment. It is also used as a basis for review, study, and evaluation of the care rendered to the patient; as an adjunct in the education of many personnel and often as a reference source; as a source of statistical data, such as births, deaths, or hospital admissions; as a basis for making plans for the future and for anticipating needs; as a legal protection for all concerned; and as subject material for comparative studies and research. The medical record system must be organized to accord services to many groups: patients, professional staff, administration, and the community [20].

The nursing department plays a major role in the compiling of high-quality patient records. The nursing record greatly contributes to the medical record, providing a historical, documental record that assists the physician in the diagnosis and treatment of the patient insofar as notations are accurate and carefully made [20].

Problem-Oriented Recording

Lawrence Weed, M.D., has introduced a method of organizing the medical record or chart as an ongoing audit of the management of the patient's problems. The problem-oriented system developed by Dr. Weed provides a systematic method for planning and evaluating nursing care; the emergence of the problem-oriented medical record (POMR) on the health care scene gives tremendous impetus to the use of the nursing process [92].

Problem-Oriented Medical Records. The problem-oriented medical record — a type of documentation designed to improve the adequacy

and organization of clinical information for effective patient care —
is an integrated system focusing on the patient's problem. The
problem-oriented record is a patient care plan, not a physician's care
plan or a nursing care plan. It has four basic components:

1. *Data base.* History, including, but not limited to, chief complaint,
   present illness, patient profile (expansion of traditional social
   history), physical examination, and laboratory reports.
2. *Complete problem list.* The front sheet of the chart during hospitalization. It is a numbered and titled list of every problem the
   patient has or has had, as noted in the data base. A problem is defined as anything that requires management or diagnostic workup,
   including social and demographic problems.
3. *Initial plans.* Each numbered and titled problem is detailed in three
   ways.
   a. More information for diagnostic workup (the "rules out," with
      specific and detailed plans for each diagnostic possibility and
      management (parameters to be followed to indicate course of
      disease, response to therapy, and toxicity from therapy).
   b. Therapy. Statements not only on drugs and procedures but also
      precise statements of goals, end points, and contingency plans.
   c. Patient education. The plan for educating the patient and his
      family about each problem.
4. *Progress notes.* Notes numbered and titled to correspond to the
   specific problem to which they refer.
   a. Narrative notes: symptomatic, objective assessment plan (SOAP).
   b. Flow sheets.
   c. Discharge summary [7].

The problem-oriented medical record is described as effecting the
following:

1. Encouraging the use of sound logic in thoughts about patients.
2. Enabling one to use the record as efficiently as a medical
   dictionary.
3. Allowing the physician to communicate his thoughts to nurses and
   other members of the health care team who are assisting him in
   the immediate care of patients.
4. Enhancing the continuing education of the physician and all who
   assist him in the care of the patient.
5. Preparing students, physicians, and others for the computer world.

6. Establishing a common bond among several physicians and a patient.
7. Evaluating the critical thinking of the practitioner by allowing an audit of the record to determine what care was given and the logic behind each intervention [7].

Problem-Oriented Approach in Nursing. Nursing has modified and applied Dr. Weed's basic concept to nursing practice. The problem-oriented record offers a logical way to organize the data and to support one's conclusions. A problem-oriented approach in nursing: (1) offers one way to care for people with problems, in and out of the hospital, and a means to evaluate care so it can be improved; (2) serves as a guide to organizing nursing care around patient needs; (3) provides a systematic method of problem solving within a definite framework that helps to guide and support the nurse in problem solving and decision making; (4) allows nursing the freedom to make independent judgments about problems and actions; (5) makes explicit and effective use of the nursing process not optional but expected, since nurses will participate in recording with a problem-oriented format; (6) provides a logical, precise list of all the patient's problems, the current treatment, and the plans of the health care team relative to each problem; (7) ensures that the patient and his problems become the focus of health care; the method of recording data requires that one approach the patient in terms of health problems rather than in terms of disease, procedures, or specific professional orientation; and (8) should improve communication within nursing as well as with the patient, his family, and others on the health care team.

The focus of the nursing process and the problem-oriented thinking and recording system will be to address problems in nursing's territory of coping with daily living in health-related areas. Problem-oriented record keeping will pose problems for those nursing personnel who have avoided involvement with the thinking patterns of the nursing process, the knowledge base of nursing's diagnostic concepts, and the art of communicating in writing.

The problem-oriented system of record keeping also provides a common approach for nursing, medicine, and other health care teams. This mutual orientation enhances collaborative attempts toward defining and developing congruent roles. Likewise, problems can be categorized and used to study the care given by the interdisciplinary health care team [74]. Problem orientation provides a common language among health disciplines and may help to bridge the gap between nursing and medical approaches to the patient/client [59, 61].

The components of the POMR may be applied to nursing as follows:

1. On admission, or as soon as possible thereafter, patient information is collected (the nursing history), which serves as the basis for planning nursing care.
2. Following the initial collection of data, a numbered list of problems is formulated, including patient problems identified from the nursing history and from data recorded by health care professionals; new patient problems are added to the patient's list record as they are identified.
3. A plan is prepared for the solution of each patient problem that has been identified and recorded. The plan consists of one or more of the following:
   a. Collection of additional relevant data.
   b. Transmission of information to patient or others.
   c. Statement of nursing care objectives and orders designed to solve or manage a specific problem.
4. This phase is comprised of the chronological sequence of notes pertaining to the evaluation of nursing progress in the management of each patient problem; additional data; new plans; and modification or deletion of old plans.
5. This phase is a summary of the patient's nursing problems; notes are made of those problems that were resolved, with recommendations for the management of those problems still present; discharge or the final note represents a final progress note [87].

Role of the Nurse Director. As the nurse director reflects on her responsibility and accountability for nursing services, problem-oriented charting is a management tool that requires her attention. Strict adherence to the guidelines proposed by Dr. Weed does not limit thought and creativity. The guidelines simply represent the framework within which excellence can be pursued, achieved, and measured. The system provides the nurse director freedom to make independent judgments about nursing problems and their management within a definite framework to guide and support the decision-making process. She must determine how she can set up conditions for her staff so that they may become skilled at recording and organizing data in a problem-oriented manner.

Assuming that hospital administration plans to implement the problem-oriented approach, the nurse director must plan for its development and implementation within the nursing department as well as the hospital. If there is no current plan by hospital administration to move in this direction, the nurse director must consider setting a goal to achieve it. What the nurse director believes about the problem-oriented approach as a management nursing tool will determine her commitment to this trend in care. She will find ways to get her staff to develop statements of belief regarding the problem-oriented approach and to establish objectives about the approach; then she and her staff can strive together to translate those beliefs into action.

The literature is growing with stimulating writing about the problem-oriented format in the delivery of nursing care. Published sources should be purchased for the hospital library and made available to the nursing staff and other members of the health care team. A second means of implementing a problem-oriented format is through an in-service educational program. The program content and learning experiences should be built around systematic planning and critical thinking; problem-oriented charting is not separate from the whole problem-oriented process. The learning experience can be started by teaching problem-oriented charting as an impetus to reinforce a problem-solving process already present in the individual practicing nurse. All nursing personnel, regardless of their role, should participate in the educational experience; it is hoped that the staff will obtain a common frame of reference for viewing the problem-oriented approach. After the nursing staff has completed an educational program designed to explain the concepts, opportunities need to be provided for the staff to practice problem-oriented recording. If a school of nursing uses the clinical facilities of the hospital, it is desirable that the nursing service director find a way to involve faculty in the educational experience — as either participants or instructors or both. Workshops sponsored by various nursing organizations provide opportunities to learn how other hospitals or health-oriented settings utilize the problem-oriented approach. Outside change agents may be used to introduce the problem-oriented approach or to serve as consultants [87].

The process of planning and implementing changes in the nursing department through the application of the problem-oriented patient care system should be viewed in light of the opportunities and possibilities for overall nursing staff and organizational development [87]. The challenge of the nurse director and her nursing staff is to create a professional climate for nursing practice by being more responsive to integrating new knowledge for improved patient care.

Nursing Audit Program

A major management tool that contributes directly to the evaluation and improvement of nursing care is a nursing audit program. The nursing audit enables the nurse director to uncover inefficient care and points the way to an elevation of standards, reduces the incidence and severity of medicolegal complications arising out of inaccurate or incomplete nursing notes and practices, and broadens and strengthens the nursing services in the hospital. This technique stresses the value of, and the need for, good interpretation by the physician of his plan of therapeutics, so that nursing service will fully understand it. Thus more individual responsibility is placed on the nurse for carrying out the medical plan. As a means of evaluation, the nursing audit reduces the possibility of an authoritarian approach in order to evoke change [20].

A nursing audit, like a medical audit, provides a systematic review of the nursing records of all patients and yields:

1. A biographical index of the quality of nursing care each patient has received.
2. Valuable and pertinent information for the medical staff and other health-related professionals.
3. Improved nursing and nursing notes.
4. Knowledge of areas of strength and weakness in nursing service.
5. Better cooperation between physician and nurse as a result of improved quality of nursing notes.
6. A record of nursing staff performance.
7. A means of self-evaluation of nursing service.
8. A chance to enrich in-service programs, which can be geared to the bona fide needs of the service [20].

The nursing audit requires close cooperation between the medical records librarian and the nurse director if it is to be effective. The medical records librarian has the following responsibilities as she reviews the nursing notes of the medical record:

1. To check nurses' notes and graphic record quantitatively.
2. To ascertain that all names, dates, and hospital numbers are correct and correspond.
3. To check that all notes are signed by recording nurses.
4. To check admission and discharge notes to see that time and manner of admission and discharge are stated.
5. To check the physician's orders against nurses' notes to see that orders for treatment are carried out as ordered [20].

The task of the medical records librarian does not include determining the adequacy of the nursing notes; nor is she in a position to know whether they are qualitatively of assistance to the physician in his management of patient care. This is the responsibility of the nursing department. The many variables in rendering nursing care do not easily lend themselves to statistical analysis; however, sufficient objective information can be gathered from nurses' notes to evaluate the nursing care supplied [20].

DEFINING THE NURSING AUDIT*

What Is the Nursing Audit?

1. An administrative tool for evaluating the quality of nursing care as reflected in the Medical Record.
2. It is a comparison of the care given (as shown on the record) with the standards of care (as set up as acceptable by the individual institution).
3. Responsible only for the objective evaluation of those elements of care provided by or under the specific direction of the nurse.
4. Evaluation made after the patient's discharge will be most complete. It is completely disassociated from the patient's personality.

*Reprinted by courtesy of Helen Dunn, University of Illinois Hospitals, Department of Nursing.

What Are the Essential Elements of the Audit?

1. Written standards of care which are available as a basis for comparison with the Medical Record (policies, procedure, charting guide, etc.).
2. A workable method to provide a pre-selected group of charts to the audit group.
3. A functioning audit group and/or a functioning policy-forming and coordinating group.
4. A workable system of communications designed to ensure that the data obtained reach the desired action group.

What Departments Are Involved in the Audit?

1. All mechanical aspects of the audit are the responsibility of the Medical Records Department.
2. All professional aspects of the audit are the responsibility of the nursing staff.

Who Performs the Audit?

1. Representatives from all classifications of the nursing staff who are responsible for entering information on the Medical Record and for management of chart forms (RN, LPN, Clerks, etc.).
2. Audit may be conducted by individual clinical departments (to keep group a workable size in large institution) or as a single group in a smaller institution.

Initiating the Nursing Audit

Preliminary Steps in Initiating the Audit (First Year)
1. Establishment of a core group.
   a. Membership (Maximum size 12–15)
      1) Representatives from all categories of RN's (Number depends on size of institution)
      2) Medical Records Librarian
      3) Director of Nursing
   b. Aims of original group
      1) To structure the audit and develop appropriate audit tools

      a) Define long term goals of the audit and specific aims for the original committee

      b) Prepare in usable form standards of nursing care and charting practice (Develop guides, written policies, etc.)

      c) Set up mechanics of audit

      Department of Nursing

      (1) Develop audit form

      (2) List types of charts to be audited

      (3) Set up audit schedule

      Medical Records Library

      (1) Duplicate audit forms

      (2) Set up audit book to list discharge charts

      (3) Set up mechanism for pulling charts

      (4) Set up format for monthly and annual reports

      d) Practice auditing

2) To foster in the Nursing Staff an interest and skill in auditing

Development of the Permanent Audit Structure (After at Least 1 Year)

1. Establishment of a central policy-forming group.

    a. Membership: Six members appointed by the Director of Nursing and representing all professional nurse categories; Medical Records Librarian

    b. Purpose

      1) To coordinate the departmental audits and set audit policies, establish procedures and refine existing or develop new forms and communication tools

      2) To evaluate the results of the departmental audits and to make recommendations based upon these results for the establishment of policies, procedures, or guides that will contribute to the improvement of patient care

2. Establishment of Departmental Audit Committees (Number dependent upon the size of the institution or may remain part of the Central Committee in small institutions).

    a. Membership

      1) Professional nurses from a specific clinical area (auditors — minimum 3)

      2) Any members of nursing staff who are responsible for some phase of charting (LPN, Ward Clerk) after committees have been functioning and well established

    b. Purpose

    To determine from the patient's individual record the adequacy of the nursing care rendered and the legality of the form of the chart.

Retrospective Audit

Retrospective audit is concerned with providing quality controls through peer review. Each clinical nursing unit does audits of selected cases by nursing diagnosis, degree of illness, nursing problems, or whatever classification is adopted. Each clinical nursing unit determines its own needs. The auditor uses a form provided by the patient care evaluation committee to report her review. The audit may be developed to include recommendations from various groups.

Nursing Personnel Records

For the benefit of the hospital as well as the employee, personnel files must be kept current by the nursing department. These records are confidential, and their contents should be available only to authorized persons.

The nurse director is responsible for learning from the personnel department what information is being recorded and then for determining whether additional information is necessary for nursing needs. The personnel folder will contain:

Records	Purposes
Application Blank	1. Provide a simple test of the person's ability to spell, write legibly and answer factual questions rapidly and accurately.
	2. Provide a general picture of a prospective employee before the main employment interview begins.
	3. Provide the prospective employee with a chance to think out the answers alone, then answer the questions during the interview.
	4. Assure a prospective employee that his desire for work and some of his qualifications are on record with the hospital.
	5. Provide a useful basis for understanding and guiding the person once he has been employed.
Interview Forms	1. Evaluate information obtained from the application blank or first preceding interview by preliminary employment office interview.

2. Integrate the data with one's own impression and observation to reach a decision regarding the suitability of the applicant's employment.

3. Obtain and record information not required on the application form. When reviewed together the application and interview forms serve as a basis for a decision to employ or not to employ a person.

Reference Findings

1. Application blanks provide an opportunity to check the applicant's candor and accuracy.

2. Previous employment should be investigated.

Health Status-Physical Examinations

1. Provide a record of the pre-admission physical examination to protect the hospital against the risk of claims for compensation of persons who are afflicted with pre-existing disabilities.

2. Provide future records of employee annual physical examinations and other information pertinent to his health.

Employee Performance Appraisal

1. Provide records of employee competence and performance in his assigned job.

2. Serve as a tool to counsel and guide an employee toward his personal goals for self-improvement.

3. Act as a guide for pay raises, promotions, and new assignments.

Salary Status

1. Maintain a record of salary changes and other matters relating to a change in pay which may be due to merit raises based on performance, blanket raises, or wage garnishment.

Employment Change

1. Provide information about transfers to another nursing unit or department within the hospital; promotions, demotions, change of job classification or upper staff category; change in hours of work; change from part-time to full-time status; leave of absence, etc.

Disciplinary Action

1. Maintain documented factual information to substantiate undesirable behavior.

2. Hold copies of requests of employees for conferences or statements of the offense given to the employee.

3. Document any action of Grievance Committee.

4. Try to teach self-discipline.

Accident and Incident Reports	1. Maintain a detailed record of any accident or incident an employee may encounter including the circumstances, treatment and disposition of his case.
	2. Make a formal report for administrative purposes.
	3. Undertake to identify an accident-prone individual who might be helped.
	4. Study patient incident reports for the purpose of understanding why incidents may have occurred.
	5. Identify employees who need special counseling and guidance.
	6. Study from the standpoint of improving hospital efficiency and standards of care, and prevention of litigation.
Educational Achievements	1. Maintain information and records about employee participation in educational programs such as a tuition reimbursement program.
	2. Record attendance at workshops, institutes, college courses, etc.
Staff Activities	1. Record of an employee's participation in hospital, community, and professional activities indicates his interests and willingness to accomplish hospital objectives, and contributes toward his professional responsibilities.

Storage of Files

Wherever the nursing personnel files are stored, access to them must be carefully controlled because of the confidentiality of the contents. Personnel files are generally maintained and centralized in the personnel department, and in some instances nursing files may be maintained in the nursing service office. The choice often depends on space considerations and the availability of the files to those who maintain and use them. In any case the department of nursing has a responsibility for establishing a system that will keep the records current. In the event that a member of the nursing staff leaves the hospital, her personnel file should be closed out. It is helpful at this point to review the file, perhaps summarize the information rather than keep all the single entries that are made, and if possible prepare a statement to be used as a basis for future recommendations when requested. This procedure will help to ensure a fair appraisal of a person by those who know her best at a time when she was clearly remembered. Personnel files can be an effective administrative tool for putting the right person in the right place and finding the right place for each employee [5].

JOB EVALUATION PROGRAM

In order to implement sound policies and methods of employee compensation, some organizations adopt a job evaluation program. Such a program will establish fair differentials in pay based upon differences in job content. Job evaluation is a method of placing a value on each job in an organization. Through the use of job evaluation, job structures can be formulated, which in turn will establish sound wage structures. Job evaluation attempts to determine the relative positions of jobs and job categories within a structure so that monetary values may be attached equitably. Correct job evaluation makes it possible to classify employees properly; to control wages for new employees, transfers, and promotions within the organization; to control alterations in the wage structure; to ease the way for personnel accounting and budgeting; and to assure equitable standards among departments, so that wage payments do not get out of line [12].

Many systems of job evaluation exist today, most of them alike in certain fundamentals. First, each one calls for the analysis of every job in the organization through complete job description. Second, the factors that place one job above another in the hierarchy are determined; these factors normally include mental and physical traits, skill level, responsibility level, working conditions under which the job is performed, and educational requirements. This step establishes the means by which to relate one job to another; it is probably the most important step in evaluation. Third, the particular system to be used is chosen, in accordance with the jobs in the job structure. Several methods of evaluation are available, ranging from simple to complex, depending on the size and nature of the organization; the ranking method, the classification method, the factor comparison method, and the point method. Fourth, after ensuring that almost everyone in the organization understands what is being attempted in job evaluation, the selected system is put into operation. Last, the job structure is priced, so that a wage structure may be established. In this final step, the wages for particular job classifications are formulated [13].

WAGE AND SALARY PROGRAM

The nurse director may be asked to participate in the development of the wage and salary program. Along with other members of management, she will assist in establishing and implementing sound policies and methods of employee compensation. The wage and salary program is a basic and necessary ingredient in the building of constructive attitudes on the part of employees toward their jobs and the hospital.

A wage and salary program offers to employees: (1) salaries paid according to the job; (2) more compensation for higher-skilled jobs than for lower-skilled jobs, eliminating inequities; (3) a minimal chance of favoritism in the assigning of wage rates; (4) job sequences and lines of promotion where applicable; (5) salaries at a fair rate of pay that have a predetermined relationship to salaries paid in similar jobs by competitive employers, as shown by salary surveys; and (6) increased employee morale and motivation, because the program is explainable and based on facts — employees know where they stand [12].

Benefits also accrue for the employer: (1) Employee labor costs can be planned for systematically and controlled; (2) the program can be readily explained, because it is based upon systematic job analysis and wage facts; (3) friction and grievances over wage inequities can be reduced; (4) employee morale and motivation are enhanced, because adequate and fairly administered wages are an essential need of employees; and (5) qualified personnel are attracted to fill the available positions [12].

JOB ANALYSIS

Current information about the content and nature of jobs in nursing is vital to nursing service administration. Sound personnel management requires that each individual job be defined, recorded, and communicated to the appropriate persons. The method and procedure utilized to determine the duties, responsibilities, working conditions, and working relationships of and between jobs and human qualifications of personnel is called job analysis.

Job analysis is a detailed and systematic study of jobs; it is a procedure for obtaining pertinent job information. It plays a role in manpower and organizational planning; employee recruitment, selection, and placement; determination of equitable employee rates of pay; work method improvement; the development of a training program; and performance appraisal. Job analysis may be done by a job analyst consultant, a member of the personnel department, or a supervisor from the nursing department. An important by-product of a job analysis program is that it often creates greater understanding and common agreement between the employee and his superior on the exact requirements of a job. Getting facts about a job is the main part of a job analysis: *what* the worker does, *how* he does it, *why* he does it, and the skills involved [12].

The principal items covered in a job analysis program are:

Job Title and Location. These properly designate and identify the job. Some standardization and consistency of job titling is considered advantageous.

Job Summary. This is included in most job descriptions to give the reader a quick capsule explanation of content of job — usually one or two sentences in length.

Job Duties. Usually a comprehensive listing of the duties is included, together with some indication of the frequency of occurrence or percentage of time devoted to each major duty. Always include what jobholder does as well as some indication of how he performs the tasks.

Relation to Other Jobs. This item helps to locate the job in the organization by indicating the job or jobs immediately below the one being analyzed and the one immediately above it in the hierarchy.

Supervision Given. For those jobs possessing a supervisory responsibility, an explanation of the number of persons directly supervised and their job titles is given.

Mental Complexity. This and similar terms, such as initiative, ingenuity, judgment, resourcefulness, and analytical requirements, are used to cover the degree of mental difficulty and skill required by the job.

Mental Attention. This factor relates to the degree of mental concentration and alertness required.

Physical Demand. Commonly included under this heading is an enumeration of the types of physical activity and effort required. It may involve such actions as walking, lifting, bending, climbing, and sitting.

Physical Skills. Examples are manual dexterity, eye-hand-foot coordination, motor coordination, and color discrimination.

Responsibilities. There are many kinds of responsibilities that may be assigned to a jobholder. Examples of these are responsibility for the supervision of others, responsibility for product, process, and equipment, responsibility for safety of others, responsibility for confidence and trust, and responsibility for preventing monetary loss to the company. For certain jobs, such as high-level management ones, the responsibility factors weigh heavily in establishing the pay and status of the work.

Personal Characteristics. For certain jobs such personality attributes as personal appearance, emotional stability, maturity, initiative and drive, and skill in dealing with others are important.

Working Conditions. This item pertains to the environment in which the jobholder must work.

Hazards. The conditions of work may be such that the jobholder faces certain hazards, and their probability of occurrence must be considered [12].

Job Description and Job Specification

A job analysis results in two types of written records — job description and job specification (see Figure 11). Job descriptions generally present the principal duties, responsibilities, and organizational relationships that make up a given job or position. They define work assignments and a scope of responsibility that are sufficiently different from those of other jobs to warrant a particular title. What a job description is and how useful it is as a practical instrument are matters that depend in a large measure on who makes it and how it is made [12].

A job description should include the following:

1. A job description must be up to date and correspond accurately to current job requirements.
2. The title of a job should clearly indicate the principal demands made by the job and jobholder. It also sets each job apart from every other job.
3. The summary of primary duties gives an overview of what the job is essentially. It serves as a preview of the job description as a whole. The summary indicates what the job is and how and to what extent this job differs from the other jobs.
4. The description should be complete but not overly detailed. The main purpose is to develop a concise description and analysis, with substantiating data, of all normal job requirements, or what the worker does most of the time.
5. Standard forms should be used for all jobs within each category.
6. Job descriptions must be realistic in terms of both technical and human resources available.

Principles of organizing and writing job description data that contribute to their development are as follows:

1. Arrange descriptions of duties in some logical order.
2. State separate duties clearly and concisely, and do not go into such detail that it becomes a motion analysis.

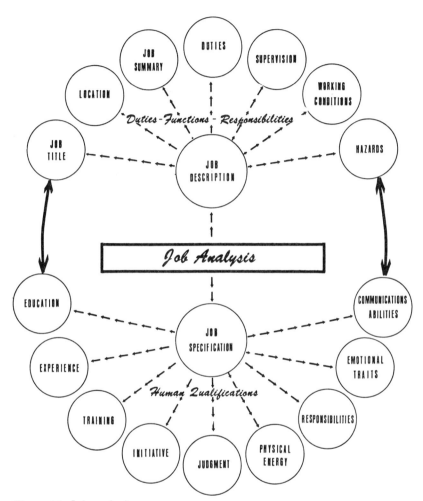

Figure 11. Job analysis.

3. Begin sentences with active, functional verbs, such as *performs, uses.*
4. Use quantitative words where possible.
5. Use specific rather than vague words where possible.
6. State duties as duties; postpone statements of qualification until later.
7. Avoid generalizations.
8. Where possible, determine or estimate the percentage of total time spent on an activity.
9. Limit the use of the word *may* with regard to performance of certain duties; the use of *routine, daily, periodic,* and *occasionally,* if well defined, will make the meaning more specific and clear [73].

The information recorded on a job specification describes the human qualities that are necessary to perform the job adequately. Although the data recorded on the job description can be rather objectively determined, those shown on the specification are subjective. The job specification depends upon the value judgments of a number of people: job analyst, jobholders, and supervisors.

Job descriptions and job specifications can be a liability if they are inaccurate, incomplete, or outdated. They can be assets if they cover every position in the organization, offering an operational view of the whole and showing that every job has been designed and analyzed as an integral part of a total effect [12].

Because of the proliferation of new knowledge and technological innovation in the health field, job descriptions are subject to frequent change and are hard to maintain. The nurse director must systematically and periodically review them in order to maintain their relevancy. She must see that:

1. Job descriptions are written for all position classifications in the nursing department, delineating the functions, responsibilities, and desired qualifications.
2. Job descriptions are reviewed and updated every six months.
3. All positions are evaluated within the year.
4. Specifications are developed for all positions.
5. Job performance criteria are established for all nursing positions.

There are two ways of ensuring that the job information is an accurate representation of current conditions in the nursing department.

One approach places major reliance upon the supervisors, who are responsible for reporting any significant changes in the makeup of the jobs in their nursing units. The second approach requires a periodic audit of the jobs in the department by a selected group of nursing personnel, the job description committee, with the assistance of a member of the personnel department.

EMPLOYEE PERFORMANCE APPRAISAL

Performance appraisal is that aspect of management concerned with evaluating the performance of employees and its relationship to the organization's goals. Strengthening the hospital's position of leadership depends on steady improvements in employee performance and an inventory of people capable of advancing to greater responsibility.

Evaluation of personnel at work is a continuous process. Employees show in their daily activities and actions how well they are meeting job requirements. Personnel know that supervisors are required to evaluate them with respect to their job as well as their potential for growth. The "how" of employee appraisal, however, is the more difficult aspect of evaluation. The nurse director and her administrative staff must develop a systematic evaluation plan and procedure and make it known to the entire nursing staff. The rating of employees, both subordinate and superior, can be a threatening experience or a motivating experience.

The leadership climate established by the nurse director sets the tone for the evaluation process. The manner in which she evaluates assistants or supervisors will influence their attitudes toward subordinates. A nurse director must know what she thinks about people and work. Does she believe:

1. The average person has an inherent dislike of work and will avoid it if he can.
2. Most people must be coerced, controlled, directed, and threatened with punishment if managers are to get people to put forth adequate effort toward the accomplishment of organizational objectives.
3. The average person prefers to be directed, wishes to avoid responsibility, has little ambition, and wants security above all.

Or does she believe:

1. The expenditure of physical and mental effort in work is as natural as play or rest.
2. External control and threat of punishment are not the only means for bringing about effort toward organizational objectives. People will exercise self-direction and self-control in the service of objectives to which they are committed.
3. Commitment to objectives is a function of rewards associated with their achievement.
4. The average person learns, under proper circumstances, not only to accept but to seek responsibility.
5. The ability to exercise a relatively high degree of imagination, ingenuity, and creativity in the solution of problems is widely distributed in the population.
6. Under the conditions of modern industrial life, the intellectual potentiality of the average person is only partially utilized [63].

The nurse director and her administrative staff must explore and determine together what they believe about people and work. They must further consider what they believe about an employee appraisal program. From such beliefs may flow objectives such as:

1. To improve employee performance in the job now held.
2. To develop people to their fullest potential.
3. To encourage imagination, ingenuity, the acceptance of responsibility, and more intelligent efforts to achieve nursing goals.
4. To provide an opportunity for employees to know where they stand [63].

A plan of action and procedure is developed based on the above objectives. The plan should be designed for all levels of personnel (supervisors to nursing assistants). For example:

1. *Clarify the job description.* The nurse director and the supervisor meet to discuss the supervisor's job description and what is involved in each of the major areas. They agree on content and on what the supervisor is accountable for.
2. *Set objectives.* The supervisor then develops objectives for accomplishing her job responsibilities by defining the "what, why, where,

when, and how." Her objectives are job oriented, department oriented, and self-development oriented. The process of setting one's own performance objectives is highly valuable both as a learning experience and as a source of personal motivation. This approach proposes placing the major responsibility on the supervisor for establishing performance goals and appraising progress toward them. The nurse director enters the process actively only after the supervisor has done a good deal of thinking about her job, made a careful assessment of her own strengths and weaknesses, and formulated some specific plans to accomplish her goals.

3. *Do a performance appraisal review.* At the end of an agreed-upon time period the nurse director and supervisor meet to discuss how well the supervisor has done in pursuing the objectives she has previously set for her work. It can be expected that some of the objectives will be attained, others partially completed, and others still far from achievement. Together the nurse director and supervisor can analyze the causes interfering with the achieving of set objectives and can develop alternative solutions. The nurse director relies on discussion rather than direct orders as a means of influencing the supervisor. She emphasizes success to build successful achievement. She helps the supervisor to relate her self-appraisals, her objectives, and her plans to the realities of the nursing department and the hospital. The supervisor is concerned with how she stands in relation to *her* supervisor's evaluation. The nurse director has an obligation to point out areas in which a supervisor can improve and explain why it is to the supervisor's advantage to undertake this improvement. The cycle of setting performance appraisal objectives takes place again and continues periodically as part of the evaluation process. The nurse director is able to evaluate the supervisor's judgment and her ability to set objectives as well as to attain them.

This approach to performance appraisal gives the nurse director and the supervisor a chance to spend time planning, organizing, leading, controlling, and motivating. Both become involved in the management process, but the nurse director does not give up her management responsibility of expecting certain results from a supervisor. As part of the process the nurse director does provide the supervisor with coaching, training, or direction as needed. If a supervisor fails to reach realistic objectives or tends to be a "doer" rather than a leader for results, the nurse director must eventually take corrective action.

Some advantages that may result from the proposed performance appraisal procedure are as follows:

1. The supervisor knows in advance the basis on which she is going to be judged.
2. The supervisor and nurse director agree on what the supervisor's job really is.
3. The relationship between the supervisor and nurse director is strengthened by this approach.
4. This approach has a self-correcting characteristic which tends to help people set objectives that are both challenging and reachable.
5. Educational needs may be identified for future self-development.
6. This approach treats as a total process an individual's ability to see a departmental problem, devise ways of attacking it, translate his ideas into action, incorporate new information as it arises, and carry his plans through to results.
7. People can and will make their greatest contribution to the organization under conditions of greater self-direction and self-control.

The success of such a program will depend on how much the administrative staff believes in it and is willing to cooperate. A person who is committed to her work and is eagerly striving to achieve specifically formulated objectives wants her work evaluated. This conclusion is applicable to all categories of nursing personnel.

The nurse director should hold her administrative staff accountable for developing good written records regarding the performance of personnel. A series of well-written evaluation records can be useful for counseling an employee relative to the type of work for which she is best suited. Decisions regarding promotion, transfer, or special guidance will be based on the written evidence and growth expressed in the records.

A written record is also significant in situations in which an employee feels that her supervisor has not been "fair." If an employee's behavior or performance is not meeting the expectations of the job, this fact should be recorded and shared with the employee. In the event that the situation persists, the supervisor or head nurse should discuss and record each incident and conference. For example, a nursing assistant was careless in her work, was slow in her performance, and had difficulty relating to other nursing personnel. She also had been to the emergency service several times because of major and minor accidents that had occurred while she was caring for patients. The supervisor maintained records and held several conferences with the assistant. When there was no apparent improvement, the nursing assistant was given a two-week termination notice. She became very disturbed and requested conferences with the nurse director and the personnel director. Since she felt she was being treated "unfairly," she wanted to appeal to the grievance committee. The nurse director reviewed with her the steps required to initiate a grievance. She eventually decided not to use the grievance procedure and terminated her services. The supervisor had maintained adequate and accurate records relating to specific incidents concerning the nursing assistant. These records would have served as supporting evidence regarding the supervisor's position. If the supervisor had failed to record each instance and had not discussed it with the employee, the latter would have had cause to be concerned. If the nursing administrative staff strives to deal fairly with employees, their records will show favorable as well as unfavorable written incidents.

Education is a legitimate sphere of activity for reaching organizational objectives. Educational activities can (1) develop the creative talents and abilities of individuals; (2) develop skill in problem solving, planning, fact finding, and exploration of alternatives prior to action; and (3) increase skill in discovering and using resources, promote teamwork, and increase acceptance of responsibility — all crucial to institutions in accomplishing objectives [40].

Staff development and promotion of educational programs are accepted practices today in most organizations. Employing agencies do not expect prospective employees to appear with all the necessary preparations for the job. In hospitals the cost must be borne by the patient along with other costs. Hence, it behooves those responsible for administering educational programs and those who attend them to see that these activities result in improved services to patients. Everyone employed by a hospital plays three important roles: first, as a worker with assigned duties and responsibilities; second, as an employee, part of the team with certain loyalties; and, last, as a person — a member of a community, taxpayer, consumer, voter, and sometimes parent. All staff education within an organization has one of three goals: to increase knowledge, to increase skill, or to change attitudes to develop a better employee or person. The ultimate objective of the educational program is to bring about behavioral changes in the employee to make him different in the future. Education, training, and development are a continuous process, designed to help individuals grow to their fullest, to keep them up to date with new knowledge and technology, to enable them to do their present jobs better, and to help them prepare for future opportunities if they should arise within the hospital.

STAFF EDUCATION

Staff education, staff development, and *in-service education* are some of the terms used to describe a planned educational experience provided in the job setting and closely identified with service in order to help a person perform more effectively as a person and as a worker. For the purposes of this chapter, the activity will be referred to as staff education.

There is some disagreement as to whether staff education programs should be referred to as "staff training" or "staff education." "Training" has been described in terms of limited programs to increase skills, whereas "education" has a more general systematic connotation. If the goal of both concepts is to bring about improvement in behavior, the difference may be of little consequence.

ROLE AND RESPONSIBILITIES OF
THE NURSE DIRECTOR

One of the most vital functions of the nurse director is giving leadership to the staff education programs of the nursing department, as well as participating in other educational endeavors sponsored by the hospital and the community. Interpretation of the philosophy and objectives of a staff education program (see Appendix 16) to the hospital administrator, department directors, medical staff, and nursing personnel is important. The degree of understanding provided by the nurse director affects attitudes toward the staff education program, its acceptance by nursing personnel, and the support it receives.

The nurse director is responsible for planning a program of in-service education for staff development of all nursing personnel. She must ascertain the hospital administration's (1) attitude toward education, training, and development of employees; (2) philosophy of education; (3) willingness to commit itself to provide educational programs; and (4) willingness to support those programs. The title of the program, the organizational plan, the position titles, and the number and kinds of positions necessary to reach the objectives and carry out the functions will be determined by the size, complexity, and philosophy of the nursing department and its in-service program.

If the program is to be dynamic and ongoing, someone must be accountable for it. The nurse director has to decide what is wanted and needed by the nursing department. A nursing staff education coordinator can serve as a valuable assistant to the director. She must be able to work with and through persons of diverse background, training, and experience in order to create an effective learning climate. She should have an interest in and an awareness of the needs and problems of nursing service. She must believe in the merit of staff education and its contribution to patient care. Other desirable attributes include teaching experience with adults, the ability to derive satisfaction from the achievements of others, and a commitment to the program and its objectives.

The responsibilities of the staff education coordinator are to plan, organize, direct, coordinate, and evaluate the staff education program of the nursing service department. These responsibilities include:

1. Providing leadership in formulating the philosophy and objectives of the program in accordance with the philosophy and objectives of the nursing service department.
2. Determining the educational requirements of the employees necessary to accomplish the objectives of the nursing service through collaboration with line and staff personnel.
3. Planning and implementing the program of instruction designed to meet the nursing service needs.
4. Communicating the plan for the program in such a way as to encourage and foster participation, involvement, and cooperation.
5. Participating in counseling and guidance of personnel in relation to their educational needs.
6. Recommending a budget to meet the objectives of the staff education program.
7. Planning and organizing the resources and facilities needed to accomplish the objectives of the program.
8. Contributing to the development of philosophy, objectives, policies, procedures, and job descriptions for the nursing service department.
9. Developing, maintaining, and utilizing records and reports pertinent to the program.
10. Supervising the nursing service educational staff and teachers in the program.
11. Evaluating study and research findings for application to educational programs.
12. Initiating and/or participating in studies and research activities related to staff education.
13. Participating in activities that further employee professional growth and development.
14. Preparing an annual report of the staff education program, including evaluation and recommendations for future programming.
15. Participating in and promoting membership, interest, and participation of others in the activities of the professional nursing association, in allied health organizations, and in supportive community activities.

BUDGET

The nurse director, with the assistance of the staff education coordinator, is responsible for the preparation of the annual budget for the nursing education program. The budget must be justified on the basis of the need for well-prepared personnel at all levels so that patients will receive the best possible care and services; it must further emphasize the need for patient and family teaching programs. The nurse director and her administrative staff need to consider what such programs will be expected to accomplish and approximately what they will cost. The educational coordinator must see that expenditures do not exceed the appropriations made for the program.

The educational costs in hospitals have always been a point of concern; the question is raised as to why patients should be charged for such costs. The nurse director and her staff must assist the hospital administration in justifying the educational costs for patient care:

1. The nursing staff members provide a variety of activities as part of nursing care directed to the teaching of patients and families.
2. Education programs lead to upgrading nursing staff job performance based on new knowledge and technology.
3. Education programs aid in the preparation of future health-oriented personnel using the hospital facilities as a clinical atmosphere for learning.
4. As a health center, the hospital conducts community health programs for its citizens.
5. Educational costs must include purchasing supplies and equipment necessary for effective teaching.

The nurse director and her staff must be able to give an explanation when asked about educational costs; consumers expect answers. With the great emphasis today on cost-effectiveness and on finding ways to reduce hospital costs, resources for educational programs may be cut; consequently, the data on educational costs should be available together with the rationale for such expenditures.

STAFF EDUCATION PROGRAM AREAS

A staff education program (in-service education) includes all those activities that are planned by the hospital or nursing service for the education of nursing personnel with the purpose of improving care to patients; the motivation of the learner (employee) is considered to be important in the achievement of her goals for her work [82]. Four basic areas that can serve as a framework for programming are orientation, skill training, continuing education, and leadership and management [67]. Most educational activities can be classified within this framework.

Orientation

An orientation program is that phase of the staff education program conducted for the purpose of helping a new employee adjust to her new environment and duties. An orientation period also provides an opportunity for the nursing service instructor to learn about a new employee and gives the new employee an opportunity to talk about her aspirations as a person. Overall orientation program objectives may include:

1. Introducing new nursing personnel to the hospital environment, in order to achieve maximum adjustment in the shortest time.
2. Giving the employee additional knowledge regarding conditions of employment.
3. Creating within the individual an awareness of role, responsibilities, and relationships in the new situation.
4. Giving the new employee information about the hospital and its purpose, the location of various departments, and the organization of the unit to which the employee is assigned.
5. Helping the new employee understand and appreciate the interrelation of allied services in the care and treatment of patients.
6. Acquainting the individual with her place and role on the nursing team.
7. Helping each employee become aware of her contribution toward the collective goal of hospital personnel.
8. Promoting an understanding of the relationship between the hospital and the community.

The nursing staff and new employees should be aware of the orientation program, its philosophy, objectives, and policies. The more the staff understands the basis for the program, the greater will be their support. The following policies can strengthen orientation program experiences:

1. All new personnel are assigned to the staff education unit until the instructors release them for duty on their assigned nursing units.
2. The staff education coordinator plans orientation programs for all levels of personnel based on the new employees' needs and assigned positions.
3. The staff education instructor plans the hours of duty for all new nursing personnel so that they are available as needed for orientation.
4. New employees are not used for service needs during their orientation period.
5. The length of an employee's orientation period will depend on her needs and the requirements of her position.
6. The staff education instructors are responsible for the clinical supervision of new personnel during their orientation periods and for making the necessary arrangements with supervisors and head nurses for any desired clinical experiences.
7. The new employee is responsible to the staff education instructor during her orientation period.
8. If an employee does not appear to adapt to her new position, the staff education instructor discusses the employee's future with the supervisor responsible for the person's employment. They must determine whether she should be retained.
9. When an employee has successfully completed her orientation period, the staff education instructor notifies the supervisor, and arrangements are made to transfer the new employee from the educational unit to her assigned nursing unit.
10. The supervisor and head nurse who receive a new employee introduce her to their specific unit according to the unit orientation plan.
11. The head nurse evaluates the performance of all new employees following a six-week period on the assigned nursing unit.
12. Each time an employee is moved from one position to another within her working environment, reorientation is needed.
13. Planned orientation programs should be developed for all levels of nursing personnel and other persons who have some relationship to nursing. Programs can then be adjusted to the needs of the individual.

Hospital Orientation. Orientation is essential for all new employees in a hospital, regardless of the position to be filled or the educational background and experience of the individual. All new personnel need to become acquainted with the physical and social environment in which they are to function, and it is the responsibility of hospital administration to provide the opportunity in a planned way. In many hospitals, orientation programs are held periodically for all new employees. The objectives of the hospital orientation program must be clearly identified. As the nursing department plans its orientation program, it must be in harmony with the hospital program. Hospital orientation programs may include topics such as introduction to the overall physical setting of the hospital, presentation and explanation of the hospital's philosophy and goals, description of the organizational structure of the hospital, review and interpretation of hospital administrative policies and procedures, and an explanation of hospital relationships with the community.

Nursing Service Department Orientation. As a new employee enters the nursing department, she learns that it has relationships, direct or indirect, to all the departments of the hospital (see Appendix 17). There is also much to learn about how the nursing department is organized and administered and how nursing relates specifically to the various departments. New employees must be assisted to see their role in relation to the department of which they are a significant part. Content for this specific section of an orientation program may include topics such as introduction to the philosophy, objectives, and standards of nursing care; description of the nursing department's plan of organization, administrative policies, and interdepartmental relationships; interpretation of departmental and unit policies and procedures; and review of the method of assigning patient care and responsibilities of the various categories of nursing personnel. The nursing service departmental orientation should be held periodically, depending on the number of new personnel employed. For example, if the program is conducted once a month, all new people employed since the last month's program attend the departmental orientation. This may also be the case for the hospital orientation.

Unit Orientation. A significant aspect of the orientation program is the introduction of new personnel to their assigned nursing unit. The staff education coordinator should assist the supervisor and head nurse in developing a unit orientation program, copies of which should be placed in the unit administrative manual and the nursing service staff educational manual. Areas that may be included in a unit

program are unit organization, types of patients, method of assignments, nursing care plans, patient care conferences, educational conferences, role of various personnel, staffing, tour of unit, records and
reports, demonstration of equipment, supplies and equipment, personnel evaluation, teaching responsibilities, and public relations.

The orientation program should include a section related to the employee's specific job. The job description may have been discussed in
general terms by a supervisor prior to an employee's appointment;
however, an opportunity should be given for the person to ask additional questions. The employee should be encouraged to strive toward
providing patients with quality nursing services. At this time she
should also learn about the criteria established for evaluation of her
performance, and the procedures and forms used.

The staff education coordinator and her instructors are responsible
for overseeing new employees during their orientation periods. While
the hospital and nursing service orientation programs are formal-
structure programs accommodating several persons, orientation to
the job and nursing unit is usually on a one-to-one basis. Regardless
of the setting for the various phases of an orientation program, opportunities must be provided in which employees feel free to ask
questions, offer comments, or share their thinking. They will do so if
the educational coordinator sets the climate for favorable conditions
of learning.

To be successful, an orientation program requires the coordinated
efforts of both the nursing service staff and the staff education instructors. It further calls for the support and leadership of the nurse
director. A well-planned program should ultimately contribute to
improved care to patients and employee self-development.

Skill Training

The skill training program is that phase of the staff education program directed toward providing employees with the skills and attitudes required for the job and keeping employees abreast of changing
methods and new techniques [67]. This operational definition may
apply to all categories of nursing personnel, those who must be
prepared in basic skills and those who need to review basic skills or
procedures in order to perform a job at the desired level of proficiency.

Formal on-the-job training programs may include providing new
skills for groups of allied health workers (nursing assistants, techni-

cians, or unit clerks) who have had no previous nursing experience. Refresher courses may be conducted periodically for professional and practical nurses who want to enhance their skills. Other newly employed nurses may need only a brief period to review specific skill areas before assuming responsibility on their assigned units. Technical programs may also be conducted to prepare persons with special skills in nursing areas such as surgery, orthopedics, psychiatry, emergency unit, or central service.

Formal skill programs should be planned and developed by the nursing service staff education instructors. As courses are implemented, members of the nursing service staff (professional or allied) should be asked to evaluate them. If, for example, a program for nursing assistants is being developed, revised, or evaluated, selected representatives from that group should be asked to participate in reviewing the program and its proposed objectives and outline. Since nursing assistants are directly involved, they should have something to say about what they are taught and how they are taught. The same thing would hold for all groups for whom programs are planned.

The ability to participate in small-group activities is a skill that is desirable for all members of the nursing department. Within the department there are many group activities that involve personnel, such as weekly meetings, team conferences, nursing care conferences, and reports between tours of duty. One of the concerns of any nurse director is getting personnel to take part as responsible group members. Time used in small-group activities is costly and therefore must be used wisely. If it is believed that personnel should be involved in the activities of the nursing department and share in making recommendations, employees must have opportunities to learn how to be responsible participants of a group.

One type of educational program, group-participation training, has as its objective to help individuals accept personal responsibility for themselves and others in a small-group experience. People learn how to learn by undertaking a series of learning experiences, by examining their participation as they proceed, and by helping to improve the learning situation. This approach rests on two assumptions: that adult learners should have the freedom to assert their individuality and that adults can learn how to work and learn cooperatively without injuring the dignity and respect due fellow learners [17].

This type of participation training program has the following benefits:

1. Staff members of the group learn to plan, and take part in, a series of small-group discussions that deal with topics agreed on by the staff members.
2. The staff learn more about themselves — how they are seen by co-learners, how their participation affects others, what some of the educational problems and needs of a group are, and how to deal with those needs.
3. The staff learn how to help others in a group-learning situation.
4. The staff learn how to develop disciplined freedom of expression.
5. The staff learn, through experience, what helps and what hinders productive learning through group discussion.
6. The staff learn, through experience, group educational skills and concepts such as goal setting, interpersonal communications, evaluation, consensus, disciplined observing, leadership, focusing on topics, and discovering and meeting educational needs [17].

Group-participation training offers sound educational experience in each group role — leader, co-leader, observer, recorder, resource person, group participant, and trainer. As each staff member, including the leader, learns how to play each role, the base of leadership broadens because all members become less fearful of taking on the job of leader or any other group responsibility [17].

Participation training should not be thought of as a form of group psychotherapy; it has no treatment function. In psychotherapy groups the therapist often interprets patients' motivation and accounts for present problems by tracing back through their past life experiences to discover the underlying cause of their behavior and unconscious motives. The educational participation trainer does not get involved in these issues. The therapist helps people analyze their personality structure (psychodynamics); the educational trainer does not. In a participation training program, the educational emphasis is on a problem common to the nursing staff members, and there is no analysis of individual personalities. Evaluation in a training group of staff members is confined to factors in the present group situation. Emphasis is placed on present relationships among group members (sociodynamics), not on the workings of individual personalities (psychodynamics) [17].

In order to introduce this type of program into a nursing service staff education program, selected members of the nursing staff must learn to be trainers. As they learn and train others, the concept of participation training can be directed downward to the basic unit of the nursing department — the clinical nursing unit. This approach allows all levels of nursing personnel to share in the training. Moreover, it encourages the involvement of many people with varied backgrounds in sharing and discussing a subject relevant to a specific need. The success of nursing services is dependent, to some degree, on the ability of nursing personnel to plan together for the care of patients over a 24-hour period. It is also dependent on the ability of nursing personnel to participate in other group activities outside of the nursing department directed to planning and coordinating patient care. As people are able to relate in the group as responsible participants, it becomes less burdensome to arrive at decisions regarding the welfare of patients and others.

Continuing Education

The continuing education program is that phase of the staff education program aimed at helping the employee keep up to date with new concepts; increasing knowledge, understanding, and competence; developing the ability to analyze problems; and working with others. If it is believed that the personnel who are already a part of the organization constitute the most promising manpower, then efforts should be directed toward their uninterrupted self-development.

The responsibility for a continuing education program, in a sense, is every employee's concern in the nursing department. If this is an accepted belief and it is acted on, the end results will contribute toward quality nursing services and employee self-development. Continuing education for improvement of service permits the greatest opportunity for choosing what kind of program to maintain. With it the staff can use imagination and experimentation in planning programs to meet the changing needs and demands of the various clinical nursing areas.

The use of small groups as the focus for staff education has potential for individual self-actualization. Small-group activities and instruction tend to promote rapport among members of the clinical unit. Within each nursing unit, personnel may carry on programs that they believe serve continuing education needs. When the staff of one unit is invited to an interesting continuing education program with staff of another unit, personnel learn to share and plan together.

Each level of nursing personnel, such as nursing assistants, unit clerks, licensed practical nurses, staff nurses, head nurses, or supervisors, may hold monthly meetings, at which time an educational program is presented on a topic of interest, usually selected by the group.

Continuing education can include programs conducted within the hospital as well as those held outside the hospital. Attendance at each program may motivate the staff to call for new and different experiences, to try for more individual fulfillment of their needs, to enter other educational activities, and to increase their interest in things outside the hospital community. As an individual, an employee may enroll in correspondence courses, vocational or technical courses, or college courses relevant to her job. Many hospitals support this type of employee continuing education by a tuition reimbursement program.

Another phase of continuing education includes attendance at conventions, workshops, or institutes offered by many different national, state, regional, and local organizations in the health field. As a nurse director approves staff attendance of institutes, workshops, or other educational activities, the objectives of the program should be carefully reviewed to determine their relevancy to nursing. Those attending should prepare a written report, share it with others, and show how they plan to use what they have learned.

The hospital library can serve as a center of educational activities and a resource for individual continuing education. The well-stocked library is a laboratory where nursing personnel may do research in the literature and keep abreast of the fast-moving advances in medicine, nursing, and other areas of interest.

Planning programs on a community-wide basis with other hospitals and health care agencies is another approach to expanding continuing education for health workers. An area-wide in-service education committee might be made up of representatives of hospitals and nursing homes. Funds and resources can be brought together. For example, one of the hospitals in a community receives a new piece of equipment and plans to conduct a program to acquaint the personnel with its use; perhaps neighboring hospital personnel could be invited to attend. Better understanding of continuity of patient care can be promoted by better understanding of the services (social and health agencies) available within the community. Hospitals and other health care agencies can plan programs together to enhance continuity of patient care and increase the skills of their respective health workers.

Leadership and Management

A leadership and management program is that phase of the staff education program directed toward equipping a selected group of employees for growing responsibilities and new positions in nursing [67]. The nursing service administrative staff and staff education coordinator should identify those persons who show leadership potential. It is also helpful to know which nurses really aspire to positions of greater responsibility in nursing service administration. The hospital education department, the local colleges, or the universities may offer management development programs in areas such as fundamentals of supervision, building effective communications, developing creative-inventive ability, effective listening, labor relations for first-line supervisors, and the art of human relations. The staff education coordinator should devise a specific program for each level of managers — supervisors, head nurses (see Appendix 18), assistant head nurses, and team leaders — for the purpose of widening their understanding of their role in the administration of nursing care within the clinical unit. Program objectives should be developed in conjunction with selected nursing service administrative personnel serving as resource people.

PROGRAM PLANNING

Program planning is a process by which the nature and sequence of future educational events are determined and organized; it is a flexible means through which a group of people can share in planning in an organized way. It should be used creatively, not slavishly [64]. The following are some of the general principles of program planning:

1. The overall objectives of the health care agency should be considered.
2. The educational needs of the potential program participants should be considered.
3. A wide range of resources (human and material) should be used.
4. The planning group should include people (resource persons) who are potential participants in the group.
5. Democratic processes should be utilized wherever possible in planning the staff program.

6. Various methods that might be used in reaching the objectives should be explored in the planning.
7. The program planning should allow for flexibility.
8. Provision should be made for appraisal and evaluation of the staff education program.

Educational activities may be planned by a staff education instructor or by a supervisor, head nurse, or staff nurse. This type of planning is most likely to take place when the person doing the planning knows a great deal about whatever is to be taught whereas those for whom she is planning have little or no knowledge of the subject. For example, the staff education coordinator may plan some learning activities to introduce new employees to the nursing department and its operations. Sometimes it is practical and effective for an entire group to plan its learning activities. The group should not be very large. Its members should know how to plan, and they must be able to plan in an efficient and productive manner. Each person in the group can be involved to the extent that each accepts active responsibility for the learning venture. Because it may be impractical for a whole group to assume responsibility for planning, committees can set up learning activities. Even when one individual is primarily charged with doing the planning, she often uses a committee to help her identify the needs and interests of the learners.

According to McKinley and Smith [64], one flexible procedure for planning effective education programs includes finding an interest or need expressed by the greatest number of those who will take part in a program, breaking down the interest or need into a group of related topics, setting goals for the learning activity, selecting appropriate resources, selecting appropriate educational techniques, and outlining each session and the various responsibilities to be carried out.

IDENTIFYING EDUCATIONAL NEEDS
AND INTERESTS

It is essential to give employees opportunities to identify their educational interests and needs in order to help motivate them to participate actively in programs. When they are consulted, they tend to accept responsibility for learning. Inexperienced people often plan programs by selecting *how* information is to be acquired and goals achieved before they determine *what* is to be learned and achieved. Logic dictates that the *how* come after the *what*. This is the reason it is necessary to begin the planning process with the consideration of needs and interests of the learners [64].

An interest is something a person would like to learn about or understand better. People may say, "I am interested in learning about the nursing care of patients with an artificial pacemaker" or "I am interested in knowing how a pacemaker is inserted." They may be identifying an interest that can serve as a basis for planning.

An educational need is characterized by a lack or deficiency that can be satisfied through learning experiences. People tend to seek activities through which they can meet their needs. Needs and interests are interrelated; interest points toward a need and is an expression of a need. When a person's needs and interests coincide, he is generally motivated toward a learning experience [64].

There are various types of needs. For example, it is helpful to differentiate between a *felt need* and a *real need*. A person cannot always tell which need is felt and which is real. A staff nurse may feel that she needs to improve her care to patients, whereas her real need is to learn how to organize her work assignment so that her nursing care is effective. Understanding that felt needs are sometimes mistaken for real needs, those involved with programs for adults can help them to identify their needs [64].

When personnel are asked to identify their needs, they tend to mention broad, general, or impersonal things. For example, a nursing supervisor has been having difficulties with some of the personnel she supervises. She may need to learn to understand herself in relation to the employees with whom she works. But she will identify her need as the developing of a smoother working system or the selecting of better personnel. People may resist recognizing their real needs. They sometimes prefer to deal with vague or impersonal symptomatic concepts because they have not learned that cooperative educational experiences can bring about desirable group and personal change. A factor in program planning is the effort to change people's behavior in a desirable direction through legitimate learning experiences.

It is not always possible to distinguish a real need from a symptomatic one. Instructors or leaders must proceed on the basis of a need the participants have identified; they must begin where people are, recognizing the learner's present intellectual and emotional condition as the logical starting point for an attempt to help her grow and mature. Interests and needs can be identified by means of interviews, checklists, group sessions, program observation, and informal discussion [64].

As nurse directors assess and respond to the needs of nurses, health providers, and consumers, they are in a position to work and cooperate with educational institutions and, it is hoped, to create the curricula needed by them. The nurse director can ask assurance for: (1) adequate dissemination of clinical content for health care providers; (2) inclusion of sufficient content about social conditions of consumer families and the community culture; (3) training skill development for group participation of health care providers; and (4) adequate programs in leadership and administration for present and future health team leaders, including content in organizational structure, decision making, team building, group participation, career development, the management process, planning and managing change, behavioral science concepts, systems theory, community and organizational development, leadership development, and methods of teaching.

PROGRAM EVALUATION

Most people responsible for educational activities agree that it is important to evaluate them. Many organizations spend a great deal of effort, time, and money conducting educational programs for their employees. It is hoped that this kind of experience will, in appropriate ways, modify the employee's attitudes and behavior. Generally, programs are justified on the assumption that the educational experience does effectively change the views and reactions of persons in attendance.

McKinley and Smith [64] believe that evaluation is not a single process but an intrinsic part of the interrelated activities of reviewing past educational experiences, establishing learning objectives, planning the staff education program, and measuring results. Planning for evaluation should begin in the initial stage of these activities.

All types of staff education programs must be evaluated to determine the worth of each as reflected in job performance. The evaluation process may involve the participants, staff education instructors, supervisors, head nurses, or a combination of these four. The evaluator is attempting to learn what has occurred in terms of (1) the effectiveness of the training methods and program contents, (2) changes in behavior of participants, (3) changes in on-the-job performance, and (4) improvement in the achievement of work unit goals, measured on a group basis.

Evaluation is important for the future to establish guidelines, to justify, improve, and determine the effectiveness of programs, and to improve behavior and select and shift personnel.

Some general principles for evaluating educational programs are as follows:

1. All programs can be evaluated in some way, because they are aimed at change.
2. All programs should be evaluated because management cannot be expected to accept them on faith.
3. Each program must have clearly defined objectives, so that the program planner can determine whether they were reached.
4. Dollars and cents evaluation is impressive but is not always possible, because attitudes have no price tag.
5. Results are most significant and meaningful when comparisons are made between:
   a. Trained and untrained groups.
   b. Groups trained by different methods.
   c. The same group before and after training.
6. Evaluations should be specific in terms of a particular program.
7. The effects of complex training programs can be studied more productively if each part is evaluated.
8. Evaluation of training is most effective if built into a program.
9. The evaluation procedure may include technical phrases (statistics), which sometimes will require the help of professional experts [50].

The evaluation of a program may fall into four steps: (1) to determine how the staff feels about the program, (2) to determine how much the staff has learned in the form of increased knowledge or understanding, (3) to measure the changes, and (4) to determine the effects of these behavioral changes on the objective criteria [50].

After building in the evaluation process as a part of a training program, there is a need to interpret the data and to plan appropriate follow-up action. Here are some suggested questions to ask in planning follow-up of a program:

With management
1. To what extent do you feel this activity is helping to improve the performance of personnel?
2. What specific benefits has this activity shown in time, effort, and money invested in training?
3. What suggestions do you have for improving the activity?
4. What additional help do you need?

With personnel
1. How useful has this training been to you?
2. What has helped you most on the job and what has been the least help?
3. What suggestions for improvement do you have on any phase of your training or program?
4. What additional help do you need? [50]

UNDERSTANDING THE ADULT AS A LEARNER

When developing educational programs for adults, it is important for the teacher or leader to know something about the nature of adults as learners — what motivates them, what conditions underlie their effective participation, and what conditions help promote the acceptance of personal responsibility for learning [16].

Teachers — and adult learners too — have not always understood how adult learning differs from childhood learning. There is, however, a growing awareness of the differences in the field of adult education, out of which is evolving a uniquely adult approach to the learning-teaching transaction. Many adult programs use the formalized structure to which youngsters are regularly exposed in their daily school life — which is effective largely because children have not lived long, their experience is limited, and they have had few practical opportunities to test ideas. A rather natural teacher-learner relationship develops in which the child is dependent upon someone who he thinks knows the facts. The child often recognizes that he doesn't know, and he tends to accept information, training, and ideas [16].

As an individual moves into adulthood, his feelings of dependency decrease and he begins to think he knows. He usually sees himself as a responsible, self-directing, independent personality. He resists reorganizing of his attitudes and behaviors, which have grown out of his response to many years of experience, and he is likely to resist someone else's attempt to force him to reorganize himself. The teacher-student relationship in adult groups, therefore, must be modified if the program is to be most successful. It has to be recognized that adults are both dependent and independent. Extremes could be dangerous. Adults have a deep psychological need to be treated with respect, to be perceived as having the ability to run their own lives. They tend to avoid and resent being placed in situations in which they feel they are treated like children, told what to do and what not to do, talked down to, embarrassed, punished, or judged. They resist learning under conditions that are incongruent with their self-concept as autonomous persons [16].

In areas in which adults do not know the facts, certainly one who does should guide them to pursue their inquiry purposefully. Even in this circumstance the adult brings more in experience and maturity to the learning situation than the child does. Adults ordinarily have some firmly fixed ideas, which they have lived with for some time.

It takes more than simply *telling* in order to help an adult who has cherished misconceptions for decades. He does not usually make rapid adjustments. And since the adult does not respond so quickly to adjustment as the child in school, methods must be used that are more appropriate to the problem at hand. If creative learning is to take place, adult learners must be treated differently from children in the usual class [16].

Because adult learning is a highly personal experience, adult programs should be based on principles that recognize this fact. First, adults learn best when they become actively involved as persons in the learning experience. Second, if adults are to learn most effectively, they must discover a personal reason for learning about a given topic. Learning programs should begin to deal with needs that the learners recognize as needs. Third, adults must share the responsibility for the success of the learning experience. Learners can best become responsible for learning if they actively participate in some way. There is no shortcut. It is not enough to be told that adults are responsible; they must experience what it means to accept responsibility for their growth and the growth of other persons in educational ventures [16].

It has been found that there are certain conditions under which adults learn most productively. These conditions, however, were developed as a result of the following assumptions about the nature and task of adult education:

1. Adult education should be in keeping with the nature of the society in which it takes place.
2. Three important tasks of adult education are to help all interested persons to know more about themselves, to understand their relationships with their fellow men, and to better understand their vocations as citizens of a free society.
3. People need to become intimately and personally involved in the learning process.
4. People are at their best when doing what they are able to do and what they like to do.
5. People deserve the privilege and responsibility of having something to say about what and how they learn [15].

The educational conditions under which adults learn best are: when they accept responsibility for learning and helping others to learn; when they overcome fear and timidity and feel free to express themselves; when they can relate new ideas, skills, or experiences — see new relationships; and when they have opportunities for experimentation and creativity [16].

Today's nurse, regardless of her position, recognizes her responsibility to teach. She finds herself conducting staff education programs for personnel or planning them for patients and their families. She needs to be a teacher or a learner, or both, on a continuing basis. Increased understanding of a pattern of learning that leads to change (see Appendix 19) should help her to be more comfortable and successful in her teacher-learner role.

AUDIO-VISUAL INSTRUCTION

With the rapidly changing scene in medical technology, nurse directors are faced with preparing, as well as maintaining, the competence of nurses and supportive nursing personnel. Ways must be found to extend continuing education over the 24-hour period and to use the instructional staff members to their fullest. With the development of a variety of audio-visual resources and devices (see Appendix 20), it is possible, at any time, to provide learning experiences that have important educational significance. Teaching with the assistance of audio-visual devices has been shown to enhance the quality, quantity, and duration of learning. Developments and improvements in optical and electronic engineering have provided easily operable audio-visual machines to meet any identifiable educational objective.

The tremendous surge of activity and interest in new educational media may be discerned in the growing numbers of educational television stations, closed-circuit television installations, and self-instruction laboratories. It is also reflected in increased numbers of teaching machines and programmed materials, portable videotape recorders, and vastly improved devices for the swift and economical production of a variety of graphic materials.

Many commercial firms and educational institutions have turned their attention to the development of more effective teaching apparatus. Thus, use of nonbook media for instruction has increased dramatically in the last ten years and will continue to increase rapidly.

The nurse director must therefore recognize the need for technical innovation and be willing to advance its concepts into staff education programs. The nursing administrative staff and the instructors must both be knowledgeable about the various instructional aids. Together they must also acknowledge the need to evaluate audio-visual devices and products, prepare everyone to know how to use them, be able to justify budgetary requirements for them, and share in maintaining and caring for them.

It is fortunate that science and technology have provided tools and knowledge to make learning possible. Still, there can be no guarantee that staff members will grow or change in desirable ways simply because their learning experiences are conducted through the use of educational media, old or new.

The ultimate responsibility for creating a favorable learning environment in order to achieve desired educational objectives rests, as always, with the instructor. There is as yet no adequate substitute for the instructor's unique ability to plan and organize learning experiences and to select, adapt, and appropriately relate instructional devices and materials for the achievement of learning [19].

TRENDS IN HOSPITAL EDUCATION

Today there is a trend toward coordinated hospital-wide educational departments. Hospitals are striving to organize their resources, both external and internal, to fulfill their commitments to continuing education. Responsibility is lodged in the central administration rather than within the various departments, and the director of education crosses departmental lines. Some authors believe that this system is a more efficient means of using resources, effecting innovation, improving and upgrading employee performance, and creating a liaison with other institutions and agencies [39].

Hospitals are sharing educational services with one or more other hospitals in a form of cooperation that they find advantageous. Some hospitals share educational services through informal agreements, others through formal contracts or by setting up corporations; still others share services through organizations to which they are related. A group of institutions may organize a consortium to sponsor educational services. Components of a consortium may include hospitals, health centers, educational institutions, extended care facilities, or state associations. Any one of the components of these organizations may serve as the coordinator of the consortium.

A nurse director must be aware of the trends in hospital education and of their implications for nursing and patient care. Hospital organization and policy determine the educational structure in light of their philosophy.

The human resources of any organization constitute one of its most important assets. Indeed, its successes and failures are largely determined by the caliber of its workers, including managers, and the efforts they exert. Therefore, the recruitment policies and techniques an organization adopts to meet its manpower needs are of vital significance. There is much to be gained from the adoption of carefully worked out, stable policies in the area of employment; they can be positive management tools to shape the entire recruitment and selection program.

PROMOTION POLICIES

As vacant positions occur within the nursing department, it must be determined whether they will be filled from within the department or whether new personnel will be recruited from the outside. A policy that encourages promotion from within the department or hospital tends to enhance the morale of the staff. Most people expect to advance to positions offering higher pay and status during their work careers. As one employee moves into a higher-level position, this move may cause a succession of advancements for other employees. However, promotion from within sometimes causes problems and limitations. For example, it may prevent the introduction of new ideas and knowledge into an organization and perhaps may perpetuate outdated practices. It sometimes leads to organizational inbreeding.

Perhaps the most fruitful guideline of action is to fill the majority of vacancies from within, but to go outside when qualified persons are not available inside the organization. In order to introduce new ideas, consideration should be given to filling a moderate percentage of management positions from the outside.

SOURCES

The means by which people are recruited vary, depending on such elements as hospital management policy, the type of positions open, the supply of labor in relation to demand, and the nature of the existing labor market. If internal recruitment is a practice, vacant positions can be posted on bulletin boards, and employees who feel qualified can be invited to apply. Nursing vacancies can be announced at departmental meetings. If the hospital has an official publication, space could be allotted to announcing job openings. Sometimes employees will pass the word to their friends and relatives who may be seeking work.

Other sources for recruitment include the use of public employment agencies, private employment agencies, and advertising in newspapers, professional journals, and magazines. Schools and colleges can be informed of job opportunities. The American Nurses' Association Professional Credentials and Placement Service supplies nation-wide personnel services. State professional counseling and placement service offices, while offering nation-wide services, tend to encourage filling of vacancies in their respective states. This practice may limit both the director and the potential employee, for neither is made aware of broader opportunities.

There are a number of private placement agencies. The extent of services they offer varies; some are relatively well known. The nurse director should select agencies she knows are reliable. She might inquire from her colleagues and gather information that will help determine which private placement agency to use.

Since management consulting firms become intimately acquainted with the personnel of numerous client companies, they are often in a position to recommend an individual as a likely candidate for top positions in nursing. At the annual conferences or meetings that all professional associations hold throughout the country, employers and job-seeking members of the association can almost always meet and discuss job opportunities.

The nurse director should work closely with the director of personnel in planning for manpower needs. A recruitment committee can be formed for the purpose of establishing recruitment policies and procedures and developing an action program to recruit qualified nursing staff.

LEGISLATIVE ENACTMENTS

Today people are aware of their rights through legislative enactments, and a nurse director and other persons responsible for recruitment should be equally prepared. There are federal and state laws relating to minimum wages, child labor, assignment to hazardous operations, and antidiscrimination.

The Fair Labor Standards Act, as amended in 1966, contains provisions and standards concerning minimum wages, equal pay, maximum hours, overtime pay, record keeping, and child labor.

The Civil Rights Act of 1964 requires no job discrimination based on race, color, religion, sex, or national origin.

The Age Discrimination in Employment Act of 1967 promotes the employment of the older worker based on ability rather than age, prohibits arbitrary age discrimination in employment, and helps employers and employees find ways to meet problems arising from the impact of age on employment.

The Federal Wage Garnishment Law, effective July, 1970, limits the amount of an employee's disposable earnings that may be made subject to garnishment, and it protects him from discharge because of garnishment for any one indebtedness. The term *garnishment* means any legal or equitable procedure through which earnings of any individual are required to be withheld for the payment of any debt.

STAFF SHORTAGE

Many nurse directors are faced with a shortage of personnel. Some believe it is due to the distribution of manpower; others feel it is due to improper utilization of the manpower on the job; still others regard it as being caused by a combination of distribution and utilization of staff; and some believe that nurses lack a personal commitment to nursing.

The problem of turnover of nursing personnel continues to plague the nurse director. The nursing profession is characterized by high mobility, as are some of the other women's professions. The tenure of the majority of nurses in staff positions tends to be short. The issue of retaining married nurses in active full-time careers is as pressing as in earlier years. Whether it is realistic to expect this group to contribute more is debatable. The reentry of married women into nursing depends upon many variables, of which commitment is one. The nurse director is faced with the dilemma of providing patients with continuous nursing care when the services of the nursing staff are discontinuous. Nurses are assigned for eight hours a day, five days a week, and the tenure will probably be short. The movement of a large number of staff, by season, by marriage, and because of pregnancy, is ever present.

With the shortage of nurses in various parts of the country, inactive nurses are being begged to return to work. Many who do so find some difficulty in adapting to the changing scene in nursing. Nursing practice is more complex than ever before and will continue on this course at an accelerated rate. Scientific discoveries, technological changes, and radical new treatments in recent years have changed health practices. The knowledge needed by the nurse practitioner today is vastly different from that called for only a few years ago. She is required to master an intricate body of knowledge beyond the immediate concerns of nursing and to make independent judgments about patients and health services.

The shortage of professional nurses since the end of World War II has stimulated hospital and nursing administration to seek new ways of extending nursing services. One way is to employ professional nurses on a part-time basis. The use of part-time personnel provides considerable flexibility in meeting the staffing needs of the nursing department. The nurse director is generally able to maintain a permanent full-time nursing staff consistent with the size of the hospital's work load; part-time workers can then adjust the size of the working staff to fit the hospital needs at any particular time. Part-time nurses can take over full-time positions when difficulties are encountered in employing full-time staff. For example, evening and night shifts may be staffed with a high percentage of part-time nurses.

Excessive use of part-time staff, however, can create serious administrative problems. The fragmented pattern of services of part-time nursing makes continuity of patient care difficult. Moreover, part-time workers increase and complicate the administrative and supervisory work load, especially in scheduling and communicating and in maintenance of performance standards.

Nurses who are married appear to have strong ties with their profession, but home life and family are first priorities. They want to keep in touch with nursing and are sometimes able to work part-time for a given period. The nurse director who is able to utilize these persons, provided a mutual agreement can be worked out on scheduling hours, may be paving the way for nurses who will perhaps return to full-time active duty when family obligations allow it. Keeping the part-time nurse's skills updated requires imagination and innovations on the part of nursing administration. An investment in part-time nurses can ultimately result in a stable full-time staff for the future.

Refresher courses must be made available to those who have given up nursing to raise families and need to brush up their skills. Teaching faculty are therefore required who are prepared in the area of employee development.

The problem becomes one of quick preparation of people to assume nursing care responsibilities when availability of staff is limited and when those competent to teach cannot be released from patient care duties. There is a disjointedness between the time new personnel are available and the times the other employees leave, resulting in gaps in patient care delivery.

Standards should be developed by which people who are on the various levels of nursing could advance from one level of preparation to another, allowing for career mobility. Through this type of advancement more people could be prepared to take on more responsibility and more complex tasks. Unfortunately, rigid ideas have been maintained about the roles and obligations of various members of the health team.

Shortage of personnel may be due to a lack of clearly defined activities for the various categories of health workers, partly because of an increasing number of categories and considerable overlapping of functions. Sometimes there is a tendency on the part of nursing administration to deviate from job descriptions, which are specific, and to encourage employees to expand their activities into areas for which they are not prepared and which could be dangerous to patient welfare.

If a shortage does exist in a nursing department, the director must decide how the staff will be utilized, how they will be assigned, and how much orientation and training will be needed for the job. All this is part of management determination. The nurse director must confront the hospital administration with the manpower problems and suggest ways in which she needs its support to provide sufficient care to patients. Because of the grave responsibility the nurse director holds for the coordination of patient care, she must impress upon the administration that a lack of staff or a lack of proper utilization of the present staff can endanger the lives of patients, and in some instances lead to legal proceedings.

TURNOVER

The nurse director should know how the nursing department stands in relation to its labor turnover activity. A study of attrition figures will help her to determine the extent of turnover and when and where it is occurring. It will further pinpoint labor turnover within the nursing personnel categories. She will want to know whether changes in hospital or departmental policies, organizational structure, or administrative procedure have had an effect on the rate of turnover. Turnover computation may be done by the personnel department or, in some instances, by the nursing department.

Labor turnover may be defined as the total number of separations that occur during a specific period. Many separations are beyond the control of management (such as the death of an employee). Some separations can be planned in advance (such as retirement). The largest group of separations, however, is that of employees who quit.

High turnover is sometimes viewed with alarm because of its cost to an organization. Obvious direct costs of attrition are those of employing a replacement for the person who leaves and the cost invested in her training, salary paid to the replacement during her nonproductive training period, and errors in efficiency that can be expected during that period. Indirect attrition costs are in areas such as the impact on recruiting when potential employees are aware of a high rate of attrition in a prospective employer-organization, lowered morale of present staff when they see people leaving all around them, and increased work load and demands placed upon managers, who must generally supervise inexperienced replacements. On the basis of these costs alone, a persuasive case can be made for effective control of attrition.

On the other hand, some organizations have found that a moderately high rate of attrition can be an asset rather than a liability. If attrition is selectively controlled to ensure that the right persons are remaining and the marginal ones are leaving, it can have these positive effects: (1) ensure a constant infusion of new blood and fresh thinking and thus maintain the organization's vitality; (2) provide assurance against obsolescence; and (3) ensure relatively constant availability of high-level talent for movement into managerial ranks.

Since costs can be high either in attrition or in little attrition of the wrong people, management must know who is leaving, why she is leaving, and whether her leaving is a net plus or minus for the organization.

The causes of turnover are numerous and varied, but what may not be recognized is that, given adequate compensation practices, a basic communication problem lies behind them — the average person is frustrated, at least to some degree, because she does not know what she is supposed to do, and her work may be evaluated according to an unknown (to her) set of standards. The communication confusion shows up first in recruitment and selection practices. If a manager cannot sit down with her present employees and clearly outline what is expected of each one, how can she possibly determine what qualities she is looking for in potential employees? Turnover statistics may be improved if the following managerial rules are observed:

1. Employees should be qualified before they are assigned to a task.
2. Employees should be trained to do the work that is assigned to them.
3. Managers should make time available to employees who indicate the need for guidance or counsel.
4. Managers should let people know what is expected of them and not keep them unaware of things they should know.
5. Employees should be told how they are doing — whether well or poorly.
6. Managers must be fair and consistent in their actions, their decision making, and their behavior.
7. Managers must allow their employees to speak freely and to criticize openly.
8. Managers must be constantly alert to the possible presence of employee dissatisfaction and take prompt steps to correct such a situation if it exists.

EXIT INTERVIEW

A well-planned exit interview serves as a management tool because it produces valuable information and improves employee attitudes. Even if the exit interview were only a ventilation session in which the employee had an opportunity to get a few things off her chest, this would be a beneficial activity and would justify the time devoted to it. The employee, having expressed any resentments, may then speak better of the hospital in the community at large. Both the resigning employee and those who remain behind will be aware of the fact that their opinions and their perceptions are considered of value by management.

The nurse director and her administrative staff have a responsibility to determine why people are terminating their services. The training and development of personnel are costly, and turnover in staff affects the patient's care and his hospital costs.

In an exit interview, an outline of salient points can serve as a guide for the interviewer. The content of an exit interview may include the following:

1. How does this employee rate on attitude?
2. How does this employee rate on performance?
3. Did this employee present any supervisory problems?
4. How did the employee get along with others?
5. Would this employee be reconsidered for employment?
6. Was her attendance satisfactory?
7. What are the employee's strong points?
8. What are the employee's weak points?
9. Does the employee have a new job? Better salary? Better opportunity?
10. What did she give as her reason for leaving?
11. What is the real reason for termination?
12. Was the employee dissatisfied with
    — Supervision,
    — Working conditions,
    — Promotional opportunities,
    — Salary,
    — Employee benefits,
    — Location,
    — The job itself, or
    — Fellow employees?
13. What did she like best about her work?
14. How does she rate morale in the department?
15. Would she like to work here again?
16. Does she have any suggestions for improving her job or other aspects of the department?

The exit interview provides feedback from employees concerning their attitudes and dissatisfactions. It also offers the possibility of salvaging an employee who intends to quit, and provides management with information regarding reasons for leaving. However, this technique has its limitations, since it requires skilled interviewers to persuade employees to talk, as well as to get to the real meaning behind what they say and what they do not say.

18. Research

The nursing profession is concerned with providing the best possible nursing care to people, contributing toward solving the health care problems of society, and formulating a scientific base for the practice of nursing. One way to contribute to the achievement of these goals is through research. The nursing profession has arrived at the point where it must assume responsibility for doing its own research.

The need for nursing research has arisen rapidly, as a result of: (1) the changing world of nursing and health care; (2) the public's discontent with health services; (3) the need to improve patient care; (4) the growing concern for establishing a scientific foundation of nursing practice; (5) the growing need for research in clinical nursing and for educational, administrative, and managerial research in nursing; (6) the expanding role of the nurse, and the demand for research that will provide a wide philosophical base for health care; and (7) the need to increase the pool of potential researchers [1, 85].

MEANING OF RESEARCH

Research is defined as a systematic inquiry to discover facts or test theories in order to obtain valid answers to questions raised or solutions for problems [70]. Nursing research is concerned with the systematic investigation of nursing practice itself, and with the effect of this practice on patient care or on individual, family, or community health [70]. Nursing research has as its subject the care process and the problems that are met in the practice of nursing, such as maintenance of hygiene, rest, sleep, and nutrition; relief from pain and discomfort; and counseling, health education, and rehabilitation [32]. Research in nursing has as its subject matter the profession itself — its practitioners and the characteristics of their practices, and the utilization, costs, administration, career patterns, and educational levels of nurses and student nurses [32].

Research is essentially a method; it begins with a question in the mind of the researcher. Man is a curious person. Everywhere he looks he sees phenomena that arouse his curiosity, that cause him to wonder, to speculate, and to ask questions. He discovers situations whose meaning he does not comprehend. By asking relevant questions man creates a favorable attitudinal climate, an inquisitiveness regarding pertinent fact that is a basic prerequisite for research itself; for research arises from a question intelligently asked in the presence of a

225

phenomenon that the researcher has observed and that puzzles him. By asking the right question, the researcher finds both relevance and direction in his quest for truth [53].

Look around you. Consider the unresolved and baffling situation that compels you to ask "Why?" What is the cause of the situation? What does it all mean? Observe the nursing care being given in your department. If nursing problems seem to be present, you would normally say that something ought to be done about them; your chance is through research. These are questions that reveal man's need for knowledge and suggest points of departure for research.

For some people in nursing, research has been perceived as something done by university professors or scholars in ivory towers; this concept has now faded away. We now know that research, and particularly nursing research, requires the talents and experiences of a variety of people to be successful. In nursing research, there is very little a nurse investigator does alone; she needs others to assist her in the achievement of research goals. The role each person plays in contributing toward nursing research varies and is proportionate to that person's understanding of research and other factors in the setting. All nursing personnel can share in nursing research, whether by participating in research itself, supporting research, or using the research findings. Nurses can look at happenings in nursing and identify what they can best do with available resources. The degree of research involvement in a health-oriented setting may vary, but small beginnings can lead to the larger research picture in nursing.

SCIENTIFIC BASE FOR THE PRACTICE OF NURSING

Research is the chief means of expanding the scientific boundaries of nursing. The profession of nursing has the responsibility of carrying forward research activities that will provide the basis for the professional practice of its members. There is a need to gain the necessary support from nurse practitioners and nurse clinicians in the actual setting where the research is being done. Each profession, through its community of practitioners, educators, administrators, and researchers, must determine its own goals, and the most appropriate means of achieving those goals for the greatest good of society [49]. Nursing research is important, not only for the survival of nursing but also for the well-being of those who are served by nurses. In a period of change and transition, research and research findings are essential in building a sound foundation in nursing.

Nursing recognizes its responsibility as a profession to search for and build a broader and sounder knowledge base for its professional practice; such a knowledge base can be achieved only through the systematic efforts of research. While research conducted in the various biological, physical, and social science disciplines has a bearing on questions relevant to nursing practice, the profession of nursing itself must assume the full responsibility for studying those questions that have direct relevance to the conduct of the profession.

NURSE DIRECTOR'S ROLE

The nurse director is in a strategic position to provide the leadership to augment the research endeavors of nursing. She can begin by examining her own beliefs about research, evaluating her own understanding, knowledge, and skills in the area of research. If the nurse director has had educational and practical opportunities to expand her knowledge and skills in research, she is in a desirable state to promote research. Those directors who have not yet had opportunities to broaden their understanding of research are encouraged to begin expanding their visions of the meaning of research. The nurse director is in a position to plan deliberately for the development of research activities within the nursing department. If the hospital and nursing service philosophies identify research as one of their major concepts, the nurse director can then carry out this commitment and translate its meanings into action.

The nurse director sets the climate for the research environment. This is evidenced by her commitment to the research effort. She strives to encourage hospital administrators and other department heads to share in and support nursing service research activities; she capitalizes on promoting, when possible, an interdisciplinary approach in solving research problems in nursing or health care. Once a positive attitudinal environment has been created, the hospital by its commitment can assist the nursing department in the research process by providing, for example, release time for nursing personnel participation, financial support, access to data, help with data collection, physical facilities, a library, laboratories, office space, equipment, computer services, statistical devices, and other services needed.

It is important that the nurse director identify the hospital's statement of philosophy and policy regarding research; nursing will then develop its policy and procedural statements in relation to the overall hospital policy (see Appendix 21). A nursing service research committee can be established for the purpose of achieving nursing's objectives (see Appendix 22). The committee should identify guidelines for obtaining approval for nursing studies (see Appendix 23).

What can a nurse director do to promote research endeavors? Some suggestions are:

1. Plan deliberately for the development of research activities.
2. Demonstrate a positive attitude toward research and a general commitment to inquiry.
3. Enroll in research classes at a university.
4. Develop a research course through in-service education to acquaint the nursing staff with the meaning, process, and use of nursing research.
5. Learn how to use research findings in daily practice.
6. Identify the role that the nursing staff can play in the support and promotion of research.
7. Participate in activities related to research that are promoted either within the hospital or by other disciplines.
8. Read and evaluate research.
9. Keep abreast of new knowledge coming out of research.
10. Identify within the nursing setting or the community those nursing problems for which research is needed, and communicate this need to researchers.
11. Cooperate when research projects are initiated in the nursing department or hospital by researchers within or outside of the setting.
12. Provide opportunities for the nursing staff to develop skills to carry out simple but carefully defined studies in their nursing unit or in the nursing department.
13. Stimulate and guide the nursing staff in conducting studies.
14. Encourage staff members to view themselves as participants in, contributors to, and replicators of research.
15. Determine if findings in research have any significance for nursing care.
16. Allow staff to attend conferences and workshops on research.
17. Obtain budgetary support for research education and activities.

18. Share research findings of any studies with others.
19. Make research publications and journals available to the nursing staff.
20. Encourage replication of studies reported in the literature.
21. Hold annual research conferences to study problems identified by the nursing personnel [1, 47, 56, 78, 85].

HUMAN RIGHTS

As the nurse director supports the advancement of scientific knowledge toward the achievement of improved health care, she must be aware of what is involved regarding human rights. A ready source that should be in her library is *Human Rights Guidelines for Nurses in Clinical and Other Research*, published by the American Nurses' Association [9]. The human rights of the participants/consumers as well as those of nurse investigators who engage in research must be considered. The relationship of trust between patient and nurse requires the nurse investigator to assume special obligations to safeguard the patient in several ways:

1. The patient needs to be assured that his right to privacy will not be violated without his voluntary and informed consent.
2. The nurse investigator guarantees that no risk, discomfort, invasion of privacy, or threat to personal dignity beyond that initially stated in describing the subject's role in the study will be imposed without further permission being obtained.
3. The patient is assured that if he does not wish to participate in the study, he will not be subjected to embarrassment, nor will the quality of his care be influenced by this decision [9].

In most institutions that are engaged in research, a committee is charged with the responsibility for an initial and continuing review of projects and other activities that involve human subjects; membership should be representative of all groups whose members are likely to be involved in the implementation of the study undertaken. A list of all research projects approved by the hospital committee must be sent routinely to nursing and other departments that are involved in the implementation of the studies. The nursing service department can establish a committee (see Appendix 22) for the purpose of carrying out its research endeavors and providing leadership in the identification of nursing problems. The nurse director has a responsibility to support and enforce the committee's policies and procedures governing the rights of prospective subjects. She also needs to become informed about various legal parameters affecting nurse-patient relationships. With respect to human rights, legal accountability focuses on evidence that the professional nurse has not failed her responsibility by either intentionally or unintentionally withholding relevant information that might have altered the patient's decision. Knowledge about the scope of nursing practice and the ethical issues affecting all practitioners in emergency situations is a necessary requirement for the nurse director [9].

The development of scientific knowledge in nursing will increasingly involve nurses in clinical research; other nurse practitioners in hospitals can find themselves participating in clinical research developed and implemented by nursing or other health professionals. Ethical concerns about potential violations of human rights become crucial whenever new and untried procedures are to be used and when the outcomes are unknown. The concept of informed consent applies not only to patients but also to nurses, who are expected, as part of their daily tasks, to implement activities that potentially carry risk or have uncertain outcomes [9].

It must be recognized that risk is potentially present in all situations where untried procedures are involved; the patient must be given all relevant information prior to participation in activities that go beyond the established and accepted procedures necessary to meet his personal needs. Nurses must be concerned about patients who by reason of their illness are not able to protect themselves effectively from externally imposed threat or injury [9].

The nurse director is responsible for the development of specific guidelines, policies, and procedures (see Appendix 23) for research activities carried on either by the departmental nursing staff or by outside nurse researchers or graduate students. Investigators, for example, are obligated to communicate in advance to the hospital administration or the director of nursing service, or both, the purposes and strategies of the research and to provide usable feedback upon completion of the research project. The hospital must be assured that the investigator's findings will attempt to support the major effort of the institution, which is the improvement of services.

RESEARCH PROCESS

The nurse director must possess some basic understanding of the research process, since nurse investigators will approach the director for support in achieving certain research goals. The various steps of the research process may include: (1) selection of a nursing problem, (2) search for and a review of literature, (3) theoretical framework, (4) hypotheses, (5) research methods, (6) data collection, (7) analysis of data, (8) findings, (9) conclusion, (10) recommendations, and (11) written report. Several references that are listed at the end of this chapter elaborate on the research process in depth for those directors who may need this information.

The nurse investigators will present to the nurse director, for her consideration, a nursing research proposal. A proposal (see Appendix 24) is a written plan; it is as essential to successful research as an architect's drawing is to the building of a house. The heart of all research planning or design is the research proposal. Investigators are very aware of the importance of the proposal, since major research projects are frequently approved or rejected on the basis of the proposal. A well-written proposal stands a better chance of obtaining financial grants and subsidies.

An investigator's proposal affords an opportunity to evaluate the total research plan before an inordinate expenditure of effort, time, and money is invested in the project. A careful review of the proposal will reveal the degree to which the researcher has thought through the details of the investigation. The proposal will show whether the investigator has envisioned the dimensions of the task and considered the problems involved in the acquisition of the data and their subsequent treatment and interpretation [70]. Sound proposals generally prevent mistakes. The proposal, as a prospectus, plan, outline, statement, or draft, sets forth the research problem clearly; it indicates precisely the manner in which an investigator proposes to resolve a problem within the framework of the scientific method. The proposal also assists the nurse director to consider important details with implications for the nursing service department or the hospital.

ROLE OF NURSING PERSONNEL

The nursing staff members are encouraged to expand their visions of the meaning of research and to perceive themselves as participants in, contributors to, and replicators of research as well as users of research findings. It is desirable that all nursing personnel have some basic understanding of research. As their understanding expands, they will see that their nursing practice should be based less on imitation and intuition than on validated scientific inquiry [88]. Through research, nursing personnel can establish the relative effectiveness of various nursing interventions as well as the conditions that enhance or impede desired patient outcomes. Nurses will then question their practices, explore the outcomes, and contemplate new interventions. Each one will bring to her nursing services the intellectual curiosity and creativity essential to research [88].

The collection of data is a significant part of the research process, and all levels of personnel may share in this aspect of research. However, staff members must understand fully the reason for their participation, since participation without understanding can be disastrous to the research activity [88].

What can nursing personnel do to promote research endeavors?

1. Understand the need for research.
2. Understand the research process.
3. Develop a positive attitude toward research.
4. Develop a genuine commitment to inquiry.
5. Learn to question, to probe the unknown areas.
6. Possess a feeling of responsibility relative to the advancement of knowledge.
7. Become consumers of research.
8. Learn how to use the findings of research.
9. Learn more than they now know about research.
10. Develop a growing respect for evidence and for the value of inquiry as a means for achieving continuous learning, the advancement of knowledge, and the improvement of practices.
11. Read critically; value the research contributions of nurses who are engaged in inquiry.
12. Identify how all staff members can best utilize their talents to make an impact on transforming nursing into a scientific, humanistic, learned profession.
13. Collaborate with others in generating nursing research [1, 47, 78, 88].

Nursing personnel should be encouraged to identify research problems in nursing that they believe need to be investigated for the future. Fox [27] has developed a model for identifying research problems in nursing; this model is based on the nursing process and identifies the following types of studies that relate to:

1. The health needs of people.
2. The decisions inherent in the nursing process.
3. The professional role and the legal limits of nursing practice.
4. The setting in which the nursing process is utilized.
5. Utilization of the nursing process by nurses with varying experience and education.
6. Role of the client, his family, and professional and other health personnel in implementing the nursing care plan.
7. Impact of direct nursing care on the client.
8. Communication of data [27].

Yura [94] says that research plays an important role in the development and refinement of the nursing process and in the development of nursing science. Since the nursing process provides a common base from which many nursing actions can proceed, it also requires investigation into topics such as:

1. Utilization of the nursing history in the development of the nursing care plan.
2. Number and kinds of decisions made based on data of the nursing history.
3. Definition of the client's role in the development of the nursing care plan.
4. Rationale used by nurses in selecting a specific nursing action to resolve a problem.
5. Determining factors inherent in the nurse's decision as to whether or not to refer a client problem to another health care professional or another agency.
6. Rationale for delegating actions to be performed by members of the nursing team rather than by the nurse herself.
7. Impact of agency policies on the number, kinds, and quality of decisions made by the nurse relative to assessing, planning, implementing, and evaluating care.
8. Development of tools to evaluate the impact of nurse actions on client behavior.
9. Determining the client's role in evaluating the nursing care rendered to him.

10. Determining how nurses use research findings and incorporate them into their use of the nursing process [97].

Research is an integral part of nursing. More and more practitioners are becoming nurse researchers, with the result that we can look forward to an acceleration of nursing research. It is therefore timely to consider the implications for the nurse director and her need to become associated, involved, and supportive of nursing research projects. Research involves not only knowledge and skills but also a commitment to its purpose. The nurse director is in a strategic position to assist both the nurse practitioner, who is responsible for action in nursing, and the nurse researcher, who builds knowledge in nursing. Both the nurse practitioner and the nurse researcher are interested in solving nursing problems; their efforts can be supported by a nurse director who views research as a means to achieving nursing and health care goals and providing a scientific base for the practice of nursing.

1. Abdellah, F. *Better Patient Care Through Nursing Research.* New York: Macmillan, 1965.
2. Adeho, E.   Identifying problems for nursing research. *Int. Nurs. Rev.* 54:1, 1974.
3. American Hospital Association. *Nursing Department Reports to Administration* 3:1, 1965.
4. American Hospital Association. *Nursing Care Plans: The Role of the Director of Nursing* 6:1, 1967.
5. American Hospital Association. *Maintaining Nursing Staff Personnel Files* 8:2, 1969.
6. American Hospital Association. *Nursing Service Department Organization* 9:1, 1971.
7. American Hospital Association. *The Patient's Medical Record: Problem-Oriented System.* Chicago: The American Hospital Association, 1973.
8. American Nurses' Association. *The Nurse in Research: ANA Guidelines on Ethical Values.* New York: The American Nurses' Association, 1968.
9. American Nurses' Association. *Human Rights Guidelines for Nurses in Clinical and Other Research.* New York: The American Nurses' Association, 1973.
10. American Nurses' Association. *Peer Review — Guidelines for Establishment of Committees.* New York: The American Nurses' Association, 1973.
11. Batey, M.   Conceptualizing the nursing process. *Nurs. Res.* 20:296, 1971.
12. Beach, D. *The Management of People at Work.* New York: Macmillan, 1967.
13. Bennett, A.   Departmental policies — guides to action. *Hosp. Top.* 45:44, 1967.
14. Bennett, A.   Setting departmental objectives. *Hosp. Top.* 45:49, 1967.
15. Bergevin, P. *A Philosophy for Adult Education.* New York: Seabury Press, 1967.
16. Bergevin, P., and McKinley, J. *Design for Adult Education in the Church.* New York: Seabury Press, 1958.
17. Bergevin, P., and McKinley, J. *Participation Training for Adult Education.* St. Louis: Bethany Press, 1965.
18. Block, D.   Evaluation of nursing care in terms of process and outcome: Issues in research and quality assurance. *Nurs. Res.* 24:256, 1975.
19. Brown, J., Lewis, R., and Harclerood, F. *A-V Instruction — Materials and Methods.* New York: McGraw-Hill, 1964.
20. Browning, V.   The nursing service audit as a tool for the improvement of nursing. *Hosp. Manage.* 101: 94, 1966.
21. Carter, J.   The nursing process and hospital administration. Unpublished paper, University of Evansville, Indiana, 1974.
22. Daubenmire, M., and King, I.   Nursing process and models: A systems approach. *Nurs. Outlook* 21:512, 1973.
23. Donnelly, P. *Guide for Developing a Hospital Administration Policy Manual.* St. Louis: Catholic Hospital Association, 1974.
24. Drucker, P. *The Objectives of a Business: The Practice of Management.* New York: Harper & Row, 1954.
25. Felton, G.   Pathway to accountability: Implementation of a quality assurance program. *J. Nurs. Admin.* 6:45, 1976.

26. Felton, G., and McLaughlen, F. The collaborative process in generating a research study. *Nurs. Res.* 25:115, 1976.
27. Fox, D. *Fundamentals of Research in Nursing.* New York: Appleton-Century-Crofts, 1970.
28. Froche, D. Scheduling by team or individually. *J. Nurs. Admin.* 4:34, 1974.
29. Froche, D., and Bain, J. *Quality Assurance Program and Controls in Nursing.* St. Louis: Mosby, 1976.
30. Furst, E., et al. *Fundamentals of Nursing.* Philadelphia: Lippincott, 1974.
31. Gestgey, D., and Metz, E. A brief guide to designing research proposals. *Nurs. Res.* 18:139, 1969.
32. Gortner, S. Research for a practicing profession. *Nurs. Res.* 24:193, 1975.
33. Greenough, K. Determining standards for nursing care. *Am. J. Nurs.* 68: 2153, 1968.
34. Gunn, M. *A Method for Developing a Master Staffing Plan for the Nursing Service Department.* St. Louis: Catholic Hospital Association, 1960.
35. Hansen, R. Research in nursing service. *Nurs. Outlook* 19:520, 1971.
36. Helger, E. Developing nursing outcome criteria. *Nurs. Clin. North Am.* 9:2, 323, 1974.
37. Hill, S. Ground rules for people who make policies. *Mod. Hosp.* 3:87, 1958.
38. Hooper, F. C. *Management Survey.* London: Isaac Pitman, 1948.
39. Hospital Research and Educational Trust. *Programmed Instruction and the Hospital.* Chicago: The Hospital Research and Educational Trust, 1967.
40. Hospital Research and Educational Trust. Planning programs for the adult learner. *Bulletin on Hospital Education and Training.* July, 1968.
41. Hospital Research and Educational Trust. The process of evaluation and follow-up in training. *Bulletin on Hospital Education and Training.* November, 1968.
42. Howell, J. Cycling scheduling of nursing personnel. *Hospitals* 40:77, 1966.
43. Howell, R. A fresh look at management by objectives. *Business Horizons.* Indiana University, Bloomington, Fall, 1967.
44. Inservice education: Hospitals use new technology of training to teach new technology of care. *Mod. Hosp.* 117:83, 1971.
45. —— Is the pyramid crumbling? *International Management,* July, 1971.
46. Jackson, B. Participant observation in nursing research. *Supervisor Nurse* 4:30, 1973.
47. Jacox, A. The research component in the nursing service administration, masters program. *J. Nurs. Admin.* 4:35, 1974.
48. Jameron, K., and Nailen, R. Homemade videotapes train staff and help patients understand hospital procedures. *Mod. Hosp.* 117:87, 1971.
49. Johnson, M., and Okundi, A. Roles that nurses in the community care play in nursing research. *Int. Nurs. Rev.* 20:286, 1973.
50. Kirkpatrick, D. Techniques for evaluating training programs. *J. Am. Soc. Training Directors* 14:18, 1960.
51. Langston, A. Why primary nursing? *Nurs. Clin. North Am.* 10:3, 283, 1974.
52. Lawney, S. Committees — a key to group leadership. *North Central Region Extension Publication* 5:1, 1965.

53. Leedy, P. *Practical Research — Planning and Design.* New York: Macmillan, 1974.
54. Lerda, L., and Cross, L. Performance-oriented training — results, management, and follow-up. *J. Am. Soc. Training Directors* 16:19, 1962.
55. Likert, R. *The Human Organization.* New York: McGraw-Hill, 1967.
56. Lindeman, C. Nursing practice research: What's it all about? *J. Nurs. Admin.* 5:5, March–April, 1975.
57. Little, D., and Carnevelli, D. *Nursing Care Planning.* Philadelphia: Lippincott, 1976.
58. Mantheny, M., et al. Primary nursing. *Nurs. Forum* 9:1, 1970.
59. Marram, G., et al. *Primary Nursing: A Model for Individualized Care.* St. Louis: Mosby, 1974.
60. Marriner, A. *The Nursing Process — A Scientific Approach to Nursing Care.* St. Louis: Mosby, 1975.
61. Maslow, A. *Motivation and Personality.* New York: Harper & Row, 1954.
62. McClure, M. Quality assurance and nursing education: A nursing service director's view. *Nurs. Outlook* 24:367, 1976.
63. McGregor, D. *The Human Side of Enterprise.* New York: McGraw-Hill, 1967.
64. McKinley, J., and Smith, R. *Program Planning: A Handbook.* Bloomington: Bureau of Studies in Adult Education, Indiana University, 1957.
65. Mitchell, P., and Atwood, J. Problem-oriented charting as a teaching-learning tool. *Nurs. Res.* 24:99, 1975.
66. Moore, L., and White, G. Search or research? The pilot study — its value to researchers. *Nurs. Outlook* 13:43, 1965.
67. National League for Nursing, Department of Hospital Nursing. *In Pursuit of Quality Hospital Nursing Services.* New York: The National League for Nursing, 1964.
68. National League for Nursing, Department of Hospital Nursing. *Self-Evaluation Guide for Nursing Service in Hospitals and Related Institutions.* New York: The National League for Nursing, 1967.
69. Newman, W., and Summer, C. *The Process of Management.* Englewood Cliffs, N.J.: Prentice-Hall, 1961.
70. Notter, L. *Essentials of Nursing Research.* New York: Springer, 1974.
71. Odiorne, G. Management by objectives: Antidote to the future shock. *J. Nurs. Admin.* 5:27, 1975.
72. Paetznick, M. *A Guide for Staffing a Hospital Nursing Service.* Geneva: World Health Organization, 1966.
73. Patton, J., and Littlefield, C. *Job Evaluation.* Homewood, Ill.: Irwin, 1957.
74. Phaneuf, M. Model for quality: A matrix. *Assoc. Oper. Room Nurs.* 23:759, 1976.
75. Phaneuf, M., and Wandelt, M. Quality assurance in nursing. *Nurs. Forum* 4:329, 1974.
76. Porterfield, J. Quality assurance in the provision of hospital care. *Hospitals* 48:47, 1974.
77. Price, E. *Staffing for Patient Care.* New York: Springer, 1970.

78. Rinehart, E. L. *Management of Nursing Care.* New York: Macmillan, 1969.
79. Schaff, W. Making the most of the annual budget presentation. *Hospitals* 39:60, 1965.
80. Schechter, D. *Agenda for Continuing Education: A Challenge to Health Care Institutions.* Chicago: Hospitals Research and Educational Trust, 1974.
81. Smith, P. *Philosophy of Education.* New York: Harper & Row, 1965.
82. Sommer, D. *In-Service Education Manual.* St. Louis: Catholic Hospital Association, 1966.
83. Staton, J. Nursing process and basis of professional nursing. The nursing process — an eclectic approach. Unpublished paper, University of Evansville, Indiana, 1974.
84. Toffler, A. *Future Shock.* New York: Random House, 1970.
85. Treece, E., and Treece, J. *Elements of Research in Nursing.* St. Louis: Mosby, 1973.
86. Valentino, M. A philosophy of the nursing process. Unpublished paper, University of Evansville, Indiana, 1974.
87. Walter, J., et al. *Diagnosis of Problem-Oriented Approaches: Patient Care and Documentation.* Philadelphia: Lippincott, 1976.
88. Wandelt, M. *Guide for the Beginning Researcher.* New York: Appleton-Century-Crofts, 1970.
89. Watson, A., and Mayers, M. Evaluating the quality of patient care through retrospective chart review. *J. Nurs. Admin.* 6:17, 1976.
90. Watson, T. J. *A Business and Its Beliefs.* New York: McGraw-Hill, 1963.
91. Weber, H. Improving Quality of Nursing Care. In *The Nurse Consultant and Hospital Nursing Service.* New York: The National League for Nursing, 1965.
92. Weed, L. *Medical Records, Medical Education and Patient Care.* Cleveland: The Press of Case Western Reserve University, 1967.
93. Woody, M., and Mallison, M. The problem-oriented system for patient-centered care. *Am. J. Nurs.* 73:116, 1973.
94. Wooley, F. *Problem-Oriented Nursing.* New York: Springer, 1974.
95. Wortman, M., and Randle, C. *Collective Bargaining.* Boston: Houghton Mifflin, 1966.
96. Young, E. *Nursing Service Self-Evaluation Guide of Nursing.* Exchange No. 22. New York: The National League for Nursing, 1963.
97. Yura, H., and Walsh, M. *The Nursing Process.* New York: Appleton-Century-Crofts, 1973.
98. Zimmer, M. A model for evaluating nursing care. *Hospitals* 48:91, 1974.

Part IV. Establishing and Maintaining the Physical Environment

In meeting the needs of patients, the hospital's obligation is primarily an environmental one. The environment is divided into two types of resources, physical and human. The hospital administrator and department directors are responsible for working together and coordinating their efforts. Establishing and maintaining the physical environment of the hospital require informed and imaginative participation by everyone concerned. Each department director must manage his areas so as to contribute to the efficient maintenance and operation of the total physical plant. Environmental factors, physical and other, create the climate within which patient care takes place. Furthermore, it has long been recognized that the patient's perception of and response to his environment are important to his progress and recovery.

The nursing staff plays a significant role in establishing and maintaining the physical environment of a hospital. Because the staff members are so aware of the varied services needed for the proper therapeutic plan for patient care, they should be involved in the overall planning of a hospital facility. As the coordinators of the patient care units, nursing staff members should participate in detailed planning of the units from the very onset of discussion. Nursing involvement in design and structure research is crucial to the improvement of patient care. With the knowledge and experience gained through interaction with patients and their families, the nurse can be a most helpful colleague of the architect. She may well help to humanize the hospital environment and alter the structure to meet the patient's needs better [7].

As members of a multidisciplinary team planning for modification or new construction, the nurse director and her staff have the opportunity to work closely with representatives of other disciplines. Taking part in the cross-fertilization of ideas that results from the thinking of these other professionals can be a highly stimulating experience [7].

Today's hospital environment must be designed and maintained for complete flexibility so that it will be able to accommodate change without disrupting the entire health care facility. Advances in medicine, patient care, and hospital management, as well as changing employment problems, changing educational needs, growing research problems, new community expectations of hospital care, rapidly shifting populations, changing cultural and sociological conditions, effects of hospital insurance, group practice, and government aid programs — all these exert influences on hospital maintenance and design and the functions they fulfill [7].

Before a nursing unit can be designed, its objectives and functions must be clearly defined. There is a need for discussion and planning among the administration, medical staff, nursing personnel, department heads, and other concerned individuals. Once the objectives and functions are identified, the architect can become involved.

A nursing unit design should seek to achieve objectives such as:

1. Maintaining quality care for patients.
2. Achieving the lowest possible cost of building.
3. Functioning at the lowest possible cost.
4. Providing adequate space for patient services.
5. Promoting job satisfaction for the medical and nursing staff, as well as other hospital personnel who provide services to patients.
6. Considering needs of families of patients or other visitors.
7. Allowing work to be done with the greatest ease and the least waste of personnel time.

Whenever a nursing unit is being designed, opinions among those responsible for its construction may vary, despite agreed-upon objectives. Ultimately it is the responsibility of hospital administration to make final decisions. The nurse director, however, must continue to stress the need for a nursing unit that is "oriented toward people." Sometimes it may be perceived that nurses are exaggerating regarding the need for a specific space requirement or design, but the nurse director must keep in mind the many human actions that occur within the nursing unit. In order to justify her position on nursing unit requirements, she must gather data to substantiate her requests.

The nursing staff should be acquainted with the general regulations set by official hospital licensing bodies relating to the physical plant and its environmental considerations. Other sources of information are the American Hospital Association, the American Association of Hospital Consultants, and the Joint Commission on Accreditation of Hospitals. The nursing staff members must strive to increase their own general knowledge of building requirements in order to contribute effectively during the planning stage.

SIZE

Should the nursing unit be large or small? Present-day trends indicate that larger units are being constructed consisting of 40 to 80 beds.

Hospital administrators and consultants say that the larger unit is more economical to build and maintain. The nursing staff must be cognizant of this fact and they must further consider the implication of largeness relative to providing and coordinating patient services.

As units become larger, the team-nursing approach provides a method of assignment that will allow patients to identify with a specific group of personnel. It must also be recognized that the larger unit requires a higher quality of nursing supervision and administrative responsibility. The director must recruit nurses who are able leaders and can manage these areas. Larger units also mean greater distances and, therefore, consideration must be given to the use of automated devices.

SHAPE

The shape of the unit will depend on the planners, their objectives, and the functions needed to achieve their operating philosophy. Geometric nursing unit design varies and can be found in shapes such as a circle, square, rectangle, ellipse, double corridors, E shape, T shape, U shape, Y shape, or a combination of these.

Nurses will be concerned with the shape of the unit from the standpoint of the activities they perform. Distance from one point on the unit to another is of significance for the sake of economy and proficiency, as well as for the patient and his welfare. Shape can be affected by the services performed by other departments on the unit. The transportation of patients to other areas of the hospital will have some bearing on the design.

The shape and design of the unit may well have some effect on recruiting and retaining good employees. Travel distance for the nursing staff on the unit to serve patients should generally not exceed 75-90 feet.

THE PATIENT'S ROOM

The design and construction of a patient's room will depend upon such factors as the types of patients to be served and the severity of their illness, the changing patterns of medical and nursing practice, and the design and size of equipment and furniture planned for patient care.

The general trend is to accommodate patients in private or semi-private rooms. A private room should be approximately 100 square feet, and a semi-private room area should allow approximately 80 square feet per bed. Private rooms should be flexible enough so that — in case of an emergency — a second bed can be placed in it temporarily. The shape of the room should provide three feet of usable space on two sides and end of the bed. Sufficient space must be available around and near the bed in order to use specialized equipment (such as an oxygen tent); space must also be sufficient to accommodate a cardiopulmonary resuscitation team and the necessary emergency-lifesaving cart of equipment and supplies.

A hand-washing lavatory, trimmed with valves that can be operated without the use of hands, should be in each patient's room. This type of lavatory, if properly used, could minimize cross-infection. Some lavatories are placed in an adjoining toilet room.

A toilet room should be accessible from each patient's room. A bedpan flushing device should be provided on patient toilets. Patient handbars can be placed on the wall near the toilet as an aid or support. An emergency calling system should be available in the area in case a patient is in need of assistance.

Bathing facilities for patients may include tubs or showers, or both, depending on the types of patients to be served. Hand-washing facilities should be available in all bath areas used for patient treatments. An emergency nurses' calling system and suitable grab bars should be included. Doors to the toilet rooms and bathroom should be wide enough to admit a wheelchair.

Lighting in a patient's room should include a fixture for general illumination. This fixture, with an extension arm, can be attached to the bed, over the head of the patient. A multiple-purpose lamp that can be used by the patient for reading or detached from the head of the bed and used as an examining light should also be included. At least one light should be available for night lighting; the switch control can be placed at the doorway. All light switches in patient rooms should be of the quiet-operating type.

There should be at least one window that will allow a patient to view the outside. The sill of the window can be used as a place to store the patient's flowers or other personal gifts.

All doors to patient rooms should be wide enough for beds and stretchers to be moved through; the minimum width should be at least forty-four inches. Doors should swing into the room rather than the corridor. In an emergency, doors to patients' rooms should be equipped with hardware that will allow access.

A clothes closet is needed to store the personal belongings of a patient.

A nurse's call system should be available for each patient. It may be an audible communication system, or in some instances, a one- or two-way audio-visual system. Communication can take place between the patient's room and the nurses' station; at the same time a visible signal light should appear above the patient's room door and in the clean and soiled utility rooms to serve as an additional visible signal.

Each patient bed should have duplex receptacles, located as follows: one on each side of the head of each bed and one receptacle on another wall. Parallel adjacent beds require only one receptacle between the two beds. If motorized beds are used, receptacles are necessary.

THE NURSES' STATION

Most hospitals appear to support a centralized nurses' station. Other hospitals may locate a mini-station within or next to the patient's room. The centralized nurses' station is an area in which major medical treatment and nursing care planning occur. Because it serves as a focal point for bringing health-team members together, it must provide the space, equipment, and supplies necessary to promote coordination of patient care.

Sufficient space must be available for both physicians and nurses to perform necessary recording functions. Because of the major activities and traffic patterns that occur within this area, two separate charting and recording areas are desirable — one for physicians and the other for the nursing and other authorized personnel. A separate space, adjacent to the nurses' charting area, should be reserved for a unit secretary, if there is one on the staff. In many situations the unit secretary serves as a receptionist and coordinates activities within the nursing unit for the nurse in charge. Careful consideration should be given to the space requirements necessary for the unit secretary's functions. The area should be well lighted for the charting function.

An adequate number of chairs must be available for the medical and nursing staff members.

The communication system within the nurses' station generally may include telephones, nurses' call system, paging system, pneumatic tubes, and computer terminals. The placing of each system must be carefully planned in terms of space so as to receive maximum utilization for patient services.

Patient charts may be stored either within a permanent part of the nurses' charting desk or in a charting rack. In some instances a combination of both methods is used. Some physicians may need a mobile chart rack to transport patient records as they make rounds to the bedside.

Bookcases or shelves are needed to store books, journals, policy manuals, procedure manuals, and other reference readings needed within an arm's reach. Bulletin boards for time schedules, assignments, memos, and other types of communication should be centrally located.

Because the nurses' station is the focal point of planning and involves the interaction of many people, it can become noise generating; every means must be used to decrease this annoyance. An acoustical ceiling should be installed. Some nurses' stations are glassed in all the way up to the ceiling.

SPECIAL ROOMS

The medication room is generally centrally located within the nurses' station. The size of the nursing unit and the method of assignment (such as the team method) will generally determine how many medication rooms are needed. Each medication room should have sufficient space for storing of important medicines and supplies. Narcotics and other selected medications should be stored in a locked area. Sufficient space must be available so that the nursing staff can work with ease and minimal interruption within the area.

A clean workroom (utility room) is necessary on each nursing unit. This space provides an area in which necessary supplies and equipment can be assembled in order to carry out a medical or nursing procedure. The area should also include a work counter, storage space, and hand-washing facilities.

A soiled workroom is also needed so that used equipment, supplies, and other materials can be separated from the clean area. It should include a sink, work counter, waste receptacles, and hand-washing facilities.

One kitchenette on each nursing unit is required; it should include a refrigerator, ice machine (preferably drop ice), work area, storage space, three compartment sinks with drainboards (if glasses are washed here), hot plate, toaster, and hand-washing facilities.

Each nursing unit needs a treatment room for various examinations and therapeutic procedures, for consultation, and for providing privacy for patients, if privacy is required in a semi-private room.

A small, quiet room should be available for families of acutely ill patients. This space permits the physician or clergyman to confer with families. The room should include a telephone, comfortable chairs, a light, and bathroom facilities.

A solarium is needed on every floor where nursing units are located. This area can afford patients opportunities for socialization, physical exercise, recreation, or health teaching. Locker space should be available to store recreational and occupational supplies and equipment.

Space must be made available on each nursing unit for educational activities to be carried on. The amount of space and the number of conference rooms will depend on the number of patients, personnel, and allied health workers involved. If an institution is conducting its own educational programs and also providing experiences for university programs, space for students and instructors must be of prime concern. If clinical experiences are to be meaningful and educationally sound, the learning atmosphere must be planned for. The conference rooms should include comfortable desks, bulletin board, blackboard, lectern, audio-visual aids, and television circuits. These areas can also be used for patient-teaching programs.

A lounge for visitors is needed. Patients who are ambulatory may want to visit with their relatives or friends, particularly if they are in a two-bed room.

Employee facilities, rest space, showers, and toilets may be decentralized on the nursing unit or centralized in an area remote from the unit. It is desirable to have small individual lockers on the nursing units, which allow the staff to store their nurses' caps, purses, sweaters, or other small items in close proximity.

The facilities of the nursing department must be periodically evaluated by the nurse director and her staff to determine what is lacking and to set the stage for eventually supplying it. This can be done by encouraging the nursing staff to observe daily what is happening to patients, themselves, and others within the clinical setting. What improvements can be made to give patients the greatest comfort? What would patients recommend in the construction and furnishings of a new building? [3]

Sometimes nursing personnel become so conditioned to the unchanging arrangements, the type of furnishings, and the upkeep or lack of upkeep of hospital patient units and rooms that they do not seem to consider how space and its contents can best be used for therapeutic purposes. The patient unit should be so arranged that it will assist the patient in accepting and being comfortable in, at best, an apprehensive environment. A hospital is an artificial environment, and the nurse director and her staff must be concerned with the patient's response to it [3].

Nursing units should be designed or remodeled so that they will improve patient satisfaction, improve the morale of patients, and improve patient confidence in the hospital, the medical staff, and nursing personnel which in total are so important to recovery. Patients' rooms should be designed and equipped to meet the physical and psychological needs of the patient and to provide a setting in which required medical treatment and nursing care procedures can be performed. Hospital facilities should be designed so that they will give patients psychological comfort and reduce the anxiety, boredom, frustration, and loss of identity that frequently accompany hospitalization [3].

PRIVACY AND EFFICIENCY

The importance attached to preserving patient dignity varies from one department to another. It should be remembered that many procedures by their very nature tend to assault the dignity of the patient. Facility adequacy in terms of patients deserves serious consideration. The preservation of human dignity implies, among other things, the safeguarding of the patient's right to privacy, not only at certain critical moments, but at all times. Probably the most discerning judgment will result if the evaluator asks herself, "How would I feel if I were the patient?"

The individual's dignity is reflected in the respect accorded by others to his need to maintain the privacy of his body. To the extent feasible, given the inescapable exposure entailed in the provision of needed care, the patient should be aided in maintaining this privacy. The design and furnishings of examination and treatment areas, in the emergency department and outpatient facilities as well as in other parts of the hospital, should be so planned as to facilitate defense of the patient's privacy and, as far as possible, to shield him from the view of others [6].

The nurse director and her administrative staff must identify what changes can be made to promote a better working environment for physicians, nurses, and others who render services to patients. The physician, for example, needs to know that in this nursing unit his orders will be carried out promptly, that he will have maximum contact with other physicians and nurses, that there will be privacy for his contact with patients and with their relatives, and that the nursing unit is designed to conserve his time in charting, writing orders, and dictating summaries [3].

EXPANSION AND MAINTENANCE OF FACILITIES

New services to patients may require expansion of facilities, remodeling of clinical areas, or new construction. For instance, the staff of the orthopedic service may ask that a recreational area be provided for patients. When requests are made for new or expanded facilities, the nurse director must provide guidelines to personnel for preparing their justification:

1. Identify the need.
2. Summarize the purpose of the request.
3. Determine whether the request requires interdepartmental collaboration and, if so, plan how this will be accomplished.
4. Describe the proposed plan.
5. Determine the tentative cost.
6. Submit a written proposal and justification to the director.

As the nurse director reviews the justification, she has sufficient information to study the need. If the justification requires clarification, she may choose to revise the written request or return it to the per-·

son who submitted the plan. A sound plan for improvements, with recommendations and justification, should be developed and then submitted to the hospital administration.

The hospital administrator must be regularly informed of the adequacy or inadequacy of facilities used in the nursing care program. The nurse director should expect the same regular reporting from the supervisors and head nurses who are accountable for clinical care.

In this technological age, the need for solid substantiation by scientifically collected data cannot be overestimated. It is desirable to plan for a realistic program of data collecting in relation to a project, whether there is to be a new building or remodeling of the present structure. This approach does require personnel to carry out a sufficient number of in-depth studies to validate justification for a specific request. A study will stimulate objective, creative thinking and replace superficial planning.

How can a plan of modernization or construction of health facilities be developed that will be adaptable to future needs? This question was answered by Eleanor Lambertsen, Vice-Chairman, Commission on Nursing Services, American Nurses' Association, in an address to the National Advisory Commission on Health Facilities in 1968.

To plan the development of modernization of construction of health facilities that will be adaptable to future needs, one should gaze as far into the crystal ball as 20/20 vision permits. The study of present demographic trends, of current morbidity and mortality statistics, and of changes emerging in the technologic, academic, and business worlds, close examination of present health programs and facilities that are innovative and forward-looking — these would seem to be the methods by which to predict at least the outlines of future needs.

According to Mark Blumberg, "Hospital planners should decide for each activity what the chances are that the hospital now being planned will not be doing that activity (laundry, baby formula, sterilization, food preparation, laboratory processing, and so forth) in ten or fifteen years." He suggests that "if a certain activity in the hospital does not involve physical contact with the patient (or maintenance of his hospital environment), then planners should ask themselves if there is a better place for that activity" [2]. James Moore of Medical Planning Associates states that the following are achievable objectives of a master plan that leads to rejuvenation rather than obsolescence of health facilities:

1. Built in flexibility for replacing nursing units from the ground up as they become obsolete (total obsolescence occurs in 10–20 years).
2. Built in flexibility for expanding or altering the adjunct paramedical and service facilities easily, inexpensively, and often (in six- to twelve-month intervals).
3. Accomplishing these objectives with no obvious and logical circulation pattern.
4. Keeping facility in operation during entire process [10].

The plant operations department plays a significant role in maintaining the entire hospital structure. Its program should provide preventive maintenance through qualified inspection.

The nurse director or her representative should meet regularly with administrative personnel and plant operations staff to discuss the adequacy of facilities used in the nursing care program. Nursing should participate in joint planning sessions regarding expansion of hospital facilities and services or the remodeling of existing facilities. As patient care becomes more and more specialized, the coordinator for the continuity of care is the nurse, the stabilizing force who remains close to the patient 24 hours a day.

Nursing can contribute and share in this objective by utilizing the plant operations staff: (1) to assist in the training of employees in the safe operation of equipment, which is necessary to keep breakdowns to a minimum as well as for understanding when equipment is not operating properly and should be shut down; (2) to assist in keeping an environmental equilibrium among such elements as noise, ventilation, safety, and lighting; and (3) to assist in all modernization programs relating to nursing areas in the development of long-range programs for capital equipment, and in new construction planning.

The safety of patients, employees, and others within the clinical facilities should be a major concern. The administrative staff can express and invite mutual responsibility, stress the aim of education and prevention of harm or disaster, and show concern about making the work place safe for the employees. Communication about safety should emphasize that every employee is obliged to share in the responsibility for safety in the nursing department. The administrative staff members have specific kinds and degrees of responsibility for providing a safe environment.

Continuous interest in the welfare of patients and employees can be demonstrated by developing adequate policies and programs as the means to a safe environment. Policy statements regarding safety, for example, should be available to personnel in the nursing service policy manual, which:

1. Asks all nursing personnel to be safety minded for themselves, toward each other, and for patients.
2. Encourages cooperation from all nursing personnel who have ideas about how to promote safety in the nursing department and the hospital.
3. Refers to the written hospital and nursing procedures that are designed to implement the hospital administration's purpose to make the clinical areas safe.
4. Defines the responsibilities of nursing service administrative staff and other personnel to promote safety.
5. Provides for an analysis of accident and incident reports.
6. Defines educational programs.

The structure and functioning of safety committees could be used advantageously in a model for participation in managing by organizational members of different levels and functions who work together productively toward shared objectives. A hospital safety committee composed of departmental directors may be delegated the responsibility to ensure a safe environment. Committees may vary in different hospitals according to size and functions and depending on hospital administration plans for a safe environment. This committee may develop a comprehensive safety program covering activities and practices of personnel and patients, as well as a checklist for use in periodic inspection of the physical plant and any observable hazards. Written reports of hazardous practices and plant conditions should be reviewed and corrective action taken.

A second type of safety committee may be formed within the nursing department, in order to channel interest down toward the level where most of the action takes place. A third type of safety committee may be composed of hospital management and employee representatives from various departments. When committee membership is rotated among hospital personnel who share and participate in planning for safe and adequate facilities, everyone's interest in safety is aroused.

The entire hospital should strive to function in a safe and sanitary manner. Although the development and implementation of an active safety program should be assigned to one or more qualified persons, all employees should have knowledge of its provisions. A preventive and corrective maintenance program should be established, and those responsible for putting it into effect should receive appropriate training. Written procedures should be readily available for employees to follow in the event of a breakdown in mechanical systems, or a lack or inadequacy of any utilities [13].

All personnel must be made aware of the fact that the use of electricity introduces the hazards of burn, fire, electric shock, and power failure. Special precautions must be taken when the care of patients requires the utilization of any electrically operated devices. All appliances, instruments, and installations must be tested to determine compliance with current leakage, proper grounding, and other safety device requirements to ensure protection of patients and employees. There must be strict prohibition of extension and indiscriminate overloading of electrical systems. Expert advice concerning electrical systems must be readily available at all times [13].

Certain devices are essential for patient safety. Each patient should have a readily available and functioning nurse call system. Grab bars, emergency call system, and similar safety devices should be installed in the patient toilet and bathing areas. Side rails should be available for both sides of beds for use when a patient's condition warrants it. The hot water supply should be regulated by thermostatic control or by other control devices so that the hot water used by patients, by hospital personnel, and by the public has a maximum temperature that cannot cause personal injury. The control devices should be inaccessible to patients and to the general public.

Written regulations governing smoking in the hospital must be adopted and should be made known to hospital personnel, to patients, and to the public. These regulations should include at least the following provisions:

1. Smoking shall be prohibited in any room, unit, or area where flammable liquid, combustible gas, or oxygen is being used or stored, and in any other hazardous area of the hospital. Such areas shall be posted with NO SMOKING signs.
2. Smoking by patients classified as not mentally or physically responsible for their actions shall be prohibited.

Safety from fire and disaster in a hospital is an ever-increasing challenge; it cannot be met by any system that does not place responsibility on management. Prevention of fire outbreak, early detection, prevention of spread, prompt extinguishment, and evacuation may be done through emergency instructions and training. Each individual employee must be instructed as to his part, including how to use fire-fighting equipment. Periodic fire drills should be scheduled to keep employee skills updated.

A fire plan should be posted in appropriate locations (for example, on bulletin boards) for all personnel to see easily. A more detailed procedure should be available at the nurses' station. Patient evacuation should be carefully planned with special attention to the evening and night tours of duty.

INFECTION CONTROL

Hospital-associated infections are potential hazards for all persons having contact with the hospital. Therefore, effective measures for the control of infections must be instituted, directed, reviewed, and changed as needed. Responsibility for this function can be given to a committee made up of representatives of the medical staff, the administration, the microbiology laboratory, and the nursing department. The chairman of the committee should be someone with knowledge of and a special interest in infection control. Representatives of other departments, such as pharmacy, dietary, central service, housekeeping, and maintenance, should be consulted when necessary and may be invited to committee meetings [13].

To carry out its responsibility, the committee should do at least the following:

1. Develop written standards for hospital sanitation and medical asepsis. These standards should include a definition of infection for the purpose of surveillance, as well as specific indications of the need for and the procedures to be used in isolation. Copies of the standards should be distributed and made readily available to all appropriate personnel.
2. Develop, evaluate, and revise on a continuing basis the procedures and techniques for meeting established sanitation and asepsis standards. This should include the routine evaluation of materials used in the data supplied from reputable sources or upon in-use tests performed within the hospital.
3. Develop a practical system for reporting, evaluating, and keeping records of infections among patients and personnel in order to provide an indication of the endemic level of all nosocomial infections, to trace the source of infection, and to identify epidemic or potential epidemic situations. Such a program is important not only for the protection of the patient, but also for the protection of the medical staff, of hospital employees, and of visitors.
4. Review periodically the use of antibiotics as they relate to patient care within the hospital.
5. Provide assistance in the development of the Personnel Health Service [13].

At each meeting the committee should review data obtained since the previous meeting. Such review may include reports of hospital-associated infections that include identification of patients requiring isolation; reports of tests conducted on sterilization devices; and reports of bacteriological studies of patients, of personnel, or of the environment. Pertinent findings and recommendations should be submitted to the medical staff, to the chief executive officer, to the director of nursing, and to other appropriate personnel. Written minutes of the meeting must be maintained [9].

Provision must be made within the hospital for the isolation of patients when necessary. Accommodations for isolated patients should enable them to receive care of the same quality as is provided throughout the hospital. Whatever the accommodation, there should be isolated work areas and equipment to assist in the control of the disease. Facilities for hand washing and for implementing good isolation techniques are a basic requirement. Isolation facilities should be available for all clinical services. For example, adequate provision is necessary for patients in labor who have confirmed or suspected infection and for the delivery of obstetrical patients with infection. There must also be facilities for the separate care of newborn infants with confirmed or suspected infection [6].

Techniques should be developed in central service to prevent the indirect transmission of infectious disease to patients by material issued from this unit. There should be written procedures for the decontamination and sterilization activities performed in central service or elsewhere in the hospital, and such procedures should be followed by all persons responsible for these activities. Although initial orientation of employees should be sufficient to enable them to carry out the tasks outlined in their job description, they ought to have additional on-the-job training. Personnel assigned to environmental tasks in special areas, such as the surgical suite, obstetrical units, emergency service, special care units, and respiratory therapy service, should receive additional training in the execution of procedures that are unique to these departments.

The nurse director must strive to mesh the nursing department's program with that of any other department whose operations maintain a high level of environmental control in the hospital. The role of the service departments is crucial in helping to prevent infection, to control fire and safety hazards, and to increase patient satisfaction.

OCCUPATIONAL SAFETY AND HEALTH ACT

The nurse director must assist in explaining to her staff the Williams-Steiger Occupational Safety and Health Act (OSHA) of 1970, its implications, and its significance. The purpose of this federal law is to assure safe and healthful working conditions throughout the nation and to preserve human resources. Both employer and employees have responsibilities. The act requires that each employer furnish his employees a place of employment free from recognized hazards that might cause serious injury or death; it further requires that employers comply with the specific safety and health standards issued by the U.S. Department of Labor. Employees are required to comply with safety and health standards, rules, regulations, and orders issued under the act and applicable to their conduct [14].

To ensure compliance with safety and health requirements, the Department of Labor conducts periodic job-site inspections, carried out by trained safety and health officers. The law requires that an authorized representative of the employer and a representative of the workers accompany the inspector. Workers have the right to notify the Department of Labor and request an inspection if they believe that unsafe conditions exist at their work site. They also have the right to bring unsafe conditions to the attention of the inspector. If, upon inspection, the Department of Labor believes that the act has been violated, a citation of violation and a proposed penalty are issued to the employer [14].

If nursing techniques, procedures, or actions do not meet OSHA requirements, it is the administrator of the employing hospital who is penalized, not the employee. The penalties imposed can be quite severe, with fines up to $10,000 for each violation [1].

In general, job safety and health standards consist of rules for avoidance of hazards which research and experience have proved harmful to personal safety and health. It is the obligation of all employers and employees to familiarize themselves with those standards, which apply to them at all times.

GETTING INVOLVED WITH OSHA*

Make certain the people in your organization are knowledgeable in depth about the [Occupational Safety and Health] Act and its administration — and are kept up-to-date on new developments. Consider setting up a special information service on this subject within your organization.

Critically examine existing safety and health conditions at your facilities.

Analyze and where necessary strengthen your own safety and health programs.

Maintain liaison with OSHA offices in the regions, perhaps detailing a specific person to be in charge of this liaison and letting us know who he is.

Also, maintain liaison with safety officials of your State government.

Organize seminars and meetings of your management, supervisors and employees.

If an employer has multiple plants, consider putting together a "road show"

*Reprinted by courtesy of *Action*, publication of the American Society for Personnel Administration.

consisting of a team of people such as legal counsel, safety director, hygienist, etc., to make presentations at the various plant sites.

Have someone or a group within your organization analyze the presently promulgated standards, and those to be promulgated in the future, in terms of their significance to your operation, and to make certain you remain in compliance.

Make sure you have an effective internal safety training program for employees.

If you find it difficult or impossible to employ full-time safety people, consider utilizing the services of consultation services, which may be available from your industry association or independently.

Be active in your industry associations with regard to job safety and health. Make sure they are active in this field. Participate in appropriate committee activities.

On your own, and through your industry associations, participate in the preparation of new and revised standards.

The effect of this legislation will tend to increase the responsibility of professional nursing. Practitioners should be aware of the law's provisions as they relate to hospitals and to the health care industry in general. Nurses will substantially assist in implementing OSHA mandates through upgrading programs of health and safety surveillance at their places of employment [1].

Nursing administration has been committed to the belief that "safety on the job is everybody's responsibility!" Nursing has long accepted safety as a moral obligation inherent in its services and practices. The Occupational Safety and Health Act of 1970 intends that nursing continue to reinforce itself by providing safe and healthful working conditions for health workers. Additional information concerning the law may be obtained through the Office of the Information Services, Occupational Safety and Health Administration, U.S. Department of Labor, Washington, D.C. 20210.

NOISE CONTROL

Greater patient satisfaction results from a quiet, comfortable, smooth-running physical plant. Indeed, operation of the plant has a profound impact on the hospital's reputation among the population it serves. People who are ill are frequently sensitive to loud sounds. Noise is a condition that exists in varying degrees in all daily pursuits. With patients, however, there is a need to minimize the effect of certain noises in order to create a restful environment.

A sound-level meter is used to measure the loudness of sounds within a specific area. Readings are given in units called decibels. A decibel is the smallest degree of sound that can be heard by the normal ear. The energy of the sound wave is expressed in numerical terms, the sound of average speech being 40 to 60 decibels. In such areas as the kitchen, utility room, and nurses' station, sounds should be maintained under 40 decibels. In the patients' rooms, the intensity of sound should be kept to about 30 decibels [8].

In an effort to reduce the noise level, care must be taken to avoid the total absence of sound, since this situation can have a disturbing and distracting effect upon the patient who has developed a high degree of tolerance to noise. Whispering, monotones, tiptoeing, or muffled conversation can be frightening to a patient who has mixed-up feelings about his illness.

The simplest solution to the noise problem in the hospital area is to modify or control conditions that predispose to intensified sound waves, human and physical. Suggestions for reducing the noise factor include the following:

1. The use of resilient floor surfaces of rubber, tile, asphalt, and linoleum in the patient areas, and carpeting in the strategic reception centers, such as waiting rooms and admitting offices.
2. The use of acoustical and absorptive materials on ceilings of noisy work areas and corridors.
3. The use of draperies, bedding, and overstuffed furniture with nonreflective surfaces.
4. The reappraisal of the public-address system or buzzer system with the view toward conversion to a noiseless communication system.
5. The use of double-thickness doors on friction hinges in patients' rooms to exclude the passage of corridor sounds.
6. The use of rubber-tired wheels on portable equipment and vehicles.
7. The use of rubber mats in sinks and on drainboards in all utility rooms (clean and soiled) and kitchens.
8. The maintenance of plumbing fixtures in good repair.
9. The use of rubberized plastic garbage receptacles, trash cans, and wastepaper baskets.
10. The lowering of the volume on radios, television sets, record players, tape recorders, and cassettes.

11. The muffling of the telephone rings.
12. Designing nursing units so that work areas are not in the immediate vicinity of patients' rooms.
13. The shrouding of computer terminals and imprinters on the nursing units.
14. A concerted antinoise campaign involving the hospital staff, the patients, and the public.

The nurse director has a responsibility to estimate the needs of the department of nursing as they relate to supplies and equipment. The hospital administrator depends on each of his department directors to assess needs carefully, make recommendations, and implement a system for the evaluation and control of supplies and equipment.

PROCUREMENT DEPARTMENT

The nurse director should become aware of the functions of the procurement (purchasing) department, so that she will know what services are available. Because the nursing department uses large quantities of supplies and equipment, careful coordination is necessary between the nursing and purchasing departments. The procurement department may be responsible for (1) determining what, when, and how much to purchase; (2) developing sources of supply; (3) receiving and checking quantity of supplies purchased; (4) inspecting receipts for technical compliance with specification; (5) storing and issuing merchandise; (6) providing the accounting department with the necessary information to effect payment for supplies purchased and received; (7) conducting research; (8) promoting simplification, standardization, and labor-saving ideas; (9) salvaging and disposing of undesirable merchandise; (10) maintaining a reference library of materials for hospital use; (11) evaluating products and sources so as to effect timely and economical purchase of materials compatible with economic trends; and (12) establishing and maintaining frequent personal contact with department directors to assist them with their needs.

Supplies and equipment are vital to the operation of an institution. *Supplies* refers to expendable items — articles being used periodically and reordered frequently to maintain sufficient amounts on hand. Amounts ordered will depend on the current patient census and the standards set up by the nursing administrative group to minimize the occurrence of over- or under-ordering.

Equipment describes more permanent fixtures and apparatus of a nonexpendable nature and should be further classified as fixed or movable. *Fixed equipment* refers to objects built into the walls and floors of the hospital and includes such things as sinks, sterilizers, lockers, cabinets, pneumatic tubes, cascade oxygen, and intercommunication system. *Movable items* may be subdivided into (1) articles that should last for more than five years, such as furniture, lamps, stretchers, wheelchairs, and examining tables, and (2) articles having less than five years of life, but which are capable of being used repeatedly before being replaced. Instruments, needles, syringes, linen, bathtubs, bedpans, and urinals are a few examples of the latter category. While supplies are ordered on the basis of the patient census, equipment can be ordered according to the maximum number of patients admissible to the unit.

The hospital generally establishes a policy and procedure on the supply, control, and distribution of items for which the procurement director is responsible. Department directors are responsible for the security and the procurement and economical usage of all supplies distributed to their areas.

Each nursing unit should have a formalized system for the maintenance of supplies. A written procedure should explain what supplies are available for use, and the amounts (stock levels) to be placed in the storage areas of the nursing unit. In establishing a stock level for departmental use, the procurement director reviews the last usage for each stock supply item with, for example, the nurse director or her representative. Together they establish a stock level quantity to satisfy each nursing unit's requirements. New items are added in amounts based on estimations made by the nursing department. Stock levels are periodically reviewed and adjusted. Stock supplies are generally delivered weekly or biweekly and are stored in their place on the nursing unit by the procurement department. The procurement director should be notified of any anticipated changes in usage of supplies or of any additional supplies needed. The unit clerk on a nursing unit can be delegated to spot-check the maintenance of supplies and assist the procurement clerk in the routing procedure.

STANDARDIZATION COMMITTEE

A standardization committee may be set up for the purpose of evaluating and standardizing supplies and equipment in a hospital. Its functions may include: (1) providing a program of product evaluation for the proper stocking of supplies and equipment that will be professionally and economically acceptable for hospital use; (2) providing a means for centrally controlling inventories, distribution, and costs relative to products and equipment; (3) maintaining supply communications between department directors and the procurement department by using a product evaluation sheet for documenting, evaluating, costing, and stocking of supplies and equipment; (4) promoting supply economy and savings by avoiding duplication and obsolescence of material and equipment; and (5) determining requirements for items or services and aiding in the development of standard specifications. The committee reviews all product evaluation sheets and will, when possible, be the decision-making body, with the approval of the hospital administrator, for the purpose of standardizing all types of supplies and equipment. The nurse director or her representative serves on the committee.

ESTABLISHING A SYSTEM FOR SELECTION
OF SUPPLIES AND EQUIPMENT

When the procurement department forwards an item that may be of interest to nursing, the nurse director must determine whether it can be evaluated by the experimental nursing unit, if one is available. Is it an item that should be evaluated by both the physician and the nurse? Is it an item that may be evaluated by both nursing and other departments? Is it an item that will require capital expenditures? Obviously, interdepartmental collaboration and administrative coordination are required in order to establish a system for selecting supplies and equipment.

Before any item is evaluated the following policies may be helpful:

1. The procurement department is made aware of all items received for experimentation. It can provide assistance and any information that will enhance the experimentation and possible justification for future purchase.
2. A tentative procedure is written to accompany all trial items. It eliminates the guesswork of determining how to use a new item. A suggested procedure provides a base to work from during the experimental period.
3. A product evaluation form accompanies each experimental item. A written evaluation of findings and recommendations provides a permanent record for reference.

4. Dates are established when a trial period begins and ends. Target dates serve as a control, and everyone is aware of what is happening in relation to a specific item.
5. A sufficient sampling of the item is available for testing.
6. The trial item is assigned to a specific area for testing. Someone should be responsible for initiating follow-up and reporting findings and recommendations.

Taking the preference of the evaluators into consideration, the nurse director and her staff must look at factors such as cost, availability of the item, and maintenance (if equipment is involved), and the choice that appears most satisfactory. The importance of careful selection of supplies and equipment cannot be overrated, not only from the standpoint of economics but from that of ensuring acceptance by those who must use the equipment. The selection of supplies and equipment for patient care is in many instances an interdepartmental function. The nurse director should consult the administrative nursing staff regarding recommendations of new items. If it is generally agreed that an item will be useful for patient services, the item is referred to the procurement director, who will present the request to the hospital standardization committee. When the item is reviewed by the group, the nurse director or her representative will have an opportunity to justify the need for it. The committee may then take action and, if necessary, refer the request to the hospital administrator.

If experimental items are proposed by the medical staff, the nursing staff may assist in gathering the necessary information requested. Items affecting a large number of physicians may be referred by them to their own clinical section group, and finally to the medical executive council, for approval. Once action is taken by the physicians, it can be referred to the hospital administrator. Sometimes the nursing department is directed by the hospital administrator to initiate the purchase.

The nurse director or her representative participates in the selection of supplies and equipment to be used by nursing. She should receive from the procurement office information that includes price, quality, performance characteristics, and availability of maintenance service. Items that affect nursing procedures can be referred to the nursing practice committee for consideration and review; that committee, in turn, will make recommendations to the nurse director. Since the nursing practice committee is primarily concerned with the development of written procedures to serve as standards of performance for nursing, it should become involved in the acquisition of items necessary for carrying on nursing services.

In the management of supplies and equipment, the following guidelines are recommended:

1. Equipment should be inspected to determine completeness, availability for use, cleanliness, safety, and convenience in placement.
2. With the introduction of new and unfamiliar equipment, each staff member who will use it must understand its operation, purpose, and aftercare.
3. Quantities of supplies on hand should be checked before reordering.
4. There must be a casual supervision of personnel to assure that supplies and equipment are being used for their specific and intended purpose.
5. Supplies and equipment should be checked for specification and quantity when received from the purchasing department.
6. Supplies and equipment should be conveniently located and easily accessible to all nursing personnel.
7. There must be some provision made for ordering on an emergency basis, emergencies being specifically defined and understood by all who might have to resort to this practice.

The selecting, standardizing, ordering, and maintenance of supplies and equipment are all part of the control system. A further component is educating all the nursing staff to share in the responsibility of maintaining and controlling supplies and equipment. During the orientation of new personnel, the procurement director should be invited to discuss hospital costs and what they mean to the patient and his family. A display of items and their purchasing cost is sometimes very revealing to the staff. To achieve their willing cooperation, nursing personnel should be instructed in the use of all items, informed of the program of preventive maintenance for equipment, assured that supplies will be available when needed, and given recognition for any ideas that may result in better utilization of both supplies and equipment and thus reduced costs.

The nursing staff must keep informed about innovations in facilities, supplies, and equipment described in hospital and nursing literature and displayed at conventions and other meetings. The nurse director must encourage the nursing administrative staff members to keep themselves aware of what is new in their particular areas of responsibility.

1. Althouse, H. How OSHA affects hospitals and nursing homes. *Am. J. Nurs.* 75:450, 1975.
2. Blumberg, M. S. Panel on Planning and Programming Factors. In *Costs of Health Care Facilities.* Washington, D.C.: National Academy of Sciences, 1968.
3. Brown, E. L. *Newer Dimensions of Patient Care.* New York: Russell Sage Foundation, 1965.
4. Burgun, A. The hospital of the future: Decentralized but integrated. *Hospitals* 43:63, 1969.
5. Carner, D. *Planning for Hospital Expansion and Remodeling.* Springfield, Ill.: Thomas, 1968.
6. Joint Commission on Accreditation of Hospitals, Hospital Accreditation Program. *Accreditation Manual for Hospitals.* Chicago: The Joint Commission on Accreditation of Hospitals, 1970.
7. Katz, G. A nurse administrator and new design concepts. *Nurs. Outlook* 15:50, 1967.
8. McGibony, J. *Principles of Hospital Administration.* New York: Putnam, 1969.
9. Mills, A. *Functional Planning of General Hospitals.* New York: McGraw-Hill, 1969.
10. Moore, J. S. Master Plan: To Obsolescence or Rejuvenation. In *Costs of Health Care Facilities.* Washington, D.C.: National Academy of Sciences, 1968.
11. Pitel, M. A nurse's view — hospital design should focus on patient's needs. *Hospitals* 42:306, 1968.
12. Sigmund, F., and Coleman, M. Appraising hospital planned obsolescence. *Hospitals* 42:306, 1968.
13. U.S. Department of Health, Education, and Welfare, Public Health Service, Division of Hospital and Medical Facilities. *Environmental Aspects of the Hospital.* Vol. IV, *Administrative Aspects.* Washington, D.C.: The Department of H.E.W., 1967.
14. U.S. Department of Labor, Bureau of Labor Statistics. *Record Requirements Under the Williams-Steiger Occupational Safety and Health Act of 1970.* Washington, D.C.: The Department of Labor, 1971.

Part V. Establishing and Maintaining the Human Environment

The effectiveness of nursing service administration depends on the ability of the director and her staff to deal with the human resources within the hospital environment and those of the community. Their main goal is to furnish a departmental and hospital climate that will promote positive human relationships. The interactions of nursing service administration have many ramifications for the patient and his family, the nursing personnel, hospital administration, hospital services, medical staff, nursing education programs, and the community. The astute nurse director will capitalize on her own knowledge and skills and those of the nursing staff in order to deal effectively with others. One of her main concerns is the management of staff at work and the development of an adequate relationship with them.

Nurse directors are buffeted each day by problems involving people. Although a few days may be uneventful, when one works with people the winds and tides of human behavior are such that one cannot predict from where the personality storms will come or how light or intense they may be. The people a nurse director works with have a great impact on her; she can fall apart emotionally if she fails to understand the basic phenomena of the hidden impacts of human interrelationships. The way a nurse director regards the people with whom she works is part of her life-style as an administrator.

BEHAVIORAL SCIENCE CONCEPTS

The nurse director should examine the findings of behavioral science to see whether they can be integrated into nursing management practices. Behavioral science may be defined as the systematic measurement of attitudes and actions and of factors in the environment that can affect them [21]. It is grounded in the belief that the needs and motivation of people are their prime concern. The behavioral scientists have directed their efforts toward developing theories explaining the relationship between motivation and productivity; the connection between the two seems to represent a set of highly complex notions about the nature of people and what motivates them to increased productivity [40].

Hierarchy of Human Needs

A. Maslow, a leading behavioral scientist, defines motivation as a state of having an internal force that moves one to some kind of action

[27]. Motivation is generated from within a person and cannot be imposed upon him. People are perceived as goal seekers from the beginning of life to its end. Any action or means used to attain a goal is called a drive. The acting out of a drive is seen as evidence of one's motivation to reach a desired goal. This theory of motivation turns goals into human needs, which Maslow categorizes and ranks into a conceptual hierarchy, beginning with the most primitive and urgent and ranging upward to the apex of the hierarchy, self-actualization. While there may appear to be nuances and gradations within any given level of need, people's basic needs (see Figure 12) are physiological or physical needs, safety and security, love and affection, and their achievement needs — self-respect, social respect, and, the highest of needs, self-actualization [27].

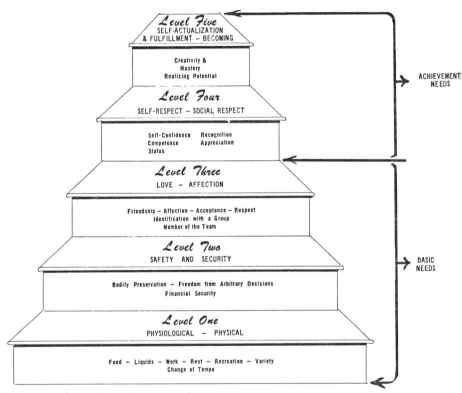

Figure 12. Hierarchy of human needs.

Throughout a person's development and maturation, these needs tend to occur in a hierarchy of preeminence, as shown in the graphic model of steps. All people have the capacity to climb up the motivational steps, and the ever-upward reaching of individuals is seen as evidence of their emotional maturity. The person who arrives at the step of self-actualization has satisfied the deficit needs and is beginning the process of becoming what he is capable of becoming. He has an inner compulsion to integrate his interests, talents, and abilities to the point that he works toward fulfilling his potential [27].

This theory suggests one stimulating approach to assessing the importance of people's needs: it provides insight into the kinds of organizational forces that may influence the behavior of people while at work. The nurse director must be sensitive to the internal and external forces that may affect the nursing staff's behavior during the performance of nursing duties. Her effectiveness depends on her ability to give others psychological room for growth — an ability that stems from recognizing employee need patterns and providing the kind of climate that will promote their satisfaction.

Motivation

Saul Gellerman [21], in his study *Motivation and Productivity*, states that motivation is not something, for example, that a manager does to influence his subordinates. Rather, the personnel are motivated by their own desire to get along as best they can in the kind of world they think they are living in. People will strive to obtain whatever values they believe are important to the extent that they feel it is safe and possible for them to do. Sometimes administrative staff members try to impose their values on others without recognizing that employee values may be different. Gellerman further generalizes that motivation problems result from the way an organization is managed rather than from the unwillingness of the staff to work hard. Managers may have a tendency to overmanage — the job of the employee is too narrow and the manager makes most of the decisions for him. The behavior of an employee can best be understood by looking at the environment the way the employee does. While both the manager and the employee may be part of the same physical environment, they do not have the same attitudes toward it. The differences, in some instances, can create severe misunderstandings on both sides. Money and its effect on an employee depend on his financial status and, more broadly, on the psychological meaning of money for him. Money can be a motivating force when financial concerns are strong, or it can serve some important psychological purpose. Positive motivation can result from challenging staff members by deliberately stretching their assigned duties, allowing them to experience the satisfaction of achievement and to develop a desire for additional expanding of duties. Management by objectives and participative management both increase the employees' commitment to work because they are actively involved in the process [21].

Frederick Herzberg [22] is best known for his "motivation-hygiene" theory. The two main components of this theory are "satisfier" and "dissatisfier" factors, which represent the content of a job.

Satisfiers (Motivators)	*Dissatisfiers* (Hygiene Factors)
Achievement	Company policy and administration
Recognition	Supervision
Work itself	Working conditions
Responsibility	Interpersonal relations (with
Advancement	supervisors, subordinates, and
Growth	peers)
	Salary
	Status
	Job security
	Personal life

The dissatisfiers (hygiene factors) represent all those factors that management has traditionally used to affect motivation. The term *hygiene* describes them because they are essentially preventive actions taken to remove sources of dissatisfaction from the environment. When any of these factors are missing, employees are likely to be displeased and to express their displeasure in ways that may hamper the organization — for example, through grievances or less productivity in output of work. If an employee is unhappy about his rate of pay, and it is corrected, a wage increase will not prevent him from eventually becoming dissatisfied with his new wage level. Hygiene needs can be satisfied only for a period of time; after a while a feeling of deficiency occurs again [22].

The satisfiers are the factors that provide employees with personal satisfaction. The key to these factors is job enrichment, which can be provided by removing some of the job controls while retaining accountability, increasing accountability of personnel for their own work, dividing the work into natural units, involving line workers in management, and increasing educational possibilities. The satisfiers tend to encourage people to work as a team [22].

For the nurse director this theory says that she must begin building more real motivating factors into her department if she hopes even to maintain the current level of nursing service productivity, let alone maximize it. She can also test the theory in the clinical setting of nursing. She may see the need to "clean" the job environment. Hygiene factors should perhaps not be used as rewards; they may seduce people away from achievement rather than reward them. If an employee is given a hygiene factor — for example, a raise in pay — it will not be a real motivator. The task for the nurse director and her administrative staff is to ask the question: How do you treat people on the job? Use of the motivators tends to produce internal generators to make people work. Motivated people will move themselves because they want to move.

Work Simplification

One example of a motivating program that has allowed employees to share in changing the nursing environment is work simplification. The concept of work simplification has been introduced into many organizations. It is downward extension of planning, organizing, and control functions that enables people at lower levels to apply their talents, individually and collectively, in managing their own jobs. In *Every Employee a Manager*, Myers suggests that work simplification replace traditional time and motion study on the assumptions that:

1. Most personnel have creative potential for improving their own job.
2. Improvements are best made by those who perform the job.
3. Self-initiated change is positively motivational, while change imposed by authority is usually resented and opposed.
4. Personnel satisfy social and achievement needs through cooperative work-improvement activities [32].

Work simplification courses are generally taught by a professional trainer, or, in some instances, a supervisor, once prepared. The course is usually about 20 hours in length and covers topics such as the principles and techniques of time and motion economy, flow chart making, cost analysis, and human relations. Most programs also include an on-the-job project for applying newly learned techniques. Development occurring through the concept of work simplification broadens employees' perspective to allow them to see their job and the organization in a responsible manner [32].

In one hospital setting a work simplification program is offered four times a year. The nursing department is allowed to send four people to each program, preparing twelve staff members with new skills. The nurse director's goal is to expose the nursing administrative team to the work simplification concept and to broaden their understanding. Once this is done, they in turn will send members of their nursing team to acquire similar skills. The ultimate aim of the nurse director is to involve all levels of nursing personnel in the program. Some of the changes that were brought about as a result of the nursing staff's attending the program include: deletion of medicine cards and treatment cards, revision of nursing forms, modification of transfer and discharge procedures affecting patients, and remodeling of the delivery room. This program receives wide acceptance because it is a productive approach for getting the nursing staff involved in improving their jobs.

Behavioral science does not draw up a simple list of what a nurse director should and should not do. However, it does reveal that the management process is much too complex to be handled effectively by approaches requiring no analysis or creativity on her part. It offers a strategy for analyzing motivational problems and, perhaps, clues as to the general causes of common problems. It is up to the nurse director and her administrative staff to diagnose specific problems that confront them and to direct action to basic causes and not merely to symptoms [40].

COMMUNICATION

Good communication is essential to the smooth operation of any organization; it is of paramount importance to nursing services, since coordination of patient care depends on it. The nurse director must create a climate conducive to a free flow of communications in all directions relating to nursing services. Further, she must provide learning experiences in which nursing personnel can acquire a basic understanding of communication concepts and their implications for everyday relationships and the care of patients.

As a nurse director and her administrative staff look at the communication effectiveness within the nursing department, they should consider the following questions:

1. How much effort is being made by the nursing administrative staff to get the opinions and thinking of the nursing teams? Responses sometimes pinpoint areas in which nursing communication has fallen down.
2. What obstacles are encountered by the administrative staff in communication? Semantic obstacles manifest themselves in thinking and language habits. Obstacles also exist in personnel themselves and in their reactions to other people and the environment, and there are obstacles in an organization as growth takes place within the institution. Growth, in and of itself, gives rise to factors that tend to complicate communications.
3. What skills and attitudes must the administrative staff strive to develop? There is a need to develop a "communication consciousness" — a better understanding and awareness of the communication process. This means that each person must gain some insight into her own thinking and language patterns. Proficiency must be developed in questioning and listening, the two most important skills involved in communication. The nursing staff must strengthen communication by attitudes and actions that will support what they say.
4. What conditions must the administrative staff strive to create in the nursing department? A communication system can be worked out by which information is transmitted horizontally and vertically, allowing for a free flow of communication in all directions. Formal structure must be strengthened and allowance made for the demands of communication; messages must be geared to fulfilling the interests of staff and networks established for feedback and follow-up. The sense of participation so vital to both employees and the nursing department's effectiveness will thus be enhanced.

As the hospital, nursing department, and patient unit continue to grow and change, their demands on communication will also change. Methods of communication must be flexible enough to keep pace with the often rapid organizational change. At the same time, the basic concepts of communication, the skills and attitudes favorable to its practice, and the conditions necessary for its success are so fundamental that they must be maintained and developed throughout organizational changes.

The great task a nurse director is faced with is improving organizational communication. Good communication is essential to the nurse director because, by virtue of her title, she is required to make decisions which should grow wholly out of assembled facts. If the facts are properly assembled, because communication has taken place in two directions — to and from everybody concerned — usually one good decision is possible. The making of a decision is thus not a function reserved only for the nurse director. In a sense, decisions are constantly being made at all levels within the nursing department. And they are made through the interchange of communication and the assembling of facts.

In establishing effective communications, here are a few points (from the American Hospital Association) to consider:

1. People have different sets of values and react to communications according to their own feelings and experiences.
2. The timing of communication must be considered; the right thing can be said or written at the wrong time.
3. The information to be communicated should be as complete as possible.
4. The method of communication should fit the occasion. Thought should be given to how a message is to be sent — written, spoken, telephoned, relayed.
5. No system of communication should be so rigid that certain messages cannot bypass established channels. If a detour is necessary, the circumstances should be explained to those bypassed.
6. Emotions are involved in communications. Meaning is transferred by attitudes, facial expressions, body movements, tone of voice, as well as by what is said and what is not said.
7. Listening, not just hearing, is a potent component of verbal communications.
8. Verbal communications may need to be followed up in writing.
9. Memoranda should be written in language understandable to the group for which they are intended [3].

The director talks daily with employees and other hospital personnel, formally or informally. Each such contact can be regarded as an experiment in human relations and communication. It is also an opportunity to practice a wide range of skills needed in management of personnel. Making the most of each personal contact may well be a learning experience and a means to improve human skills in listening, observing, and interpreting. The nurse director must use these contacts as a means of assessing employee morale within the nursing department.

The director should be interested in uncovering and correcting anything that has caused less than the highest level of departmental morale and good nursing service. Careful consideration should be given to complaints and grievances and the manner in which they are handled. For example, the nurse director should know what kinds of dissatisfaction are being expressed. Where are the complaints originating? How does the complaint procedure work? Is each nursing supervisor trying her best to learn about dissatisfaction and to remove all legitimate grounds for complaints? The attitude of nursing supervisors is a significant factor in the handling of complaints and grievances. The director must provide opportunities for the supervisors to learn about and to understand the nature of complaints and grievances.

The ability of a nurse director to go to the root of problems, questions, situations, or concerns, in order to determine basic difficulties, is valuable. She keeps her mind open and alert on issues until all the evidence is in and holds her beliefs with tolerance and charity for the beliefs of others.

The greater function of the administrator is not to answer questions but to ask them. It is only by questions that problems can be defined or, more importantly, most times even be discovered. The answers the administrator gives can be little better than the answers he receives, and those answers can be little better than the questions the administrator is asking. To a large extent, the sorts of questions the administrator asks determine the sort of administrator he is. Perplexity and puzzlement are trademarks of effective administrators, and no administrator should be embarrassed to display them. Wondering for information is not a sign of ignorance, but wandering for lack of information is a pretty fair proof of it. Asking questions is such a major function of administration that if it ever becomes an organized profession its proper coat of arms should be the question mark [12].

MORALE

The word *morale* holds real meaning for the nurse director and her administrative nursing staff. It refers to something that is felt to be of great importance even if that something remains vague and elusive. It pertains to the relations of individuals in a group, or larger organization, rather than to the individuals alone. To talk of the "morale" of a person apart from the group or organization to which he contributes his services is to talk about his personal characteristics of behavior. If the goal of the hospital is to develop a cooperative setting, it must be recognized that certain individuals because of their past social experience may be unfit for cooperation. That is, the social conditioning of the personnel who are part of a department constitutes a significant factor in determining the character of hospital morale, particularly if these people have not been well prepared for cooperation and need assistance in making an adjustment [39].

Like health, morale becomes most important when it is lost. In its everyday manifestations morale is likely to be ignored and disregarded. Many aspects of daily existence have this characteristic; they include factors taken for granted, unrecognized until they are drastically changed or disappear. Routine ways of behaving tend to bind people in collaborative effort. Only when people lose a customary way of doing things, or when they are threatened with the loss of their customary way of life, does a person in authority realize the importance of morale. Nothing makes one feel more insecure, uncertain, apprehensive, and demoralized than to have his routine ways of behavior too quickly and too arbitrarily interfered with [39].

To understand the problems relating to morale requires a simple and useful way of thinking about people in their association with one another in the hospital. From this point of view, the problems in a hospital generally break down into: (1) the daily problems of maintaining internal equilibrium within the organization — that is, maintaining a social organization in which individuals and groups, through working together, can obtain satisfactions that will make them willing to contribute their services to the objective of cooperation; and (2) the daily problems of diagnosing possible sources of interference, of locating sore spots, of liquidating human tensions and strains among individuals and groups, of spotting blockages in the channels of communication [39].

Maintaining internal equilibrium within any setting involves keeping the channels of communication free and clear. Orders can then be transmitted downward without distortion so that relevant information regarding situations at the work level is transmitted upward without distortion to those levels at which it can best be used. This process involves getting the bottom of the organization to understand the objectives of the top. It also means getting the top of the organization to understand the feelings and sentiments of the bottom. It further involves moving people about in the organization — transferring, upgrading, downgrading, promoting, demoting, placing, and selecting — in a manner that will be in accordance with the social values of the human situation and in a manner that will support morale [39].

Morale is not a quality attached to an individual or to a group; it is a dynamic relationship of equilibrium between individuals and the organizations they serve. To invoke "morale" when cooperation has ceased to exist is, in fact, too late. In this context, the nurse director becomes the guardian or preserver of morale through the function of maintaining an equilibrium that will preserve the social values in a cooperative system. Only in this sense does a person have authority [39].

A director is confronted daily with balancing "efficiency," on the one side, and "morale," on the other. She is trying to use every method that will cut hospital costs, increase output, improve the quality of care, reduce waste and accidents, and make her department efficient. At the same time, she is trying to procure the cooperation of the staff in attaining these ends. She not only has to secure their willingness to contribute their services to these purposes but also must see to it that they thereby obtain satisfactions that make them continuously desirous of cooperating. It is a problem of knowing the technical limitations, the limitations of the human organization, and the particular objectives that can be accomplished under these restrictive conditions. It means sizing up a situation — what needs to be done and how it should be done here and now in order to attain the cooperative purpose. A constant exercise of judgment is required in striving to maintain a balance among parts of the setting, in assessing its nature, and in spotting possible sources of interference that may be unduly disrupting.

The director is accountable for the performance of all the nursing staff and must devise means of getting their willing cooperation and teamwork, as well as leading them toward sharing in nursing and hospital goals. She can create a climate of cooperative relationship by conferring with them in a way that shows consideration for their ideas and experiences. When the nurse director demonstrates receptiveness to new ideas, wherever they come from, she exemplifies an attitude that all members of the nursing department need to develop and acquire if they are to play their part in a constantly changing situation.

Morale may be described as being good in the nursing department or hospital if there is a general feeling of satisfaction, an atmosphere in which the personnel are in harmony with their surroundings and pleased to be a part of the hospital. Morale may be influenced by many factors: lack of appropriate recognition for employee accomplishments, absence of a rewards system such as merit raises or promotions, low salaries, inadequate physical facilities, lack of employee participation in policy making, and innumerable others.

DISCIPLINE

Discipline is essential to organizational life. The personnel must strive to control their individual urges and cooperate for the common good; they must reasonably conform to the code of behavior put forth by the hospital's leadership so that its objectives can be accomplished. In any organized group the main objective is to develop in the staff such an attitude that they voluntarily conform to established norms of conduct; the question is how this can be achieved. Those in charge may elect to rule with great severity. Violators can be harshly punished; workers can be forced to obey and conform. The result will be negative discipline or rule through fear. The other approach is to elicit in people a willingness to obey and abide by the rules and regulations, not out of fear of the consequences of disobedience, but because they want to. This is positive or constructive discipline [9].

Generally, discipline arises out of the fact that management must have some control over its operations and must attempt to gain employees' compliance with established standards. Management usually disciplines an employee for not meeting prescribed standards of performance, for violating the rules or policies of the organization, or for insubordination [9].

Employees should be made aware of the standards against which they are being measured. Management rules for employee conduct on the job should be reasonable. Educating employees to the desired regulations will bring about better performance. Discipline should be used primarily to reinforce self-discipline within individuals and work groups, penalties being applied only after educational methods have failed. Effective discipline does include the principle that its policies must be enforced with firmness and impartiality. If substandard performance or inappropriate behavior is ignored, the staff will feel that management's announced regulations are merely words. If constructive discipline can be applied, it may save the hospital money by restoring employees who would have been dismissed [45].

Rules of conduct must be communicated to the staff. Personnel handbooks may be published and distributed to the staff, or the regulations may be posted on an employee bulletin board. Verbal explanations can serve to clarify the meaning of these regulations.

A system of progressive discipline should be developed by management, involving: (1) preliminary investigation, (2) a friendly discussion with the violator employee and a brief warning as to why further violations cannot be tolerated, (3) a stronger oral warning to the employee after a further infraction of a regulation, (4) a formal warning in written form, (5) a written warning accompanied by suspension from the job for a prescribed number of days, (6) suspension from the job for a longer period of time, and (7) discharge. This approach provides an opportunity for the employee to make amends for the violations of the rules [45].

A director and the nursing administrative staff must look at their own performance as it relates to the staff. Do we inhibit productive effort by the way we work with people? Do we constructively motivate them or destroy their motivation to reach desired patient care goals? Do we sometimes cause or allow countless individual emotional strikes to occur every day as a result of the way people are treated by those who direct their work?

When an employee appears to be a problem, how do the director and her administrative staff handle the situation? They can be sure that the rest of the nursing staff will be watching with interest. There are two ways of firing someone. The first is simply to discharge the employee — to let her go. This is the line of least resistance and is often the easiest apparent solution. But unless the employee is absolutely hopeless, discharging her only exchanges one set of faults for another. The new person will not be perfect; she too will require training and fashioning to her job.

The second way to fire a person is to fire her mind and spirit with the determination to make good. Instead of letting her go, we set a fire under her so that she will make herself go — with enthusiasm! If the employee has basically good qualities, even though she has many faults, this second way of firing is often the better. The good is conserved and the person is inspired to grow and do a better job.

In order to maintain an equitable disciplinary program, the nurse director must provide opportunities for the supervisory staff members to learn how to administer it; training programs should be available to increase their skills in applying concepts of discipline. They must learn to do the preliminary investigation if an employee fails to meet established standards of performance or conduct. It should be proved on the basis of fact that an employee was disciplined for a good reason. If supervisors are unable so to prove, the employee may have recourse to higher management, an internal employee grievance policy, or, in some instances, a union representative.

Most personnel want to do what needs to be done, at work and in their conduct, in order to achieve hospital goals and accepted standards of behavior. Even before they start work, mature persons have accepted the idea that following instructions and abiding by fair rules of conduct are responsibilities of every employee in the hospital. If the employment relationship is a good one in other ways, most persons can be counted on to exercise a considerable degree of self-discipline. They tend to respond to positive leadership and need not be threatened. Wherever effective teamwork exists, group discipline can be counted on to supplement self-discipline.

The nurse director and her administrative staff want to make sure that all disciplinary action taken is fair. The action must be consistent with sound principles of personnel relations. It must be in accord with general statements about discipline that are clear and familiar to everyone concerned, and must implement ideas that have been developed in consultation with representatives of those who are subject to discipline. Administering discipline is one of the most unwanted tasks. However, it must be recognized that nursing administration has two responsibilities: (1) to provide staff personnel who can give safe care to patients and (2) to help employees grow as individual human beings. In the light of these two goals, the task of disciplining takes on a more rewarding meaning.

 T he nurse director must be aware of her role as it relates to employer-employee relationships. The problems that arise between management and the worker are by no means unique. Realization that sound employee-employer relationships result in better patient care is reason enough to strive for the cooperation of the employee. The nurse director has to relate to people of diverse interests and emotional structure, work with and help them individually and collectively, and build on their strength for total management effectiveness and efficiency.

WHY EMPLOYEES JOIN UNIONS

It must be recognized that employees are starting to and will continue to place increased pressure on management to obtain an opportunity to influence their work environment. If this is not permitted through the formal line of authority, attempts will be made to substitute union contract change that will require it [33].

A nurse director and her management staff must understand the role and function of labor unions and in some instances learn to work with union officials toward shared objectives. It must be an accepted fact that there are employees who want to join labor groups to bargain collectively for terms and conditions of employment. Employees have the legal and moral right to form unions; this is a feature of society but could lead to embittered labor relations and possibly a strike. The easiest way to instigate a strike is to dismiss or discriminate against staff members who desire to exercise their right to form a union.

A number of reasons are given as to why employees join unions. The following list (taken from an employer's guidebook published by the Indiana State Chamber of Commerce) is a composite made from studies, surveys, and the experience of businessmen, labor lawyers, educators, and consultants representing both private industry and hospitals:

Lack of security
　No complaint or grievance procedure.
　Management too busy to listen to gripes.
　Management too busy to investigate and obtain answers.
　No observation of seniority principles.

No warnings before discipline and arbitrary discharge.
Frequent layoffs with no reason given.
Wages
  Not competitive with like jobs in other companies or in the same
    industry.
  No increases either on merit or on a general basis.
  Not informed about wage scales and how to make income increase.
  Favoritism, with different workers receiving different rates for same
    job.
Benefits
  Not competitive with other firms in same industry.
  Adequate, but not equal to or better than other firms.
Do not know what is expected of them
  No periodic appraisal of performance by supervisor.
  No uniform rules or regulations, or not made known.
  Unfair standards.
Don't have a say on things affecting job
  Suggestions not given consideration.
  Changes made without being informed; not consulted.
Poor working conditions
  Poor ventilation.
  Poor lunch or break areas.
  Poor or inadequate parking.
  Substandard cleanliness, lighting, washup areas, and safety.
Not kept informed on things
  Wages and benefits.
  Expansions, subcontracting, new management, new supervisors.
  Company plans, products, finances, future.
Lack of advancement
Poor personnel policies — not written or disseminated
Inconsistent and unfair administration of policies, rules, and
    regulations
  Favoritism, broken promises.
  Apparent harsh treatment, no consistency.
  Lack of identification with employer.
  No recognition [18].

Employees are motivated to join unions because they feel that individual bargaining power is limited. The desire for self-expression is
fundamental in most people; they want to communicate their feelings, desires, and hopes to others. The union does provide a means

through which these thoughts can be transmitted to management. Formalized grievance procedures are established by unions to handle employee problems and concerns and bring workers to join and become members of the group. Union recreational and social activities are attractive to members. When a person feels his progress up the organization ladder is blocked, he turns to the union to fulfill his needs [9].

WHY EMPLOYEES REJECT UNIONS

Some employees reject participating in unions because they distrust unions and what they stand for; or they feel that people should stand on their own feet and get ahead on their own merits. They read or hear that a powerful union has closed down an essential service and that the public is penalized. Persons in professional positions tend to reject unions but join their own professional organizations, which have functions similar to those of unions [9].

The success of unions within hospitals, as in any industry, depends largely upon the treatment of employees. If employee wages are comparatively low in terms of the marketplace, if employees are not treated fairly, or if they do not have the fringe benefits enjoyed by the overwhelming number of American workers, unionization is easier to promote. If hospital management is autocratic and arbitrary, the task of organization will be expedited.

Unions seek to fulfill their goals by means of collective bargaining and the influencing of government legislation. Collective bargaining involves the union serving as a representative of the employees in the negotiating of a formal written agreement with management, which in turn represents the employer. Collective bargaining also includes handling the daily administration of the agreement, the enforcement of the agreement, and the resort to collective action such as striking.

UNION OBJECTIVES

Wortman and Randle [46] note that there are specific objectives of unions that are raised in collective bargaining:

Wages
　Employees and their union can be expected to ask for wages that are comparable to those in similar jobs in the local market.

Like work should be paid for on a similar basis so that employees doing the same work are not discriminated against.

According to some agreed-upon formula, employees can look forward to a wage increase.

Promotions

Unions will insist that length of service be a factor in promotions — not a straight seniority system for promotions typically, but seniority along with qualifications.

Layoffs

The union will insist that seniority play a part in regulating layoffs; qualifications being equal, the junior service employee will be laid off first.

Discipline

Employees will be disciplined for just cause; this is standard in all labor agreements.

Grievance procedure

The union will insist that a grievance procedure be established whereby management decisions will be reviewable by representatives of management and the union; if there is still disagreement, the dispute will be referred to arbitration.

Fringe benefits

Pensions, vacations and holidays, social insurance, and general welfare programs will be part of the negotiations, with an attempt to make them comparable to the trend in our society.

Union shop

Unions generally will request that all employees who are covered by the labor agreement be required to join the union [46].

Richard Hacker conducted an attitude survey of more than 18,000 hospital employees. His report ("Organizational System for Change Offers an Alternative to Unions," *Hospitals*. December, 1976) describes practices that put hospitals in a vulnerable position with regard to union objectives.

Some vulnerabilities:

Shift rotation — A major concern of hospital respondents was that the personnel department does not regularly audit schedules to ensure that weekend, evening, and night shifts are rotated fairly and equitably.

Performance appraisals — Hostility and charges of unfairness can easily arise because of a supervisor's failure to conduct regular and proper evaluations, a common occurrence despite the dictates of hospital policy.

Personnel policies — Because licensed and contracted personnel often gain benefits more rapidly, nonlicensed entry-level workers may become disenchanted with a hospital administration's policies regarding their positions.

Grievance procedures — While most hospitals provide some channel for settling grievances, resolutions tend to favor management. The prospect of a union steward may appeal to the majority of workers.

Wage and salary plans — Even with sophisticated pay structures, many hospital employees feel they are not being paid fairly, either for the work they perform or in comparison to similar workers. This indicates a communications failure.

Promotion and transfer opportunities — The inherent limitations on movement in specialized hospital careers, coupled with management's seeming lack of concern for career development, could create an issue for union emphasis.

Training and development opportunities — Programs offered by the hospital's education departments are unsatisfactory to most employees, and nonprofessional, nontechnical employees express some level of dissatisfaction with every phase of their training.

Hacker offers suggestions in three areas. First, personnel policies, procedures, and practices should be reviewed periodically by a group composed of top management, department heads, supervisors, and representative employees. Second, an information system should be set up to obtain employee opinions and attitudes on aspects of work and the organization, as well as the data necessary for early problem identification and corrective decision making. Finally, hospitals must be willing to invest in developing managers and supervisors who will more effectively carry out their responsibilities within the framework of Taft Act regulations.

In order to be aware of changing laws, a nurse director may seek current legislation information from the Bureau of National Affairs, Washington, D.C. 20037. Its publications cover in detail the laws and their policies in relation to personnel management, labor regulations, fair employment practices, wages and hours, and payroll-pay policies. The personnel director generally subscribes to these publications. Other legislative information from the Bureau is contained in the *White Collar Report* and the *Summary of Latest Developments.*

THE LEGAL FRAMEWORK

Today's manager is hardly free to deal with the union as he pleases. A growing body of federal and state laws and the judicial and administrative interpretations of these laws now govern the employer at every turn. Not only have the laws become extensive, but they have become complex and often nebulous. No study of the collective bargaining process would be possible without an understanding of the basic tenets and extensions of some of the major labor legislation. The following is a brief summary of some of these laws:

The Morris-LaGuardia Act (1932) restricted the use of injunctions in strikes, made peaceful picketing and assembly lawful, and permitted payment of strike benefits. It guaranteed the freedoms of the individual employee.

The Wagner Act (1935), also known as the National Labor Relations Act, banned management interference in union organizing, formation, or administration and prohibited discrimination against employees for union activity or for filing unfair labor practice charges. It forced management to recognize and to bargain with the duly chosen representatives of the union. It also established the National Labor Relations Board (NLRB) to investigate unfair practices and to conduct representative elections.

The Taft-Hartley Act (1947), Labor-Management Relations Act, prohibited many unfair union labor practices, including restraining or coercing, discrimination, refusal to bargain in good faith, certain types of boycotts, charging excessive initiation fees, and featherbedding. Basically, it dealt with the rights of individuals and employers. It also restricted strikes in national emergencies. It included a provision that professional employees could not be organized in the same bargaining unit with the nonprofessionals unless a majority of the professional employees voted for such an inclusion. Among the amendments was the exemption of hospitals from coverage under the Act and from the obligation to bargain collectively with their employees.

The Landrum-Griffin Act (1959), Labor-Management Reporting and Disclosure Act, marked the beginning of detailed regulation of the internal affairs of unions. It was a "bill of rights" for union members. It guaranteed them equality of rights in nomination, voting, and meeting attendance. It placed restrictions on dues and gave members the right to sue the union. It set rules for union elections governing time, place, and secret ballot procedure. Recognition picketing was restricted — it forbids picketing where an employer recognizes the existing union or if the picketing union has lost an election in the last 12 months, or where picketing has occurred for 30 days without the filing of an election petition with the NLRB.

In 1974 the Taft-Hartley Act was amended to ensure protected collective bargaining activity for employees in nonprofit institutions; it defined the rights of the employees to organize and to bargain with their employers through representation of their own choosing.

The Age Discrimination Act of 1975, prohibits unreasonable discrimination on the basis of age by recipients of Federal financial assistance. The Act was signed by President Ford, November 28, 1975, part of a comprehensive package extending funding under the Older American Act of 1965. The Act, which will have no effect on the enforcement of the wider ranging Age Discrimination in Employment Act of 1967, does not specify age limits for coverage. (From *Fair Employment Practices*, Bureau of National Affairs, 1975.)

MANAGEMENT-UNION RELATIONSHIPS

If a union becomes a part of an organization, the management role in the handling of employee relationships changes. To some degree, management's freedom of action is restricted, and a labor relations program will be conducted within the framework of collective bargaining. However, this does not mean that management cannot operate successfully and effectively. Another effect of the union upon management is pressure for uniformity of treatment of all employees. The presence of a union encourages management to become conscious of employees' needs and desires. In a sense the union simplifies management's problems in dealing with employees because it can look to elected union leaders as spokesmen for the employees [33].

If employees desire to organize a union, management has a right to tell its side of the story to the employees but should not do so in a way that is coercive or threatening. Once a majority of employees vote in a union, the union is established from that point on. Conditions of employment will then be determined by a collective bargaining agent. Employees are not eligible to deal with management as individuals once the election has been held.

Before the election, management should share with employees the facts of the current policies of employment; show how wages compare with those in like jobs in the community; explain the hospital's financial condition as far as ability to pay is concerned; explain what benefits are in existence; explain the organization's promotional policies; and describe the working of the disciplinary policy, the procedure used to discharge people, and the right of employees to appeal before higher levels of management. This presentation should be made in a factual and straightforward manner and not with the implication that management is antiunion. If unions win an election in an organization, management has a responsibility to bargain collectively and to bargain in good faith.

If the hospital administration and its managers strive to understand the personnel and their needs, employees are less likely to seek outside assistance to represent them. There must be new ways of managing people. Managerial practice is by far the greatest determinant of the fate of labor unions. Unions will continue with unabated strength in organizations in which people need a protector or medium for dissipating hostility. But to the extent that managerial sophistication continues to provide greater opportunity for individuals to manage their work and determine their destiny, there will be less incentive for them to apply their talents in antiorganizational behavior.

As nursing administration looks to the future, it becomes evident that profound change will take place in the way management deals with personnel. There will be greater concern for the deeper drives of human motivation — needs, hopes, pleasures, beliefs, a focus as wide-angled as life itself. A new move toward humanism is playing a dominant role in management thought. Management will be a matter less of delegating limited responsibilities and more of motivating open-ended creativity. People will perform less out of duty and more for the self-satisfaction gained. The hours of work will be fewer and will allow more flexibility in working schedules. Managers will strive to get the best productivity from their staff by being tolerant, kind, and empathetic. This attitude will require a kind of introspection and a creative instinct to achieve the goal of maximum productivity. Managers will experiment and take chances to loosen their minds from the bonds of considering traditional solutions; they will think boldly and consider daring solutions.

Employees of today are better educated and have different needs and values from those of their predecessors. Consequently, motivational methods that may have worked well in the past are ineffective today. For the nurse director this means a greater challenge to change nursing management patterns, attitudes, habits, responsibilities, and interrelationships of her staff.

THE HOSPITAL ADMINISTRATOR

The hospital administrator bears the heavy burden of putting together all the hospital departments into a coordinated, contributing whole. He must know by what means communication can best be established with all departments in order to avoid friction, nonproductive overlapping, waste of time, waste of money, loss of empathy, and loss of respect within the group. Recognizing that the nursing department is entrusted with the coordination of patient care, in addition to providing nursing care, he depends on the nursing staff to contribute a great deal toward the establishment and maintenance of the human environment.

Recognizing that people are the key to attaining patient care goals, the nurse director strives to achieve results by using all the available strengths of people — her superior, her association, and herself. She knows that one cannot build on weakness. Making people's strengths productive is much more than an essential of role effectiveness; it is a moral imperative, a responsibility of authority and position. To focus on a person's weakness is irresponsibility. Superiors owe it to their organizations to make the strengths of each subordinate as productive as they can be [17].

Above all, the effective nurse director tries to make fully productive the strengths of her own superior. In so doing, she strengthens her own effectiveness and contributes in such a way that the administrator tends to be receptive. One does not make a superior's strengths productive by toadying to him but by starting out with what is right and presenting it in a form that is acceptable [17].

A superior is a human; he has his strengths as well as his weaknesses. He has his own ways of being productive, and he looks for these ways. They may be only manners and habits, but they are facts. To build on his strengths — that is, to enable a superior to do what he can do — will make him effective and will make the subordinate effective. The nurse director must ask herself: What can my superior do really well? What has he done really well? What does he need to know to use his strengths? What does he need to get from me to perform?

In some instances the hospital administrator receives calls from the public regarding inadequate hospital services; he may be approached by staff personnel or their families regarding the inappropriate treatment accorded hospital employees by their supervisors; he may be faced with concerns relating to medical staff activities. These and other human situations that occur in the hospital require concentrated effort on the part of the administrator and his department directors — particularly the nurse director — to examine what is happening. Since nursing branches out in so many directions within the hospital and into the community, it is in a strategic position to be sensitive to the elements that disrupt the human environment. The nurse director can contribute significantly to the hospital administrator's good management by identifying specific situations that need his attention and handling the ones that she can deal with, in order to lighten his burden.

The nurse director should evaluate her services to the hospital administrator. How well does she help the administrator carry out his programs to achieve his objectives? How much confidence does she have in his ability to accept greater responsibility? She can help him by studying his responsibilities so that she knows what he is supposed to do, what his goals are, and what methods are being used to achieve those goals. She should look for areas where assistance can be offered in the form of ideas, suggestions, opinions, and facts and figures — information and viewpoints that will help the administrator make his decisions. The nurse director should carry out assignments and meet deadlines; she can also identify areas that might have been overlooked where trouble could begin and where early work could prevent the trouble from developing [34].

A hospital administrator faces problems similar to those encountered by a nurse director, such as making effective decisions, finding the right personnel to get the work done, seeing that special assignments are completed on time, getting people to work cooperatively with each other, being accountable for all work done under his supervision, and finding accurate information on which to base decisions and judgments. In addition, he has a need for a source to help him sense the directions in which the hospital is going; the need to keep his emotions under control; and the desire to gain the approval of his superiors and others.

An effective hospital administrator, like the nurse director, demonstrates certain human characteristics:

1. Is interested in the people who work.
2. Keeps well informed about what the people under his control are doing.
3. Keeps abreast of what is going on in health care, hospitals, and society in general.
4. Listens to others and wants input from people.
5. Understands people, and knows that some days are better than others.
6. Knows that job satisfaction is vastly important to nearly everyone, and tries to contribute to the job enrichment of others.
7. Understands "the art of change" [34].

A nurse director can put the administrator's knowledge and talents to work for her performance. She can seek his assistance in the following situations, for example: checking her decisions with him from time to time; sharing with him the way she arrived at a significant decision, and asking his advice if he sees something that she may have missed; assessing how he feels about human conflicts that come up in her department; asking for suggestions as to what she can do to better herself as a nurse director; asking if he believes she is headed in the right direction. When the administrator gives her a task that is going to be particularly difficult, the nurse director should spend enough time asking questions until she understands every facet of the assignment. She should ask questions at appropriate times and show the administrator that she needs assistance and is pleased to get it from him [34].

The qualities that hospital administrators do not like to see demonstrated in the performance of a nurse director are as follows:

1. Isolation — not easily available to others.
2. Abrasiveness — keeping everyone upset.
3. Dullness — lack of flexibility, adaptability, curiosity.
4. Impatience — getting upset with others when they don't perform so fast as desired.
5. Lack of direction — not knowing where one is going.
6. Boorishness — behaving in a manner overbearing to others by reason of one's sense of importance.
7. Softness — inability to stand up for what one believes in.
8. Brittleness — being unable to change, with a desire to maintain the status quo.
9. Complacency — being satisfied that someone else can do the work.
10. Negativeness — a closed mind about anything and everything [34].

The task of accomplishing the goals of a hospital requires the strengthening of human relationships and of the organization. The nurse director must strive to move herself toward mastering this idea. The responsibilities of the hospital administrator can best be carried out by a nurse director who builds on the strengths of others to provide quality patient care.

HOSPITAL DEPARTMENTS

While the hospital administrator is the chief coordinator of hospital services, he depends on the department directors both as individuals and as a group to accomplish hospital goals, and he delegates the authority to enable them to do so. The nurse director must determine how far she can go with coordinating activities with other departments. For example, if a nurse director has business to transact with another department director, she clearly has a right to deal with him independently. The extent to which the two can make binding decisions to adopt a new course of action depends upon the scope of authority each possesses. Generally, higher management expects such interdepartmental coordination and cooperation to be extensive. The degree to which coordinate individuals in separate departments of the hospital can make commitments depends upon the philosophy and policies of top management. If the policy of the organization is one of centralized control of decision making, the two directors will have to consult their immediate superior on every issue. If the policy is one of decentralization and liberal delegation of authority and responsibility, the department directors will have wide latitude in initiating and coordinating important actions.

The place of coordination of nursing services with hospital departments and other groups should be high on the hierarchical scale of functional importance for the nurse director. Nursing service personnel make up the one group that relates all the various service areas of the hospital for the patient. Because nursing is a focal point of hospital services, it affects and is affected by what other departments do. The impact may be more or less direct, but all departments touch the nursing service in some way.

Many types of human activities take place in the nursing department, involving the efforts of a variety of specialists. Some help to make the environment livable and attractive; others participate in diagnostic, therapeutic, and preventive activities. Each contributes to the patient's welfare.

Effective unity is the aim of organizational engineering, and it is accomplished by the nurse director, who adapts and integrates the functioning of its parts. She coordinates — that is, unites — ideas of others with her own. Control is attained by the interaction of individuals, and it measures the self-direction that is part of the process. As the nurse director communicates with her supervisors, peers, and subordinates, with the patients, and with the community, so she should expect the nursing staff under her supervision to perform in suitable fashion.

People in organizations tend voluntarily to coordinate their actions when necessary. Each person, at his own discretion, adjusts to the needs of other workers. Such voluntary coordination is more likely to work smoothly if there is common agreement on a set of objectives. Through mutual recognition of objectives, the work of all persons will probably become more effective.

As a nurse director tries to coordinate the functions of the nursing department with those of all other departments of the hospital, she must discover whether these groups clearly recognize common objectives, sufficiently well stated to assure coordination for patient care. Are the objectives in writing? Do the groups see a mutual bond that directs their attention and services toward desired ends? Or is there a lack of clear-cut, acknowledged common objectives that makes coordination difficult?

As a member of top management, the nurse director participates with other department directors in hospital management. Ordinarily the hospital administrator determines the organizational structure through which this is accomplished. Regular meetings may be scheduled with agenda prepared and minutes maintained. In other situations the nurse director and selected department heads may meet periodically for coordinating patient care services. The important point is that, whatever the arrangement, the nurse director must be an active member in activities involving interdepartmental policies and functions.

The object of coordination is to identify the points where the functions of nursing and those of other departments meet, and to assure that they meet at the right time, in the right place, and without conflict or a gap. The nurse director should therefore study the functions of other departments, in order to have a real understanding and appreciation of the activities and responsibilities of all groups in the hospital. She should provide opportunities for personnel from other departments to become acquainted with nursing functions. On the basis of knowledge about the functions of other departments, she is able to make wiser decisions or recommendations to bring about better departmental coordination — perhaps through changes in policy or procedure, through improved ways of sharing and exchanging information, or through provision for consultation between the nursing department and another department when necessary. As a nurse director and her staff learn about the functions of other areas, it becomes apparent which ones relate most closely to the nursing department [4].

In some hospitals the nursing department performs duties that are the responsibility of other departments. Grouping of functions varies among hospitals because of variations in hospital size, resources, and personnel, and although nursing functions and those of other departments may not be too difficult to identify and separate, coordinating them sometimes presents difficulties [4].

Areas of disagreement inevitably arise, since much of the success in operating a nursing service department rests upon methods of working with other people. Because their routes of preparation vary and concepts of care differ, there may be conflict between the nursing service and personnel from other departments. To solve such problems, those involved must share a common concept as to the responsibility of the hospital for the care of patients.

In order to provide effective coordination between nursing service and other departments, the nurse director must lay the groundwork for it and create a climate in which coordination is possible. She will have to:

1. Cooperate with other departments and staff in carrying forward the work of the hospital as a whole.
2. Assist other departments in working out routines closely related to activities of the nursing department.
3. Study the functions and activities of other departments and interpret them to the nursing personnel.
4. Participate in joint professional meetings to plan for patient care, organized as a committee for the improvement of patient care.
5. Participate in departmental and other meetings to discuss common hospital problems: department directors' meetings or nursing service laboratory coordinating meetings.
6. Invite representatives from other departments and groups to participate in staff education programs and nursing unit conferences of the nursing department.
7. Encourage nursing staff to participate in meetings with other departments.
8. Arrange joint staff education programs.
9. Use individual conferences.
10. Use written memoranda [4].

MEDICAL STAFF

The continued achievement of high standards of patient care depends upon a harmonious, collaborative relationship between medicine and nursing [14]. Nursing and medical practice are interdependent and require full communication to assure quality care. The Committee on Nursing of the American Medical Association made the following assumptions: "(1) Nurses have a separate and distinct professional status and their contributions are those of co-workers; (2) the medical profession supports and endorses high standards of nursing education and nursing service; (3) each of the various levels of academic and technical accomplishment in nursing makes its own unique contribution to the total health care of the public" [14]. Based on these assumptions are the following objectives, developed by the AMA for its Nursing Committee:

1. To expand and strengthen liaison activities between organizations representing the medical and nursing professions at the national, state, and local levels.
2. To study and report to the medical profession on current practices and trends in nursing and on developments among nursing auxiliary personnel.
3. To stimulate, initiate, and, where feasible, support research in areas pertinent to the nurse-physician relationship in professional practice.
4. To offer advisory services to both professions on interprofessional matters.
5. To provide support and assistance to the nursing profession and its non-professional auxiliary personnel in their efforts to maintain high standards.
6. To encourage physicians to accept invitations to serve on nursing school facilities [14].

Because of the growing demand for health services and the need for manpower, the physician and the nurse recognize their full potential as a highly coordinated and mutually effective team. The AMA approved a position statement on medicine and nursing in which the following objectives are to guide the Association's activities in the area of physician-nurse relationships:

1. Increase the number of nurses.
2. Facilitate the expansion of the role of the nurses in providing patient care.
3. Support all levels of nursing education.
4. Promote and influence the development of a hospital nursing service aimed at increased involvement in direct medical care of the patient.
5. Delivery of medical care is, by nature, a team operation.
6. In order to implement these objectives, constructive collaboration of medicine with the various elements of the nursing profession is essential [14].

The physician, as captain of the health team, is responsible for bringing the highest degree of scientific competence to his task and for developing his skill as a coordinator. He recognizes his limitations, appreciates the skills of others, and is sensitive to his patient's need for services other than his own. The physician is responsible for the competence of those to whom he delegates functions. He consults his team associates and recognizes that his role is sometimes primary and sometimes secondary, and that it varies with the phases of the patient's illness [35]. Nurses are professionals in their own right, and physicians cannot justly control their clinical operations. The AMA Code of Ethics indicates that the nurse is responsible for both independent and dependent functions. She is obligated to refuse to participate in actions deemed harmful to the patient or against his interest. As a coordinator, the physician must yield some of his individualism and accept the discipline of a conjoint effort in which he is the captain of the team but without absolute prerogatives. This must be the case, too, with other professionals if the physician coordinator role is to have real significance [14].

The nurse director must identify ways in which physicians and nurses can plan and coordinate patient care activities. Alexander and colleagues [1] give these examples:

1. Doctors and nurses can work together and insist on organizational structures that will free the time of nurses to care for patients.
2. The chief of the medical staff and nurse director can work closely in developing improvement in patient care. With both groups having similar concepts of clinical practice, there would be more likeness in the manner of giving care and less disturbance in communicating.
3. Physician-nurse committees can be established to assess professional problems and take remedial action.
4. Departmental physician-nurse committees for various specialty areas are helpful.
5. Joint planning on the various nursing units on either a formal or an informal basis is in order.
6. Both groups can share educational programs.
7. Joint clinical workshops may be set up on a state-wide or district-wide level.
8. Joint research for the improvement of patient care is called for.
9. Both groups can strive toward obtaining the appointment of a physician and a nurse to the board of directors of the hospital.
10. There is joint planning for continuity of patient care.

Understanding is fundamental to establishing effective relationships. The ideas and attitudes of physicians toward nurses and nursing are products of their experience with nurses. If they are uninformed about the philosophy and objectives of nursing, the knowledge nurses possess, and the skills they have developed, physicians cannot be expected to appreciate fully the nurse's role. Therefore, it is desirable to involve physicians in nursing activities so that they can see for themselves what nurses are trying to do. Physicians can take part in planning patient care committees, in-service educational programs, and selected staff meetings, or their advice can be requested on instituting change [1].

Every recent development in medical science makes the cooperative effort of physician and nurse an urgent necessity if patient care patterns are to be optimal. Optimal service to patients is the reason for the existence of the medical and nursing professions and of all the health professions. The dialogue between both groups is beginning to consider this a joint problem soluble only by combined action. Dr. Pellagrino says we are entering a period of more critical and open discussion of the human problems involved in delivering the best medical care at all levels. The unique perspectives of the nursing and medical professions demand that their actions be guided by the patient's rights, which derive from his being human. These rights take precedence over professional prerogatives and dictate that patient care must be scientifically grounded, readily available, and individually and compassionately administered. Such firm ethical imperatives should preserve these two health professions in all their discussions from jurisdictional disputes based on economic, political, and status-serving motives [35].

The attitudes of the nursing personnel toward physicians on the medical staff have profound effects on their relationships. Some nurses are reluctant to assume new responsibilities that physicians want to delegate to them on the basis that they are not part of nursing. In reality, the expansion of the nurse's role makes the nurse more valuable to the patient and consequently increases the physician's reliance on the nurse to manage patient care; this strengthens the bond between the nurse and physician and promotes a colleague relationship. The nurse director who is faced with requests by the medical staff might be wise to explore these ideas from the viewpoint of enriching the clinical aspects of nursing and management of patient care before making a decision. Changes are occurring in medical and nursing practice, and she is in a strategic position to influence the process of reallocation of functions in an orderly manner mutually agreed upon by nurses and physicians. As physicians and nurses direct their energies to improving the climate of interchange, they can effect reforms in providing quality care to patients [5].

NURSING EDUCATION

If it is part of a hospital's philosophy to provide a learning atmosphere for students of various professional and allied health groups, the nurse director has an additional responsibility. Although the nursing department may be involved in several different educational programs for students, nursing educational programs generally are the department's major focus. To facilitate student learning, relationships must be established between the nursing service staff and the faculty of the educational program.

The nurse director has a vital role to play in contributing to the education of nurses. She must establish and maintain an environment within the nursing department that supports the program. The objectives of the nursing education program and the nursing service department must be well understood by the nursing service staff and by the instructors and their students. Much misunderstanding can take place unless both groups know what each hopes to accomplish.

Convinced of the merit and soundness of a nursing education program, the nurse director needs to gain acceptance of the program by the nursing staff and, together with the hospital administrator, to gain acceptance also by the medical staff and other department directors. This implies an understanding of the program and its effect on nursing service operations. Sessions should be conducted by the nursing education director for the various groups to learn about the nursing program (since participation is a key factor in achieving acceptance of something new or different). In approaching staff members it may be helpful to emphasize the contribution of nursing personnel to the success of the program, the need for their help in interpreting the program to medical staff and others, the willingness of those responsible to consider their ideas for improving and promoting the program, the efforts that will be made to keep them informed, and the realization that the example the staff members set as nurses cannot be overestimated. Every student nurse must spend part of her time in a hospital to learn nursing. The kind of graduate nurse the student becomes is the responsibility not only of the school but also of the hospital and nursing staff that contribute to her learning [6].

Ways must be found to create the kind of atmosphere that builds rapport between nursing service and nursing education, achieved by showing respect for each other, understanding each other's responsibilities, and agreeing on how the objectives of each can be implemented. Nursing service and nursing education personnel can participate in joint committees concerned with either patient care or education. Time and opportunity need to be provided for head nurses or supervisors or both to confer with clinical faculty in regard to patient assignments for students. The school of nursing must make known its policies and procedures, and the nurse director should approve of those relating to the part of the program conducted in the hospital [6].

With the emerging standards of nursing practice and innovative patterns for health care delivery, the partnership and ties between nursing service and nursing education must be strengthened to meet these changing needs. Can nurse administrators (education and service) work together to think about tomorrow's nurse practitioners? Can they think together about what the health needs of people and the health care delivery system will be like in the year 2000? Can they determine what the role of the professional nurse would be (if any) in the system? Can they work toward a commitment to unify nursing education and nursing service? How can the nurse director of a hospital supply the leadership to answer such questions in the hospital and at the community, state, and national level?

As nursing service directors and their staff plan for the future of their services, consideration should be given to trends in nursing such as the following:

1. Nurses will practice more independently in a variety of health care settings.
2. Greater accountability for services will be expected by patients from nurses.
3. The role of the consumer is moving toward that of planner, implementer, and assessor of health care.
4. Health care services are extending beyond traditional settings.
5. Nurses are assuming greater responsibility in developing a new health care delivery system.
6. There is a continued emphasis on specialization in nursing.

7. There is a greater sense of collaborativeness and colleagueship among nurses and other health personnel and consumers of health care.
8. There is an increased emphasis on graduate education in nursing.

THE COMMUNITY

With the rapid expansion and multiplication of health care institutions, the nurse director must be cognizant of how coordination can take place between the hospital nursing service and community agencies. Hospital nursing service is likely to be viewed more and more by the way it participates and shares with the community. The director must be sensitive to the social, cultural, economic, and political community environment.

Opportunities should be provided for both the nursing staff and community health and welfare agency staffs to share their goals, services, and desires with each other. They can be offered through in-service educational programs as well as visits to the respective agencies.

With the great emphasis on community health planning, the nurse director and her staff should become involved in civic, social, political, and health and welfare groups in order to interpret the role of nursing in the community. The health care system is undergoing a tremendous amount of change, and nursing administration must be present to share in shaping the future of health care services.

THE HEALTH MAINTENANCE ORGANIZATION

A new method of delivering health services is through the health maintenance organization (HMO). A nurse director must watch this development and determine if there may be any future implications for nursing in her particular setting. The HMO brings together a comprehensive range of medical services in a single organization so that a patient is assured of convenient access to them, and it provides needed services for a fixed contract fee that is paid in advance by all subscribers. The HMO is based on four principles:

(1) It is an organized system of health care that accepts the responsibility to provide or otherwise assure the delivery of:

(2) an agreed upon set of comprehensive health maintenance and treatment services for:

(3) a voluntarily enrolled group of persons in a geographic area; and

(4) it is reimbursed through a prenegotiated and fixed periodic payment made by or on behalf of each person or family unit enrolled in the plan.

Primary care, one of the keystones of the HMO, emphasizes those services designed to prevent the onset of illness or disability to maintain good health, and to ensure the continuing evaluation and management of early complaints, symptoms, problems, and the chronic, intractable aspects of a disease; it is the entry point into the health care delivery system, from which referrals to specialists are made [42].

An HMO may be organized and sponsored by a medical foundation, a community group, labor unions, a governmental unit, or a profit or nonprofit group, or by some other arrangement. The HMO may be hospital-based or may be an independent outpatient facility or group of such facilities [42].

CHANGE

Nurse directors need to prepare themselves for change and the techniques of change in the same way that they need to know administration, management, budget, staffing, and other related areas. They need to draw upon the latest theory and tools of change. Managing change is a function of nurse directors; change is one of the most characteristic features of nursing service administration. How nurse directors will mold and adapt their professional role under the pressure of change and challenge will depend on what they value in nursing and in life in general.

A major concern of the nurse director is the extensiveness of change or the explosiveness of change in an evolving society; she is caught either in the "pressures of change" or the "challenge of change" — whichever way one wishes to perceive the situation. Rapid and drastic change is taking place in society and in technology. The transformations have necessitated significant changes in the operations of hospitals, placed new demands on nurse directors, and brought forth emphasis on the needs and motivations of the working staff. Those hospitals which have survived and are growing are those which have learned to cope effectively with the pace of change. Successful nurse directors are those who have learned to understand and to cope with change; the less successful nurse directors have relinquished the initiative and merely reacted to change. If today's and tomorrow's nurse directors are truly to function as agents of change, rather than reactors to change, they must understand the critical changes occurring in society and their implications for nursing service administration.

The nurse director must direct her attention toward expanding her knowledge of the theory of change and developing the commitment to change that is so vital. More and more, the business of management is becoming that of providing for impending change and of trying to steer inevitable change in the direction of effectiveness. At the same time that forces and knowledge become available to help a work group to go ahead, forces are building up that threaten to impede its progress. Depending on how the nurse director deals with these forces, she is either effective or ineffective in the work situation.

No organization is exempt from change. The changes facing a nurse director in a hospital today are made even more significant by the increased rate of change. The types of change and the differences in rate of change will create an organizational world filled with uncertainty and problems. The nurse director, facing the possibility of change, must be prepared and willing to accept conditions of uncertainty and conflict. As she strives to increase her understanding of the nature and dynamics of the concepts of change, she will be better prepared to deal with the changing world [28].

Meaning of Change

Change is one of the most important facts of organizational life. Change is defined as: "to alter by substituting something else for, or by giving up for something else; to put or take another or others in place of; to make different or to convert; to exchange, alter, vary, modify" [28]. Change implies either a loss of identity or the substitution of one thing for another [28]. Regardless of how change is defined, it involves people. The primary effect of change will be on people; change means that people must alter their attitudes, values, beliefs, or ways of doing things. Change is never a simple or single occurrence within a hospital or nursing service department; it affects and is affected by the total hospital system with its many interrelationships that affect the process of change.

By definition, any living organism is constantly undergoing change. The nurse director is part of this change in many ways. She is changing because of her own physiological composition; her world is constantly changing; and the people she works with are under constant conditions of change. Effecting change is an integral part of the nurse director's role. She is constantly faced with the ever-changing needs of people and a dynamic health care delivery system [28].

The process of change follows a certain pattern wherever it occurs; (1) introduction of a new idea, (2) tension between the new and the old, (3) probable compromise and alteration, (4) a decision plan for action, followed by actual implementation, and (5) feedback, which may in turn become the idea for a new cycle of change [28].

Approaches to Bring About Change

Bennis [10] identifies eight traditional programs used to bring about change in various settings:

1. The exposition and propagation program assumes that knowledge is power; people who possess knowledge will lead in a situation.
2. The elite corps program assumes that a strategic role and not just knowledge power constitutes action for change; the effective utilization of knowledge requires that persons with knowledge and ideas be put into power.
3. The human relations program assumes that a good understanding of behavioral science concepts provides power for change to take place.
4. The staff program assumes that the use of certain people in an organization to effect change is helpful; staff members observe, analyze, and plan rationally, design appropriate change responses of an organization, and actually promote their ideas at the grass roots level in a setting.
5. The scholarly consultation program assumes that scientific findings can be made useful to certain people in an organization to effect change.
6. The circulation of ideas program assumes that change can be brought about by getting to the people with power or influence in

a setting. If change is wanted, one must get the idea to the right people.

7. The developmental research program assumes that the testing out of an idea is a means to effect change.
8. The action research program assumes that solving a problem for a client ensures that change will occur.

Bennis says that these change programs rely on reason to produce change; knowledge about something does not necessarily lead to intelligent action. There is no assurance that a wise individual who attains power will act wisely. The elite change program focuses on the individual and not the organization [10]. Today it is believed that the old approaches no longer fit — today those in authority do not just tell others what to do. People are no longer impressed by superior knowledge, since they know a great deal themselves about many things, and attitudes toward authority have changed.

Massie [28] suggests the following approaches to bring about managed change:

1. Group dynamics approach — allows people to become involved together as a group; all the members have a common bond and the experiences are highly personal.
2. Formal versus the informal power approach — allows for the use of both formal power when necessary and the informal, nondirect approach, depending upon the situation.
3. Layer approach — recognizes the differences in people and their natural tendency to resist change; using this approach to change, the nurse director would relay and communicate her plan for change to her subordinates and so on down the line until two people with similar orientations would be able to communicate with each other with no distrust.
4. Gains and losses approach — allows the nurse director to analyze a situation prior to action; the question is raised: "If the proposed change were to take place, what would be the gains and losses to the personnel affected by the change?"

Other approaches to organizational change are perceived as follows:

1. Decree approach — those in authority pass changes down the organizational structure.

2. Replacement approach — individuals are replaced in an organization; new blood is injected to effect change.
3. Structural approach — organizational behavior change is effected through changes in organizational structure and relationships.
4. Group decision approach — people are asked to participate in bringing about change.
5. Data process approach — feedback of relevant data is presented to the client system either by a change catalyst or by change agents within the organization.
6. Group problem-solving approach — problem identification and problem solving through group discussion promote change.
7. Group approach — training in sensitivity to the processes of individual and group behavior assumes that change will occur [10, 26, 28, 43].

Without effort on anyone's part, people and organizations do change — even when they appear to be quite stable. Change occurs as individuals, groups, institutions, and communities are forced to respond to forces from within or without. Such change may be referred to as "organizational drift" because it takes place by happenstance. The changes are not planned or deliberated on; they just occur, with little consciousness on the part of the individual group, organization, or community affected. Changes of this kind are recognized only in retrospect; suddenly it is realized that a radical change has taken place [38].

Planned Change

Interest in and commitment to the concept of planned change are emerging both within individual organizations and within nursing as a profession; planned change is believed to be a more modern strategy and is being advocated for altering a situation. The successful introduction of planned change is considered a key administrative function. Massie [28] speaks of *planned change* and *managed change*; planned change involves all the things a manager thinks about doing, whereas managed change involves all the things a manager does. Lippitt [26] defines planned change as a deliberate and collaborative effort to improve the operations of a human system, whether it be a self-system, social system, or cultural system, through the utilization of scientific knowledge. *Deliberate* refers to a plan: to define ends and means; *collaborative* indicates that the plan and its implementation involve all those persons who are concerned with it. Lippitt's concept involves an agent of change, a person (or people) with the ability to help plan and affect change; the agent can be either a person within the hospital or an outside person. Reinkemeyer [38] states that to solve a problem of society is a deliberate and collaborative process involving a change. Frey [19] defines planned change in nursing service as that which is undertaken through a thoughtful, purposeful, analytical approach with full knowledge of the situation at hand and an understanding of the complexities of the change process and its anticipated results. Change, when planned and purposeful, is often the antecedent of progress, and generally when progress occurs, change has occurred, whether in the form of new ideas or old ones woven into new patterns [19].

Planned change may involve a client system — an individual, a group, an organization, or a community. Lippitt [26] says that the client system holds certain views of itself, sees itself as taking responsibility for change, and prefers that change not occur too rapidly. Change takes place when a client system is dissatisfied with the present system or is faced with external pressures, or when internal organizational requirements set up pressure for change. Interdependence among parts of an organization or change may begin with an individual or a group of individuals. The way people work together in day-to-day affairs is a fairly good index of how they will accept change. The degree of acceptability of change depends on the extent to which there is participation in decision making involving those affected by change, with opportunities to evaluate the results. Action is the beginning of everything. In every human activity, nothing of consequence happens until an individual wants to act. What a person accomplishes depends to a considerable extent on how much and why he wants to act; that much is obvious. Beyond that point, the nature of human motivation toward change becomes complex and subtle.

Lippitt [26] identified the following as the seven phases of planned change:

1. The client system discovers the need for help, sometimes with stimulation by a change agent.
2. The helping relationship of the change agent is established and defined.

3. The change problem is identified and clarified.
4. Alternative possibilities for change are examined; change goals or intentions are established.
5. Change efforts in the "reality situation" are attempted.
6. Change is generalized and stabilized.
7. The helping relationship ends or a different type of continuing relationship is defined.

Planned change is undertaken through a thoughtful, purposeful, analytical approach, with full knowledge of the situation at hand and an understanding of the complexities of the change process and its anticipated results. Planned change involves: the establishment of target dates in order to pace work realistically; organizing for change; and evaluating change.

Change Agents

A change agent may come from within the hospital system (using inside knowledge and expertise), or external agents may be obtained. As a change agent enters a situation, what does he try to do? Lippitt [26] suggests that he:

1. Diagnose the nature of the system's problem.
2. Assure the system's motivation and capacities to change.
3. Appraise his own motivation and resources.
4. Select appropriate change objectives.
5. Choose an appropriate type of helping role.
6. Establish and maintain the helping relationship.
7. Recognize and guide the phases of the change process.
8. Choose the specific techniques of behavior that will be appropriate to each progressive encounter in the change relationship.

A change agent, if one takes as a basis the theories of planned change, does not possess ready-made solutions that he must sell to a client system but, rather, helps to plan for change. Change agents must reckon with the value system, social structure, and technical system if important changes are to be accepted and implemented. They must be prepared to work with the healthy parts of the organization (some parts desire change; others resist).

A change agent makes assumptions about the nature of the client system, the process by which the system got into trouble, and the nature of the trouble. He further makes assumptions about his functions — the process that will lead to an amelioration of the trouble and the ways he can contribute to bring about change.

The nurse director as a change agent must learn to develop some conceptual framework in terms of which she can analyze the meaning of facts that are presented to her by a particular situation in which she is working. She must orient herself to theories and methods of change and must possess a theoretical basis for understanding the progress of the relationship between a change agent and a client system. She must further orient herself to the ethical and evaluative functions of a change agent. Ethical judgment involves making value judgments as well as improving interpersonal relationships and collaborating in establishing change goals.

Resistance to Change

The nurse director's world is changing and yet is resistant to change. Many people in the nursing situation may want change; some may want change to improve the present situation; yet the nurse director will find some resisting such change. Since change brings about the unknown, personnel may sometimes fear the unknown. The nurse director is then faced with conditions supporting change as well as conditions resisting change.

Resistance to change may arise from two possible sources: (1) The change may threaten a person's psychological safety; or (2) the change may have an economic impact. Resistance is a warning signal to the nurse director, for nearly all change brings an alteration in social patterns and individual behavior processes. It should be expected and anticipated that resistance will occur with change in most instances. Knowing how to overcome resistance begins with knowing why it exists.

A nurse director must strive to lessen resistance to change within her department and in the hospital. She may approach change through: (1) changing the structure — for example, the director who has authority and influence over a situation may change behavior; (2) changing the technology — for example, human behavior can be influenced through decisions by the nurse director about the types of work to be done in her department; or (3) changing the decision-making technique — for example, the director may make the decision herself, she may let subordinates make the decision, or the director and the nursing staff may participate together in solution finding.

Reinkemeyer [38] lists inhibiting factors or resistance forces that nurse directors must become aware of, including (1) ingrained traditionalism and (2) an educational deprivation, including inadequate or inaccurate education about the change process itself, "the rut of experience," and a weak knowledge base. Other obstacles common to all human systems include reluctance to depart from the known and tried; reluctance to admit weakness, such as a lack of knowledge, skill, or preparation; the fear of failure or awkwardness in adopting a new behavior; fatalistic expectation of failure; and the fear of losing some current satisfaction, such as prestige, power, or independence.

Bennis et al. [10] identify the following resisting forces to change: (1) client is opposed to change; (2) client is opposed to a particular change; (3) client clings to ideas or actions he is satisfied with; (4) client has poor relations with change agent; (5) client learns that the change costs more than expected in terms of personal involvement and becomes discouraged; and (6) client's attention is diverted to other projects.

Lee [23] summarizes the problem of resistance to change using Kipling's six "servingmen": what, why, how, when, where, and who.

What is the problem? Resistance to change.
Why such resistance? Habit, illusion of importance, personal identity, vested interest.
How can change be modified? Explain the reasons for the change and the anticipated benefits.
When should change be initiated? When the client system has tools and skill required.
Where should change start? In an area where ego involvement is least in other areas (reinforcement).
Who should introduce change? Someone who is respected, preferably someone within the group. Better still, get the whole group involved in planning change; no one drills a hole in the boat if he is in it.

Parting advice: In my experience, you cope with resistance best if you remain flexible; keep your sense of humor, and go slowly [23].

Change is more acceptable and less resistance is demonstrated: (1) when it is understood; (2) when the people affected by it have helped to create it rather than having had it externally imposed; (3) when it follows a series of successful changes rather than a series of failures; (4) when it results from an application of previously established changes; (5) when it is inaugurated after previous change has been assimilated rather than during the confusion of other major changes; (6) when it is planned rather than haphazard; (7) when its benefits are widespread; (8) when improvement is a constant procedure, rather than when the group is accustomed to a status quo; and (9) when opportunities are provided for people to contribute ideas, to understand the relevant facets of the problem, to have a clear definition of the objectives and goals of higher management, and to sense responsibility for the success of the change program [10, 19, 28].

As plans for change are acted upon, there is a need for constant feedback from various levels of nursing to higher levels of management (and vice versa) on the progress of the change program. Written information such as data and reports is valuable, but face-to-face contact, especially among task groups, is highly desirable. The implementation of a change program can result in some disagreements. If the disagreements focus on the substance of the problem, a satisfactory resolution can be expected; these disagreements may result in creative thinking and the synthesis of new ideas. On the other hand, disagreements sometimes cause interpersonal frictions and tend to grow if not checked.

Conflict

Recognizing the type of conflict that occurs daily in the hospital enables the nurse director to be more adept in dealing effectively with conflict and change. Much of the behavior conflict in organizations stems from conflicts in values. Few people are fully aware of their values, and they relate to values only through behavioral clashes. Values are what make the people of an organization human; they reign deep in people and are the base by which many people interpret behavior.

Conflict between people usually arises from interrelationships that depend on both verbal and nonverbal language. Three concepts to keep in mind are the following:

1. A statement of fact represents something that is either true or false. A person cannot demonstrate its truth or falsity, but there is truth or falsity, for example, in the statement, "This is a red apple." A statement is not just one of fact, but, rather, a statement of true fact or a statement of false fact; it is generally supported with information or research.
2. A statement of value can never be true or false; for example, "This

is a wonderful place to work." Statements of value lead to fair game for confrontation and fair game for interpersonal interface.

3. Statements of ideology are the statements that create pathological conflict within groups or in society; for example, "Jackson Hospital is the one and only hospital (of worth) in Cedar City!" "No, Clary Hospital is the one and only hospital (of worth) in Cedar City!" These kinds of statements, if asserted as facts, are not going to be too persuasive — who is right? "I am right because I am right."

As a nurse director deals with conflict, she needs to know what types of statements she is dealing with in various situations. Change may be viewed, in some instances, as a threat to people's values. People may have trouble adjusting to rapid change because it shakes them up. If a nurse director can manage change, she may be able to reduce, to some degree, conflict of values among the nursing staff. Conflict between organizational and personal values is a fact of life; the hospital must develop values for a world that includes many external forces, whereas the values of individual staff members tend to be personal and confined to a smaller world. The nurse director strives to be aware of her own attitudes toward conflict — including her ambivalences. The nurse director must be on speaking terms with herself before she can communicate with others.

The hospital is a human institution made up of individuals, each possessing his own unique needs or goals, which may or may not achieve actualization; it is composed of heterogeneous groups of people with diverse vested interests; it has a growing diversity of personnel. All these factors are potential causes of conflict. It is quite reasonable to conclude that conflict is a phenomenon of common occurrence in human interaction.

Implementing Change

In implementing a change program, the nurse director should be aware of certain necessary elements:

1. The hospital administration must have an understanding of the change and its consequences.
2. The change effort should be perceived as being self-motivated and voluntary.
3. The change program must include emotional value as well as in-

formation for successful implementation; it is doubtful that relying solely on expert power is sufficient.
4. The change agent can be crucial in reducing resistance to change.

Whoever is responsible for initiating or implementing the change process needs to ask certain basic questions:

1. Does the organization have internal mechanisms that are sensitive to new developments in the external environment?
2. Does the organization have any planning policies and procedures for reacting to changing signals?
3. Are the action programs consistent with policy planning?
4. Has the organization developed stabilizing forces following action programs?
5. Does the organization have realistic and meaningful measurements for evaluating the result of change?
6. Is there feedback into the organization, to allow the organization to modify past policies and to make it sensitive to future changes?

Suggested guidelines for implementing change are as follows:

1. Inspire nursing personnel to initiate and accept change.
2. Promote cooperation among the nursing personnel, which is necessary for a climate conducive to change.
3. Set environmental conditions that facilitate the nursing staff's motivation toward accepting the change process.
4. Recognize the role of the democratic process and get nursing personnel involved in the situation for successful change.
5. Promote coordination and collaboration of nursing activities with other groups to support the change process.
6. Keep an open mind to suggestions offered by the nursing personnel; this serves as a stimulus for change.
7. Accept the challenge of commitment to change in order to allow nursing to grow.
8. Support and urge change in nursing.
9. Cultivate ideas from the nursing staff; if they are viable, disseminate them.
10. Give staff members credit for their ideas.
11. Pull together and apply the creative problem-solving ability within your own organization; properly prepared interdisciplinary

groups can supply the integration of thinking and creativity necessary for effective activity.
12. Hold intergroup meetings; when problems among work groups become acute and there is a mutual commitment to deal with them, intergroup meetings are a highly relevant force for change.

A nurse director who is committed to change must engage in environmental watching. She must go out into the hospital, community, and larger systems; talk with nurse directors, nurse practitioners, nursing students, members of the health team, and consumers of nursing care; read the many reports on health, manpower, education, technology, and social issues and problems; and find the trends that are, or soon will be, beating hard on her doors [38].

The world of the nurse director is changing in subtle and dramatic ways. The world is growing smaller and more complex as each part needs the other part for existence and growth. A nurse director strives to work with and relate to all parts of the environment that interact with nursing services. There will be a greater need than before for nurse directors with the ability to see interdependence and to respond accordingly to changing situations.

A nurse director should develop her abilities to analyze critically, to confront, to negotiate, and to implement appropriate changes within the nursing department and in the hospital. When disparities exist that are incongruent with the notion of quality patient care or with the guiding philosophy that influences how nurses are to function to provide that level of care, the nurse director should intervene for change. Her task is not only to teach or prepare herself to expect and seek change but also to do likewise for her nursing staff; she needs to find ways to help them become committed to change (see Appendix 25). By her example, the nurse director could begin by professing in work and action her belief in change and progress. Nurse directors who really believe in change and who attempt continuously to adapt and readapt ideas, plans, and practices must expect sometimes to "run a messy ship"; they should not expect to know all the answers before making a move. A modern approach requires time, in a sense, for a "muddling through" style of leadership, defined as the art and science of making incremental changes; this means one small gain, followed by another and another of testing and retesting [43].

THE NURSE DIRECTOR

While the nurse director strives to establish and maintain the human resources of the hospital, she must recognize the inevitable problem of difficult relationships. Sometimes these are personal; other times they involve the whole nursing department; or the problem may externalize itself in physician-nurse relationships. To recognize that whenever a group of people work together there are bound to be frictions, hostilities, and inadequate communication — and to accept this fact — can help reduce some of a nurse director's sense of defeat and frustration. Whatever a director plans to do administratively should never be stopped by a fatalistic negation based on difficult relationships [44]. The nurse director has a great social responsibility, regardless of the existing problems, to make it possible for those who work in the hospital or nursing department to perform effectively.

The tremendous task of creating an environment in which people can work together harmoniously and with coordinated effort requires patience, persistence, and courage. The nurse director does not shoulder this task alone. She exercises leadership but engages her whole staff. She recognizes that the involvement type of organizational climate is essential to administering nursing services. Modern problems are too complex and diversified for one person or one approach. Therefore, there is a need to blend skills and perspectives in the form of problem sharing and problem solving to achieve the desired goals for patient care. However, it must be remembered that synergy through the effectiveness of people cannot be achieved instantaneously or through directives — that people require time and opportunity for the development of trust, communication, and commitment [32].

EMERGING ROLES IN NURSING

There is an emerging group of professional nurses with diverse advanced educational preparation (and with a variety of labels) who may seek employment in hospitals. Some nurse directors may welcome these practitioners as adding a new dimension to nursing services, whereas others may perceive them as impractical. Since the preparation of each of these advanced practitioners may vary, a nurse director and her staff should learn about these categories of nursing and ask what they can provide to enhance nursing services. In many situations, position descriptions that fit these roles may not exist within the organizational structure.

Even if a nurse director wanted to employ some of these advanced practitioners, the number of potential employees available at the present time would be limited. However, if they were available, the nurse director should ask herself if she would be willing to utilize an advanced nurse practitioner in nursing services. A prospective advanced nurse practitioner should be able to describe what she believes she could do for patient care, present an outline of her curriculum plan, and demonstrate a willingness to fit into the organizational structure in light of the nursing service philosophy of a setting. Successful nurse practitioners have learned that their role depends on an ability to relate well to others; no matter how well prepared a nurse is, expertise is no guarantee of entry into the nursing system.

Recognizing that advanced nursing practitioner roles can enhance nursing services, a nurse director can set the stage for their arrival by: (1) showing open trust and acceptance of the newly employed nurse; (2) interpreting the new role to the staff and the hospital personnel; (3) allowing the nurse to establish her own position description (if it does not already exist) and asking other members of the nursing staff for suggestions; (4) encouraging creativity on the part of the new practitioner; (5) serving as a sounding board for the nurse's creative ideas that could provide quality nursing care; (6) structuring the position within the organization so that the advanced practitioner will know to whom she is responsible; (7) recognizing that advanced nursing roles represent nurses who have advanced clinical knowledge, are more flexible, and are able to function more independently than in the past; and (8) sharing in the evaluation of the role within the nursing service department.

The nurse director and her staff must be attuned to the health and nursing issues of today and tomorrow. It is desirable to challenge the nursing staff, under nursing administration leadership, to develop position statements that represent individual as well as collective thinking on the following issues:

Continuing education for re-licensure
Peer review

Patient's bill of rights
Role of nurse practitioners
Independent nurse practitioners
Levels of nursing education
National health insurance
Career ladder
Certification programs (ANA)
Accreditation of nursing education programs
One professional organization
Institutional licensure
Mandatory continuing education
Voluntary continuing education
Role of nurse in health care delivery system
Baccalaureate degree as minimal qualification for the professional
    nurse
Professional rights and autonomy
Financing of nursing education programs

Many more issues can well be added. The idea is to stimulate the nursing staff to think critically about what is happening now and what can be done to plan for the future of nursing. N. Butler says: "People, it has been said, can be placed in three classes: the few who make things happen, the many who watch things happen, and the overwhelming majority who have no idea what has happened." It is hoped that nurse directors are among the many who make quality nursing care happen. The nurse director will strive to bring the overwhelming majority of nursing staff, health care providers, and consumers to share in shaping an effective hospital care system for the community.

Part V References

1. Alexander, E., et al. *Nursing Service Administration.* St. Louis: Mosby, 1962.
2. Althouse, H. How OSHA affects hospitals and nursing homes. *Am. J. Nurs.* 75:450, 1975.
3. American Hospital Association. Administrative communications. *Practical Approaches to Nursing Service Administration* 3:2, 1964.
4. American Hospital Association. Coordination of functions. *Practical Approaches to Nursing Service Administration* 6:3, 1969.
5. American Hospital Association. The nursing department's function in formalized educational programs. *Practical Approaches to Nursing Service Administration* 8:3, 1969.
6. American Hospital Association. Nurse-physician relationships. *Practical Approaches to Nursing Service Administration* 10:2, 1971.
7. Argyris, C. *Integrating the Individual and the Organization.* New York: Wiley, 1964.
8. Aydelotte, M. Gaps Between Service and Education. In *The Health Manpower Dilemma.* New York: National League for Nursing, 1970.
9. Beach, D. *Personnel: The Management of People at Work.* New York: Macmillan, 1967.
10. Bennis, W., et al. *The Planning of Change.* New York: Holt, Rinehart, and Winston, 1969.
11. BNA Films. The Cine Conference Center, Rockville, Md.
12. Brown, R. E. *Judgment in Administration.* New York: McGraw-Hill, 1966.
13. Clark, B. Economy, change, and renewal. Unpublished paper presented at the Conference on Education and Productive Society, University of Alberta, Canada, 1964.
14. Committee on Nursing. Medicine and nursing in the 1970's: A position statement. *J.A.M.A.* 213:1881, 1970.
15. Committee on Nursing. Objectives and program of the AMA Committee on Nursing. *J.A.M.A.* 213:1881, 1970.
16. Delou, G., and Gebbie, K. *Political Dynamics — Impact on Nurses and Nursing.* St. Louis: Mosby, 1975.
17. Drucker, P. *The Effective Executive.* New York: Harper & Row, 1967.
18. *Employer's Labor Relations Guidebook.* Indianapolis: Indiana State Chamber of Commerce, 1970.
19. Frey, M. Administration in nursing service: The stimulus for change. *Int. Nurs. Rev.* 18:15–50, 1971.
20. Gaynor, W. How costly is your labor turnover? *Personnel Admin.* 15:30, 1970.
21. Gellerman, S. *Motivation and Productivity.* New York: American Management Association, 1963.
22. Herzberg, F. One more time: How do you motivate employees? *Harvard Bus. Rev.* 46:53, 1968.
23. Lee, I. Cope with resistance to change. *Nursing '73,* March, 1973.
24. Leninger, M. The leadership crisis in nursing: A critical problem and challenge. *J. Nurs. Admin.* 4:28, 1974.
25. Likert, O. *The Human Organization.* New York: McGraw-Hill, 1967.
26. Lippitt, R., et al. *The Dynamics of Planned Change.* New York: Harcourt, Brace, and World, 1958.

27. Maslow, A. H. *Motivation and Personality.* New York: Harper & Row, 1954.
28. Massie, L., and Douglas, J. *Managing — A Contemporary Introduction.* Englewood Cliffs, N.J.: Prentice-Hall, 1973.
29. McGregor, D. *The Human Side of the Enterprise.* New York: McGraw-Hill, 1960.
30. Miller, M. Nurses' right to strike. *J. Nurs. Admin.* 5:35, 1975.
31. Mills, A. *Functional Planning of General Hospitals.* New York: McGraw-Hill, 1969.
32. Myers, M. S. *Every Employee a Manager.* New York: McGraw-Hill, 1970.
33. Odiorne, G. *How Managers Make Things Happen.* Englewood Cliffs, N.J.: Prentice-Hall, 1973.
34. Osterhaus, L. Union-management relations in 30 hospitals change little in three years. *Hosp. Prog.* 48:68, 1967.
35. Pellagrino, E., and Duke, M. What's wrong with the nurse-physician relationship in today's hospitals? *Hospitals* 40:70, 1966.
36. Pigors, P., and Myers, C. *Personnel Administration.* New York: McGraw-Hill, 1965.
37. Quint, J. Communication problems affecting patient care in hospitals. *J.A.M.A.* 195:36, 1966.
38. Reinkemeyer, A. An ideology of change. *Nurs. Forum* 9:340, 1970.
39. Roethlisberger, R. *Management and Morale.* Cambridge, Mass.: Harvard University Press, 1950.
40. Rush, H. *Behavioral Science — Concepts and Management Application.* New York: Conference Board, 1969.
41. Stevens, B. Effecting change. *J. Nurs. Admin.* 4:23, 1975.
42. U.S. Department of Health, Education, and Welfare, Health Services and Mental Health Administration. HMO — the concept and structure. Washington, D.C.: The Department of H.E.W., 1974.
43. Watson, G. *Resistance to Change: Concepts for Social Change.* Washington, D.C.: National Education Association, 1967.
44. Weber, H. Nursing from Reality. In *Better Patient Care from the Organized Nursing Service's Point of View.* New York: National League for Nursing, 1965.
45. Werther, W., and Lockhart, C. *Labor Relations in the Health Professions.* Boston: Little, Brown and Company, 1976.
46. Wortman, M., and Randle, C. W. *Collective Bargaining — Principles and Practices.* Boston: Houghton Mifflin, 1966.
47. Zimmerman, A. Taft-Hartley revised — implications for nursing. *Am. J. Nurs.* 75:284, 1975.

Appendixes

STATEMENT ON A PATIENT'S BILL OF RIGHTS

1. The patient has the right to considerate and respectful care.
2. The patient has the right to obtain from his physician complete current information concerning his diagnosis, treatment, and prognosis in terms the patient can reasonably be expected to understand. When it is not medically advisable to give such information to the patient, the information should be made available to an appropriate person in his behalf. He has the right to know, by name, the physician responsible for coordinating his care.
3. The patient has the right to receive from his physician information necessary to give informed consent prior to the start of any procedure and/or treatment. Except in emergencies, such information for informed consent should include but not necessarily be limited to the specific procedure and/or treatment, the medically significant risks involved, and the probable duration of incapacitation. Where medically significant alternatives for care or treatment exist, or when the patient requests information concerning medical alternatives, the patient has the right to such information. The patient also has the right to know the name of the person responsible for the procedures and/or treatment.
4. The patient has the right to refuse treatment to the extent permitted by law and be informed of the medical consequences of his action.
5. The patient has the right to every consideration of his privacy concerning his own medical care program. Case discussion, consultation, examination, and treatment are confidential and should be conducted discreetly. Those not directly involved in his care must have the permission of the patient to be present.
6. The patient has the right to expect that all communications and records pertaining to his care should be treated as confidential.
7. The patient has the right to expect that within its capacity a hospital must make reasonable response to the request of a patient for services. The hospital must provide evaluation, service, and/or referral as indicated by the urgency of the case. When medically permissible, a patient may be transferred to

*Reprinted, with permission, from *Hospitals, Journal of the American Hospital Association*, 47 (February 16, 1973), p. 42.

another facility only after he has received complete information and explanation concerning the needs for and alternatives to such a transfer. The institution to which the patient is to be transferred must first have accepted the patient for transfer.

8. The patient has the right to obtain information as to any relationship of his hospital to other health care and educational institutions insofar as his care is concerned. The patient has the right to obtain information as to the existence of any professional relationships among individuals by name, who are treating him.

9. The patient has the right to be advised if the hospital proposes to engage in or perform human experimentation affecting his care or treatment. The patient has the right to refuse to participate in such research projects.

10. The patient has the right to expect reasonable continuity of care. He has the right to know in advance what appointment times and physicians are available and where. The patient has the right to expect that the hospital will provide a mechanism whereby he is informed by his physician or a delegate of the physician of the patient's continuing health care requirements following discharge.

11. The patient has the right to examine and receive an explanation of his bill regardless of source of payment.

12. The patient has the right to know what hospital rules and regulations apply to his conduct as a patient.

CHRONOLOGY OF MAJOR FEDERAL HEALTH
PLANNING LEGISLATION

1946   The Hospital Survey and Construction Act (Hill-Burton)
provided, among other things, for the creation of a state
hospital planning council to assess the need for new hospital
construction and to develop a plan indicating priorities to
meet these needs.

1961   The Community Health Services and Facilities Act, among
other things, provided grants for voluntary health facility
planning agencies at the local level.

1964   The Hospital and Medical Facilities amendments (Hill-Harris
Act, P.L. 88-443) provided funds for modernization or
replacement of health care facilities, as well as providing
additional funds for facility planning purposes. In addition,
the law provided matching funds for the purpose of establishing health facility planning agencies in areas where there
had been none before.

1966   The Comprehensive Health Planning and Public Health Service amendments (P.L. 89-749) provided health revenue
sharing funds for state governments, plus grants for comprehensive health planning at the state and local level.

1972   The Social Security amendments of 1972 (P.L. 92-603)
added, among other things, Sections 234 and 1122 to the
Social Security Act. Section 234 requires institutional planning by hospitals, extended care facilities, and home health
agencies as a condition to participate in Medicare. Section
1122 provides, in participating states, that health care facilities and HMOs would not be reimbursed by Medicare (Title
18), Medicaid (Title 19) or the Maternal and Child Health
Programs (Title 5) for depreciation, interest, and return on
equity capital relating to capital expenditures determined by
designated state agencies to be unnecessary.

1975   The National Health Planning and Resources Development
Act of 1974 (P.L. 93-641) amends the Public Health Services
Act by adding Titles 15 and 16. Title 15 revises existing
health planning programs at the state and area-wide level as
well as encouraging the Secretary of HEW to work on the

*Reprinted, with permission, from *Hospitals, Journal of the American Hospital
Association*, 50 (June 16, 1976), p. 128.

development of national health policy. Title 16 revises the Hill-Burton program for the construction and modernization of health care facilities, linking the award of grants and loans to the mechanisms created in Title 15.

NURSING SERVICE DEPARTMENT OF SAINT LOUIS
UNIVERSITY HOSPITALS*　　277 Beds
St. Louis, Missouri

Nursing Service Philosophy, Scope and Objectives

I. Introduction:
   The Nursing Service is an organized professional department of
   Saint Louis University Hospitals. Directly responsible to Hos-
   pital Administration.

II. Purpose:
   The purpose of Nursing Service is to provide the best possible
   care for the total needs of the patient in accordance with the
   policies set forth by the administrative body and the dictates
   of Christian Charity.

III. Philosophy:
   We of the Nursing Service Department support the philosophy
   of Saint Louis University as set forth in the Credo of Saint
   Louis University. We believe that Nursing Service has an obligation to minister to the diverse needs of the patient; physical,
   psychological, spiritual and economic. That we have a duty
   toward the relatives to treat them with kindness and keep them
   informed regarding the progress of the patient.

IV. Scope:
   The scope of Nursing Service embraces:
   A. The administration and promotion of good nursing care
      based upon scientific principles and directed toward the
      total needs of the patient.
   B. Active participation in health groups for: promotion of
      health, prevention of disease, research in improvement of
      nursing care, and rehabilitation of the disabled.
   C. Continuing contribution to nursing education through the
      provision of excellent nursing care and cooperation with
      the School of Nursing.

V. Objectives:
   To provide nursing care that is safe, intelligent and scientifically
   sound.
   To provide nursing service in full accordance with the policies
   and philosophy of the Hospital.

*Reprinted by permission of Saint Louis University, St. Louis, Missouri.

To provide nursing care which meets the standards of care as established by the Department of Nursing.

To provide an environment conducive to self-development.

To engage in a continuing program of research for the improvement of nursing care.

JEWISH HOSPITAL*   441 Beds
Louisville, Kentucky

Section I. Purposes

The Jewish Hospital is open to every creed and is operated:

A. To establish and maintain a hospital for the care of persons suffering from illnesses or disabilities which require that the patients receive hospital care.

B. To carry on any educational activities related to rendering care to sick and injured or the promotion of health, which in the opinion of the Board of Trustees may be justified by the facilities, personnel, funds or other requirements that are, or can be, made available.

C. To promote and carry on scientific research related to the care of the sick and injured insofar as, in the opinion of the Board of Trustees, such research can be carried on in, or in connection with, the hospital.

D. To participate, so far as circumstances may warrant, in any activity designed and carried on to promote the general health of the community.

E. To provide facilities, conducted on Israelitic lines, wherein the sick and injured of any faith can enjoy during their illness the observance and consolation of their religion.

F. To carry out any other activity that is covered in the Articles of Incorporation of the Jewish Hospital Association of Louisville, Kentucky, as amended November 9, 1932.

Jewish Hospital Nursing Department
Philosophy

Nursing Service believes:

That man is the creation of God and that His dignity is to be respected in life and death.

*Reprinted by permission of Jewish Hospital, Louisville, Kentucky.

That the Golden Rule is basic to all interpersonal relationships.

That the needs of patients, physical, emotional, social and spiritual, must be met through coordinated efforts of nursing, medicine, and other allied health and welfare disciplines without regard for race, creed, or ability to pay, as outlined in the Articles of Incorporation of the hospital.

That nursing service is the department through which the team effort of the entire hospital organization can be coordinated to achieve its objectives for the patient. When the total organization is administered by democratic principles within the framework of sound policy the hospital emerges an entity which is something more than the sum total of its parts.

That continuing education for all levels of personnel is essential. Personal satisfaction through realization of goals helps to create stability which maintains the high standards of patient care at Jewish Hospital.

That Nursing Service creates and maintains an atmosphere conducive to learning to allow the medical and nursing programs to achieve their objectives.

MIAMI VALLEY HOSPITAL*   800 Beds
DEPARTMENT OF NURSING SERVICE
Dayton, Ohio

The Philosophy of Nursing Services

We, the Miami Valley Hospital, Department of Nursing Service, believe in the personal worth of each individual. Therefore, we are committed to administer optimum patient-centered care for each person coming to us for assistance along his illness-health continuum and to provide an environment conducive to the maximum development of each employee in the Department of Nursing Service. Accordingly, preservation of individual human dignity for both patient and employee shall be realized.

Goals and Objectives

Goals:
1. Manage and administer the highest degree of quality, individualized comprehensive patient- and family-centered care to

*Reprinted by permission of Miami Valley Hospital, Dayton, Ohio.

each person needing assistance to attain and maintain or regain his highest level of wellness.

2. Maintain an adequate and competent nursing staff who can recognize job satisfaction utilizing the employee appraisal system and through personal growth experiences.
3. Provide educational opportunities which will facilitate personal and professional growth for the nursing and allied health care personnel.
4. Promote the attainment and maintenance of a high degree of community health team cooperation and communication.
5. Support and implement the hospital policies and financial plans of Miami Valley Hospital.
6. Maintain a high level of cooperation, interaction, and goodwill between the hospital and the community which it serves.

Objectives:

1. Develop recognition of each patient's need for independence, his right for privacy, and his desire for self-awareness in relationship to his illness.
2. Provide effective patient care related to the patient's needs as much as the hospital and community facilities permit.
3. Encourage interaction and involvement with the patient and his family in order to assist him in his acceptance of and/or adjustment to his condition.
4. Carry out therapeutic measures ordered by the physician with intelligent application to the individual needs of the patient.
5. Continually study and evaluate the quality of patient care and implement improvements.
6. Create an atmosphere that is favorable to both patient and employee morale and to personnel growth.
7. Appreciate and acknowledge the contribution and worth of all personnel in assuring quality patient care.
8. Estimate the requirements of personnel for the Department of Nursing Service and recommend and implement policies and procedures to maintain an adequate and competent nursing staff.
9. Continually evaluate the competency and attitude of all employees in the Department of Nursing Service.
10. Provide an orientation program for new employees and provide for the continuing and in-service education needs of all Nursing Service personnel.

11. Develop an awareness and understanding of the legal responsibilities in nursing and practice within this framework.
12. Initiate, utilize, and/or participate in studies or research projects designed for the improvement of nursing administration and other hospital services.
13. Participate in and/or facilitate all educational programs which include student experiences in the Department of Nursing Service.
14. Encourage and provide the means and methods by which the nursing personnel can work with other groups in interpreting the objectives of the hospital and nursing service to the patient and community.
15. Maintain sufficient hospital supplies and promote their proper utilization.
16. Promote communication to nursing personnel regarding implementation of and changes in hospital policy, either patient-centered or employee-centered.
17. Coordinate the functions of the Department of Nursing Service with the functions of all other departments and services of Miami Valley Hospital.
18. Foster and maintain good public relations.

ST. JOHN'S HOSPITAL*   173 Beds
Salina, Kansas

Philosophy of St. John's Hospital

St. John's Hospital, operated under the sponsorship of the Sisters of St. Joseph of Concordia, Kansas, is founded on a belief in God and in the dignity of man as created by God; and in this creation, man is endowed with certain needs, rights, privileges, obligations and abilities.

We believe man has physical, psychological, spiritual and social needs. We believe that God and man are served in a special manner by those who strive to meet those needs regardless of race, color, creed and social or economic status.

We believe that good health is living at the highest level of wellness of which one is capable.

*Reprinted by permission of St. John's Hospital, Salina, Kansas.

We believe that people's health needs and the health care system are constantly changing, requiring innovative and effective leadership, and the greater emphasis should be placed upon the prevention of illness while maintaining quality acute care services consistent with the ethical and religious directives as promulgated by the Catholic Hospital Association.

We believe that our employees are persons of dignity and worth and must be given the opportunity and encouragement to develop both personally and professionally as well as to be appropriately involved in the operation and direction of the institution.

We believe that our medical staff, volunteer groups and community are people of dignity and worth who make significant contributions to the institution and should be appropriately supported and involved.

Mission

To provide quality health care services and programs which restore and promote good health primarily to the citizens of North Central Kansas, and to provide physicians, employees and other resources necessary for delivery of quality care within a secondary level health care organization.

Philosophy of St. John's Hospital Nursing Department

We, the members of the Nursing Service Department, believe that nursing is a service to mankind which renders the best possible care to all patients irrespective of race, creed, and status.

We believe that the emphasis of this service must be on the spiritual, physical, and emotional needs of the patient who is perceived as a person and as a member of society.

We believe that nursing care of the highest standard demands a working environment which is conducive to professional, emotional, and social growth of all persons.

We believe that cooperative human activity and wholesome human relationships with effective lines of communication result in loyal and satisfied personnel and consequent attainment of goals.

We believe that through continued educational programs, evaluation of nursing care rendered, and research activities, nursing service cooperates with hospital administration in promoting curative, preventive, and rehabilitative aspects of nursing as well as supporting health practices in the family and community.

Objectives

1. To give a high quality of nursing care for the patients in St. John's Hospital geared to meet spiritual, psychological, physical, and social needs of patients.
2. To carry out therapeutic measures as ordered by the physician, with intelligent application to the needs of the individual patient.
3. To make studies relating to nursing care and nursing service in order to improve the quality of nursing care and effective utilization of nursing personnel.
4. To provide orientation, in-service, and continuing educational programs to promote personal and professional growth of personnel.
5. To promote good personnel policies and practices to further the self-development of all groups within the department.
6. To foster and coordinate with nursing education activities which contribute to the welfare of the patients, students, and nursing personnel.
7. To participate in all programs basic to the purposes of such education and research as the hospital may carry on which involve nursing service activities.
8. To formulate and recommend policies for the improvement of patient care.
9. To cooperate with all departments of the hospital in achieving the total purposes of the hospital.
10. To foster and maintain good public relations through its personnel both in their functional capacities and as individuals in the community.

COOK COUNTY HOSPITAL*   1495 Beds
DEPARTMENT OF NURSING SERVICES
Chicago, Illinois

Philosophy of Nursing Service Administration

Nursing Service Administration believes that:

I. The patient has a basic right to expect and receive quality health care at Cook County Hospital.

*Reprinted by permission of Cook County Hospital, Chicago, Illinois.

    II. Patient care depends upon the efficient and economical opera-
tion of all of the hospital services. Toward this end, Nursing
Service Administration will function under a triad plan in
which there will be shared responsibility and accountability
with Hospital and Medical Administration.

    III. Nursing services and activities must be patient-centered.

    IV. Good human resources are an organization's priceless asset. Job
satisfaction and the general welfare of its personnel are of
sincere concern to Nursing Service Administration.

    V. Nursing is a vital service based on scientific knowledge and
should be relevant to the changing needs of society.

    VI. Nursing has the responsibility to provide and encourage a
suitable climate for varied learning experiences.

The forms in appendixes 4 through 8, 12 through 15, and 17 and 18 are used by permission of Deaconess Hospital, Evansville, Indiana. The figures cited in these forms are meant as examples and are not intended to represent actual figures. — M. D.

Objectives
Nursing Service Department

Nursing Unit _____
Quarter Dates _____
Annual Date _____

Objectives	Comments	Proposed Period for Achievement		
		Fiscal Quarter (3 mos.)	Short Range (Under 12 mos.)	Long Range (Over 12 mos.)
1. Establish an experimental unit for the purpose of study and research to improve nursing care.	Will coordinate with Hospital Research Committee.			X
1.1 Develop a plan of action to establish an experimental unit.		1st Quarter		
1.2 Identify methods other hospital nursing services use to improve the practice of nursing.		3rd Quarter		
1.3 Submit recommendations to nursing administration.		4th Quarter		
2. Study the concept of primary nursing care as a system of delivery of nursing service.				X
2.1 Develop a plan of action to study the concept of primary nursing.		1st Quarter		
2.2 Initiate a plan of action for study.		2nd Quarter		

2.3 Submit report and recommendations to director of nursing. 4th Quarter X

3. Identify activities that are non-nursing and make recommendations to hospital administration.

3.1 Involve nursing units in study of nursing activities. 2nd Quarter

3.2 Make recommendations to hospital administration. 4th Quarter

Prepared by: _____ Date _____

_____ Date _____

Reviewed by: _____ Date _____

General Ledger Monthly Expense Account Summary
Nursing Service Expenses
Department of Nursing

	Current			Year-to-Date			Account No.	Description
Feb. Expense	Actual Expense	Budget	Last Actual	Actual Expense	Budget	Last Actual		
							100	Salaries & wages
							125	Employee medical examination
							126	Employees' medical care
							135	Uniforms
							140	Supplies
							142	Books, periodicals & subscriptions
							145	Dues & membership fees
							146	Textbooks
							148	Library supplies
							151	Travel & seminars
							154	Medical-surgical supplies — chargeable
							155	Medical-surgical supplies — non-chargeable
							156	Drug & pharmaceutical supplies
							159	IV solutions and sets
							190	Telephone, telegraph, & comm. system

Continued

General Ledger Monthly Expense Account Summary (Continued)

Feb. Expense	Current			Year-to-Date			Account No.	Description
	Actual Expense	Budget	Last Actual	Actual Expense	Budget	Last Actual		
							192	Gas
							194	Water
							206	Miscellaneous repairs & maintenance
							209	Electrical repairs & maintenance
							220	Laundry service
							227	Disposal service
							232	Dairy products and formula
							241	Freight & parcel post
							245	Special lab work
							264	Other professional fees
							271	Other equipment rental
							350	Miscellaneous
							901	Provision for depreciation of equipment

Nursing Unit 34
Expense Report
Forecast versus Actual

April Month Expenses	Current Actual Expenses	Current Budget	Current Last-Yr. Expenses	Account No.	Description	Year-to-Date Actual Expenses	Year-to-Date Budget	Year-to-Date Last-Yr. Expenses
10,765	11,214	9,698	9,622	100	Salaries & wages	11,214	9,698	9,622
100	94	99	108	140	Supplies	94	99	108
189	86	80		154	Medical-surgical supplies — chargeable	86	80	
337	230	250	209	155	Medical-surgical supplies — non-chargeable	230	250	209
39	47	38	37	156	Drug & pharmaceutical supplies	47	38	37
		30		159	IV solutions and sets		30	
10	19	17	35	215	Miscellaneous repairs & maintenance	19	17	35
478	399	700	629	325	Student nurse time	399	700	629
135	135	100	73	901	Depreciation — equipment	135	100	73

Department Totals	Current April Month Expenses	Current Actual Expenses	Current Budget	Current Last-Yr. Expenses	Year-to-Date Actual Expenses	Year-to-Date Budget	Year-to-Date Last-Yr. Expenses
	12,053	12,224	11,012	10,713	12,224	11,012	10,713

NURSING DEPARTMENT
Proposed Capital Expenditure Items Requested by
the Nursing Units for the Fiscal Year 1977–1978

Requesting Unit	Item	Number Needed	Cost Each	Total
NSO	Copier	1	$2500.00	$2500.00
NSO	Typewriter	1	250.00	250.00
All Units	Addressograph Recorders	20	100.00	2000.00
SU	IV Support Hangers	6	250.00	1500.00
SU	Surgical Case Carts	1	846.00	846.00
20, 33	Stretcher Cart with Backrest	2	420.00	840.00
EU	Table, Examining	1	730.00	730.00
EU, ICU	Wheelchairs	4	250.00	1000.00
44	CircOlectric Bed	1	1500.00	1500.00
22, 30, 40	Refrigerators	3	300.00	900.00
EU, 20, 30	Portable Weight Scales	2	190.00	380.00
24, 26	Desk	2	250.00	500.00
24, 26	Chairs, Desk	2	100.00	200.00
24, 26, NSO	File Cabinet	3	100.00	300.00
Total				$13,446.00

NSO = Nursing Service Office
EU = Emergency Unit
SU = Surgery Unit
ICU = Intensive Care Unit

7. Hospital Calendar Budget

Date	Participants	Activity
January 15	Hospital Administration Budget Officer Department Directors	General discussion of budget planning for new fiscal year.
February 1	Hospital Administration Budget Officer Department Directors	General discussion of budget and presentation on anticipated activity for next year. Consider hospital objectives and capital projects.
February 2	Data Processing Director Budget Officer	Prepare personnel base information and expense work sheets for Department Directors.
February 3	Budget Officer	Distribute personnel base information and expense work sheets to Department Directors.
February 4– March 30	Hospital Administration Department Directors	Review of first draft of a departmental budget by Department Director and the administrative officer to whom he reports. Justifications for additional expense or personnel requirements are reviewed. Revisions made, if necessary.
March 1	Budget Officer	Deadline for budget forms and information from Department Directors.

Date	*Participants*	*Activity*
March 3–30	Budget Officer	Compile income and expense budget for hospital and submit to Administration.
April 1	Hospital Administration	Final approval of income and expense budget. Determine amount of funds available for capital expenditure.
April 10	Budget Officer Department Directors	Meet to determine how allocated capital expenditure funds will be distributed among the departments.
April 15	Hospital Administration Board of Directors	Review, approve and recommend revisions if necessary.
April 25	Hospital Administration	Distribute final approved budget to Department Directors.
May 1	Hospital Administration Department Directors	Administer new fiscal hospital budget.

Date	*Participants*	*Activity*
January 15	Nurse Directors Assistant Directors Supervisors Administrative Assistant Head Nurses	General discussion of nursing budget planning for the new fiscal year.
January 16	Administrative Assistant Nursing Service Office Secretaries	Prepare work sheets for personnel unit staffing requirement, expense budget, and capital expenditures.
January 23	Nurse Director Nursing Budget Committee	General discussion of the nursing budget and presentation on overall departmental anticipated activity for the coming year. Consider departmental objectives and capital needs.
January 25	Nurse Director Assistant Director Supervisors	General discussion of the nursing unit budgets and overall departmental anticipated activity for the coming year. Consider unit objectives and capital needs. Distribute budget work sheets to supervisors.
January 30	Supervisors Head Nurses Assistant Head Nurses	Plan for personnel requirements, expense budget, and capital expenditures for each nursing unit. First draft of unit budget plan.

Date	Participants	Activity
February 3	Nurse Director	Receive personnel base information and expense work sheets from Budget Officer.
February 10	Supervisors	Submit budget drafts to the Nurse Director.
February 15–17	Nurse Director Nursing Budget Committee	Review first draft of the nursing departmental budget prepared by those responsible for segments of the budget.
February 18		Director and Committee invite the Supervisor, Head Nurse, and Assistant Head Nurse of each nursing unit to present and review their budgetary needs. Revision made if necessary.
February 23	Nurse Director Administrative Assistant	Compile and prepare proposed budget. Complete budget work sheets requested by Budget Officer.
February 27–28	Hospital Administrator Nurse Director	Review first draft of nursing budget. Justifications for additional expense or personnel requirements are reviewed. Revision made, if necessary.

Date	Participants	Activity
March 1	Nurse Director	Submit budget forms and information to Budget Officer.
April 25	Nurse Director	Receive approved nursing budget from Hospital Administration.
April 27	Nurse Director	Distribute sections of budget to Nursing Administrative Staff.
May 1	Nurse Director Administrative Staff	Administer new fiscal nursing budget.

9. Nursing Definitions

I. *Nursing* in its broadest sense may be defined as an art and a
    science which involves the whole patient — body, mind, and
    spirit; promotes his spiritual, mental and physical health by
    teaching and by example; stresses health education and health
    preservation as well as ministration and spiritual as well as
    physical; and gives health service to the family and the com-
    munity as well as to the individual.

    — Sister M. Olivia Gowan: *Proceedings of the Workshop on Administra-
    tion of College Programs in Nursing*, June 12–24, 1944. Washington,
    D.C.: Catholic University of America Press, 1946, p. 10.

II. Nursing is not only a performance of skills and techniques;
    nursing is care of patients with the responsibility and need for
    the nurse to understand people, their motivation and their
    behavior. The use of this understanding throughout all of her
    care of these patients that she serves, to that ultimate well-
    being and self-realization for them, is an interacting operation
    that must be considered in the measurement of the goodness
    of care.

    — Frances Reiter Kreuter: The Evaluation of Nursing Care. In *The
    Yearbook of Modern Nursing, 1957–58*. New York: Putnam, 1958,
    pp. 193–194. Originally printed in the December, 1956, issue of *The
    Minnesota Nurse.*

III. Professional nursing is an art and a science dominated by an
     ideal of service in which certain principles are applied in the
     skillful care of the sick in appropriate relationship with the
     physician and with others who have related responsibilities.
     It is concerned equally with the prevention of disease and the
     conservation of health. Skillful care embraces the whole
     person — body, mind and soul — his physical, mental and
     spiritual well-being. Nursing encompasses:

     1. Caring for the sick and injured, bringing to bear the re-
        sources of the patient, his family and environment and
        the services of available cooperating personnel to facilitate
        his recovery and rehabilitation in accordance to the
        diagnosis made and treatment prescribed by a licensed
        physician.

359

2. Helping an individual and his family to take positive action in relief of illness and improvement of his individual, family and community health needs.
3. Training students and auxiliary personnel to function as members of the nursing team.
4. Adapting nursing service to cooperate with responsible planning authorities in emergencies due to disaster caused by disease and natural causes of war.
5. Evaluating and conducting research to continually improve methods whereby nursing in particular and health medical care adequately meet society's needs.
6. Sharing with others in the dissemination of general health information to individuals and community groups to further the cultivation of health.

— R. Louise McManus. Reprinted by permission of the publisher from R. Louise McManus, "Society's Demands of Nurses That Influence Nursing Education," *Problems of Graduate Nurse Education*, Work Conference Report No. 2. (New York: Teachers College Press, copyright 1952 by Teachers College, Columbia University), pp. 12 and 13.

IV. The unique function of the nurse is to assist the individual, sick or well, in the performance of those activities contributing to health or its recovery (or to peaceful death) that he would perform unaided if he had the necessary strength, will or knowledge. And to do this in such a way as to help him gain independence as rapidly as possible. This aspect of her work, this part of her function, she initiates and controls; of this she is master . . . She also, as a member of a medical team, helps other members, as they in turn help her, to plan and carry out the total program whether it be for the improvement of health, or the recovery from illness or support in death.

—Virginia Henderson: *ICN Basic Principles of Nursing Care* (rev. 1969). Basel: Karger, 1969. Published for International Council of Nurses.

V. Nursing is a humanistic science dedicated to compassionate concern for maintaining and promoting health, preventing illness, and caring for and rehabilitating the sick and disabled.

— M. E. Rogers: *An Introduction to the Theoretical Basis of Nursing.* Philadelphia: Davis, 1971, p. vii.

VI. Nursing is an encounter with a client and his family in which the nurse observes, supports, communicates, ministers, and teaches; she contributes to the maintenance of optimum health, and provides care during illness until the client is able to measure responsibility for the fulfillment of his own basic human needs; when necessary, she provides compassionate assistance with dying.

— H. Yura and M. Walsh: *The Nursing Process—Assessing, Planning, Implementing, Evaluating.* 2nd ed. New York: Appleton-Century-Croft, 1973, p. 14.

VII. Nursing practice is a direct service, goal directed and adaptable to the needs of the individual, family and community during health and illness. The practitioner of nursing bears the primary responsibility and accountability for the nursing care clients/patients receive.

— American Nurses' Association. *Standards of Nursing Practice.* Kansas City, Mo.: The Association, 1975.

VIII. Nursing. . . . one of the major sectors of the health care system; seen from the point of view of systems theory, nursing is a critical system, a part of an interdisciplinary effort to promote and maintain health, prevent disease and disability, and to care for, cure, and rehabilitate the sick.

— Patricia Hasse: *A Proposed System for Nursing Theoretical Framework, Part 2.* Atlanta: Nursing Curriculum Project, Southern Regional Education Board, June, 1976, p. 36.

AMERICAN NURSES' ASSOCIATION
PHILOSOPHY OF PEER REVIEW

It is the belief of the American Nurses' Association that practitioners of nursing bear primary responsibility and accountability for the quality of nursing care clients/patients receive. Standards of nursing practice provide a means for determining the quality of nursing care which a client receives and for evaluating that care. The individual nurse carries the major responsibility for interpreting and implementing standards of nursing practice and must actively participate in decision-making processes to determine, with others, mechanisms through which standards of nursing practice can be operationalized. Furthermore, it is the responsibility of all nurses to pursue some form of evaluation of nursing care.

It is the belief of the American Nurses' Association that one way to implement standards of nursing practice and to improve the quality of care is peer review. Peer review implies that the nursing care delivered by a group of nurses or an individual nurse is evaluated by individuals of the same rank or standing according to established standards of practice. The goals of any agency providing nursing care should include peer review as one means of maintaining standards of nursing practice and upgrading nursing care. In every health care facility in which nurses practice, provision for peer review should be an ongoing process.

The purposes of peer review are:

1. To evaluate the quality and quantity of nursing care as it is delivered by the individual practitioner and/or group of practitioners, the purpose being to identify the extent of consistency to established standards of practice.
2. To determine the strengths and weaknesses of nursing care.
3. To provide evidence to utilize as the basis of recommendations for new or altered policies and procedures to improve nursing care.
4. To identify those areas where practice patterns indicate more knowledge is needed.

In every health care facility in which nurses practice, there should

---

*Developed by the Ad Hoc Committee on Implementation of Standards of Nursing Practice of the Congress for Nursing Practice, November, 1973. Reprinted by permission of the American Nurses' Association.

be provision for continuing peer review as one means of maintaining standards of nursing practice and upgrading nursing care.

Peer Review Process

Peer Review is the process by which registered nurses, actively engaged in the practice of nursing, appraise the quality of nursing care in a given situation in accordance with established standards of practice.

The peer review process includes both the appraisal of nursing care delivered by a group of nurses in a given setting and the appraisal of nursing practiced by individual practitioners.

Nursing Professional Standards Review examines the sum total of nursing care delivered in a specific setting by a group of nurses. This type of review may fall into two categories:

1. A general survey to identify the usual quality or level of care delivered by the agency or group. A random sample of at least 10 percent of the cases involved should be assessed. If the number of cases is under fifty, all cases should be assessed.
2. A special purpose survey to identify the cause or results of a specific phenomenon (such as the use of specific nursing techniques, letters of commendation from clients, etc.). A stratified sample of only those cases which exhibit this phenomenon should be assessed. If the special purpose-centered survey is used, it must be remembered that it deals only with a limited population and, as a result, inferences cannot be made about the usual quality or level of care delivered by the group reviewed.

A peer review committee may find it appropriate to function using either or both approaches.

The objectives of Nursing Professional Standards Review are:

1. To evaluate the quality and quantity of nursing care delivered by a group of nurses in a specific setting,
2. To determine the strengths and weaknesses of nursing care delivered by a group of nurses in a specific setting, and
3. To provide evidence to utilize as the basis of recommendations for new or altered policies and procedures to improve nursing care delivered by a group of nurses in a specific setting.

Data collected from Nursing Professional Standards Review may be used by administrative personnel when identifying priorities. In addition, such surveys may provide input into nursing services, Professional Standards Review Organization committees and the Joint Practice Commission.

Nursing Performance Review examines care delivered by individual practitioners of nursing. This review is designed to aid the practitioner in assessing personal growth as a professional nurse and the quality of service provided. The purposes of this review are:

1. To assist the individual nurse in improving the quality of her practice, particularly in what may be identified as weak areas.
2. To offer commendation and/or constructive criticism of an individual nurse's performance when applicable.
3. To protect the nurse from ill-founded and unjust accusations.
4. To apprise the nurse of how significantly the nurse's practice deviates from accepted professional standards and, if so, to what extent.

Data collected from a Nursing Performance Review may be utilized to make recommendations to certification boards and/or provide input into the evaluation which qualifies the nurse for clinical advancement or merit increase.

Guidelines for Developing Peer Review Committees

Each peer review committee will have to determine whether its purpose will be to survey the sum total of nursing care delivered by a group of nurses in a specific setting or to survey care delivered by individual practitioners of nursing. One agency may prefer to have Nursing Professional Standards Review and Nursing Performance Review done by separate committees, while another agency will prefer to have one committee assume a dual function.

The following guidelines were developed for use by committees undertaking one or both types of review. It is the responsibility of the peer review committee to adapt these guidelines to the specific circumstances for which the committee was developed. Such factors as who instigated the committee (agency or concerned group of nurses), the size of the institution or agency and the objective for establishing the committee will affect the utilization of certain guidelines.

The intent of these guidelines is not to dictate rules for establishing peer review committees, but to provide assistance in the task of forming a peer review committee and identifying functions and policies.

Temporary Planning Committee

1. The establishment of a temporary planning committee (either elected or appointed) is a starting point in providing the careful, thorough planning needed to establish a peer review committee. It will be the responsibility of the initial committee to:
    a. Develop the guidelines and the format that all review activities will follow.
    b. Establish a pattern of accepting referrals for peer review.
    c. Develop a system for screening peer review material which may require additional investigation.
    d. Adopt established standards of practice from which guidelines for evaluating quality care may be delineated.
    e. Differentiate among situations for review; individual cases will be handled differently from a general nursing audit.
2. Although it is not essential that every activity performed by the permanent committee be outlined before that committee is established, the planning committee will want to carefully consider the following areas:
    a. Purpose and functions of the peer review committee
    b. Composition of the committee
    c. Guidelines to be utilized by the committee
    d. Scope and authority of the committee
    e. Policies and protocol of the committee
    f. Resource input
    g. Liability of the committee
    h. Nature of data and process of data collection

The temporary planning committee will also need to consider such administrative questions as time commitment, secretarial needs, financing, frequency of meetings and membership selection process. In addition, consideration should be given to conflicts which may arise from peer* evaluation. In some instances, personal relationships may make it impossible for a committee member to objectively review a co-worker.

*A peer is a registered nurse, actively engaged in the practice of nursing, who by that fact is accountable to the consumer for the plan of nursing care.

3. The initial phases of both the temporary planning committee and the permanent standing committee will involve a considerable amount of time as well as secretarial assistance. Initially, the committees may wish to schedule bi-weekly meetings and, once the committees are well established, monthly meetings thereafter. The committees will need to allow at least one year's time to develop workable tools.

4. It is recommended that agencies who have staff members participating on either temporary planning committees or permanent review committees assume this cost as part of their normal operating expenses. This recommendation is based upon the assumption that establishment of a peer review process will provide considerable assistance in maintaining a high standard of nursing care, thereby benefiting clients served by the agency.

5. When engaging in the process of identifying the guidelines to be used by the peer review committee, the temporary planning committee will want to consider:
   a. Established standards of practice (ANA Standards of Practice, SNA Standards of Practice, Code for Nurses, etc.)
   b. State Nurse Practice Acts
   c. Existing written resources that define quality of care (professional literature)

6. The importance of involving and informing as many nurses as possible, as soon as possible, cannot be overestimated.

Upon completion of the ground rules, the initial planning committee should publicize extensively the concept of peer review. In order to provide nurse practitioners with the opportunity for input regarding the mechanics and objectives of the peer review committee, open meetings should be held. Data collected from such meetings could be taken into account when the initial planning committee outlines final objectives for the permanent committee.

After the work of the temporary committee is completed, brochures should be printed and meetings held to publicize the expected purposes, functions, procedures, etc. of the peer review. Meetings need to be scheduled carefully and frequently to insure maximum attendance by nurses affected by the peer review committee.

Permanent Peer Review Committee

The following comments are meant as guidelines in aiding temporary planning committees in establishing permanent peer review committees. It should be emphasized, however, that each committee will find some aspects of its own situation to be unique. At these times the knowledge, abilities and common sense of the committee members will have to be relied on to carry the committee through.

1. Functions and Purpose:

Each committee will have to determine whether its function is 1) to appraise nursing care delivered by a group of nurses in a given setting (Nursing Professional Standards Review) and/or 2) to appraise the nursing practiced by individual practitioners (Nursing Performance Review).

Each committee will have to adapt the following purposes of peer review to the particular circumstances for establishing the committee:

a. To evaluate the quality and quantity of nursing care.

b. To determine the strengths and weaknesses of nursing care.

c. To provide evidence to utilize as the basis of recommendations for new or altered policies and procedures to improve nursing care.

d. To identify those areas where practice patterns indicate more knowledge is needed.

2. Composition and Representation:

The composition of the group will be affected by the method of selection. For example, membership may be determined by clinical expertise, administrative hierarchy or by the group as a whole. In addition, the composition of the committee will be affected by the setting in which the committee is formed.

The planning committee will need to select a system suitable to the needs of the area under consideration. In large agencies, each nursing department may establish a peer review committee with the total agency being served by a primary committee. In medium-sized agencies, one peer review committee may serve the entire agency. In small agencies or in sparsely populated areas the peer review committee may be made up of representatives from several health agencies. One agency may feel it would be best to have Nursing Professional Standards Review and Nursing Performance Review done by separate committees, while another will prefer to have one committee assume a dual function.

Nurses employed in agencies having fewer than five nurses (i.e., school, industry, physician's office, private practice) may elect their committee on a city or statewide basis. Private duty nurses who work in more than one facility may be reviewed by one institution on the basis of a sampling of the client population served.

In setting up a peer review committee the following is recommended:

1. Each health care setting should establish a democratically elected committee for the purpose of conducting peer review.

    a. The members should be elected by the total registered nurse group. These nurses may vote for their own representative (i.e., H.N. for an H.N. representative, a staff nurse for a staff nurse representative) or for the total committee.

    b. Members of the peer review committee should be representative of all major job classifications. In agencies that distinguish among levels of clinical expertise, each level should be represented. In agencies in which classification is according to administrative position (i.e., head nurse, assistant head nurse) these levels should be represented. Other factors to take into account in selecting members are shift assignments and clinical area of practice. At least a simple majority of the committee's members should be nonadministrative.

2. In committees composed of members from several institutions, there should be at least one representative from each institution.

3. The committee should consist of elected representatives. Should the expertise of another individual be needed, the committee chairman may appoint the appropriate individual. (In the case of the committee conducting Nursing Professional Standards Review, it may be necessary for the membership to have expertise in a given area in order to successfully examine a specific phenomenon.)

It should be stressed that every member of the peer review committee shall have an equal vote.

3. Membership Selection Policies:

    The success of the committee will depend in large part on the qualifications of the members selected. It is recommended that this committee be composed of *practicing* professional nurses who have demonstrated professional commitment (i.e., volunteering to serve on nursing committees, participation in professional organizations, development of specific nursing expertise).

All members selected for the committee should be involved in a group training process to prepare them for the peer review process. Areas in which development might be needed are interviewing techniques and writing of reports.

4. Committee Size:

The size of the committee will be determined by the setting, functions and utilization of subcommittees. It is recommended, however, that committee membership not exceed nine persons. It has been noted that opportunities for participation by all members in groups exceeding ten is reduced and difficulty in communication among members increases. The odd number of nine is also recommended to prevent tie votes.

5. Subcommittees:

In order not to burden one group, it may be necessary to develop subcommittees to handle specific problems. The subcommittee could be composed either of members of the peer review committee or non-members appointed by the peer review committee and chaired by a member of the peer review committee. As a member of the peer review committee, the subcommittee chairman would report to the entire peer review committee at regular intervals. In this instance, the peer review committee could act as a consultant to the subcommittee.

6. Authority:

Peer review committees are *review* bodies, not disciplinary committees. The purposes of the peer review committee are: 1) to evaluate the quality and quantity of nursing care, 2) to determine the strengths and weaknesses of nursing care, 3) to provide evidence to utilize as the basis of recommendations for new or altered policies and procedures to improve nursing care, and 4) to identify those areas where practice patterns indicate more knowledge is needed.

Each peer review committee will need to determine whether or not the results of their work should be forwarded to certification boards, nursing services or various committees. Any outcomes of the review process to bring practice up to designated standards, remove practitioners from practice, etc. are the prerogative of other groups.

Peer review committees should be given the status of a permanent standing committee in the organizational structure.

Peer review committees should work cooperatively with other standing committees. Relationships with bodies such as the District Nurses' Association, agency administration, medical staff, certification boards and committees should be delineated and documented. This information should be available to interested parties.

7. Liability:

If the peer review process is operated strictly on the basis of documented facts, the legal liability of the committee is minimized.

If any nurse should ever decide to sue a peer review committee, the suit would most likely be classified as a defamation suit. Legally, "defamation" refers to the injury of a person's reputation or character by statements made to a third party. There are two classes of defamation: libel and slander. Libel refers to a written statement while slander refers to an oral statement.

In order to avoid such suits, the peer review committee should encourage a nurse to limit comments to statements of *fact*. Moreover, a nurse should limit comments to statements relevant to the review process, which deals only with the individual's performance in a nursing capacity.

At all times review proceedings should be carried out in accordance with established rules and principles governing the committee.

The peer review committee is entitled to examine material relevant to the reason or cause for reviewing an individual nurse or group of nurses. Such material could include patient data. When examining patient data, every effort should be made to keep the information confidential. In order to avoid a lawsuit initiated by a patient, the peer review committee should attempt to conceal patient identity when reviewing records, etc.

If legal questions arise, peer review committees are urged to seek legal counsel.

8. Policies:

Policies (or methodologies) need to be developed that will guide committee functioning on such issues as confidentiality, ways of handling requests for review, feedback mechanisms, use of consultants, availability of review material for practitioner and client consumption and reliability of materials being reviewed.

One of the first questions which will have to be settled is who will initiate the request for review. Will the request come from the Director of Nursing, individual practitioners or clients? This will need to be determined by individual committees.

A second question which arises is in what form should requests be made. It is recommended that requests for review be in writing and indicate the type of review being requested (Nursing Professional Standards Review or Nursing Performance Review) and specify the purpose of the review.

The questions of the feedback mechanisms for practice reviewed and confidentiality are also important considerations. Feedback to the nurse under review is most effective when both verbal and written communication are combined. Recipients of committee feedback will, in part, be determined by who requests the review (i.e., if the Director of Nursing requests the review, one copy would go to the Director and one copy to the nurse under review). If an individual practitioner requests a review, a copy may be sent only to the individual practitioner, who has the option of sharing the review with whomever the individual chooses.

The following guidelines are recommended:
a. Utmost care needs to be taken to insure confidentiality for the nurse under review.
b. The nurse under review is entitled to full disclosure of the committee's report on her practice.

In addition, the committee will need to establish methods of insuring confidentiality for clients when patient records are utilized as part of the data base.

9. Protocol:
   The following list addresses itself to basic procedural considerations.
   1. Review of both individual performance and group practice occurs on a regular basis at specified intervals.
   2. The chairperson has the responsibility for the initial assignment of review tasks.
   3. The entire committee need not review every problem. Specific problems may be delegated to a committee member with particular expertise in the area for initial review.

4. All assignments for initial review of the situation are made by the chairperson as soon as they are received.
5. Yearly meeting schedules need to be determined.
6. The peer review committee will determine specific data to be provided by the nurse being reviewed and inform the nurse of his/her responsibilities for presenting material.
7. The nurse to be reviewed should be given an opportunity for face-to-face confrontation with the peer review committee when such an encounter is appropriate.

10. Lines of Referral and Appeal:

It is not realistic to assume that an effective peer review program will always arrive at decisions that are wholly acceptable to all parties involved. If the committee functions through subcommittees, the main body would be authorized to hear appeals. If any party is not in agreement with the decision rendered by the peer review committee, they can (within a specified time) submit the reason for disagreement in writing.

An appeal may take two forms: 1) an individual may make an appeal because the process for review was not in accordance with established rules and regulations governing the peer review committee, and/or 2) an individual may make an appeal because the individual questions the validity of the committee's judgment.

A nurse has a number of recourses for appeal such as the established grievance procedure or the utilization of a sanctioned nurse arbitrator.

Congress	*Ad Hoc Committee*
Marjorie Ramphal	Janelle Ramsburg
Marilyn Howe	Sister Kathryn Galligan
Alice Davis	Rachel Ayers
Betty Evans	Laura Hart
Corrine Hatton	Marilyn Howe
Jeanne M. McNally	Ann G. Jackson
Sister Marilyn Schwab	Lois N. Knowles
Kathleen Sward	Virginia Petralia
Elaine Wittmann	Arthur Wheeler
	Jayne Wiggins

11. A Peer Review Tool for Directors of Nursing Service*

*Source: *Quality Assessment: Program and Process,* National League for Nursing, Western Regional Assembly of Constituent League, March, 1974, and March, 1975, Forums for Nursing Service Administrators in the West. Compiled by members of the Utilizing Nursing and Planning Models Group Forum for Nursing Service Administrators in the West. Reprinted by permission of the National League for Nursing.

Standard Performance Factors	Indicators of Level of Performance	Specific Measurements Used
1. Staff development.	1.1 Orientation is provided for new staff and for staff to a new type job.	1.1 Documentation in records of department and employee file: O.J.T. and didactic orientation.
	1.2 A system exists for staff to participate; recognition given and involvement in continuing education seminars encouraged and supported.	1.2 Documentation of attendance and reports given to appropriate staff.
	Director values staff and sends staff (not just self) to pertinent programs.	
	1.3 Inservice Education in the facility is actively planned and implemented and outcomes are measured and documented.	
2. Director's position in top management.	2.1 Makes decisions for patient care by direct input to administrative policy-making body.	2.1 Documentation of involvement in top-level management planning and decision making.
	2.2 Accepts responsibility, authority, accountability in position.	2.2 Documentation of participation in policy setting, decision making.

2.3 Visible evidence in organization clearly demonstrates 2.2.

2.4 Salary and fringe benefits are commensurate with managers in organizations with similar responsibilities.

3.1 Professional outcomes are monitored.
 — staff is involved in setting standards;
 — feedback of results given to staff to move to correct/improve practice.

3.2 An audit process is defined and in effect.

3.3 Patient comfort is a concern.

3.4 Patients speak well of care.

4.1 Plans regular meetings with staff.

4.2 Staff know director of nursing is a nurse and a member of the agency's top management team.

3. Nursing audit.

4. Interpersonal relations with nursing staff.

2.3 Title and placement on organizational chart; reports directly to the chief executive officer.

2.4 Comparative findings on personal salary scales; pay equal to any other assistant administrator.

3.1 Documentation of staff involvement.

3.2 Documented standards. Documented process and outcomes.

3.3 Documented standards.

3.4 Verbal/written feedback from patients via objective tool.

4.1 Documentation of agenda of meetings.

4.2 Staff members respond to this question affirmatively, i.e., aware of a nurse representing them in administra-

Continued

Standard Performance Factors	Indicators of Level of Performance	Specific Measurements Used
		tion. (Size of some agencies may mean staff do not know the name of the director.)
	4.3 Expectations for staff performance are included in the evaluation process.	4.3 Appraisal with formal guidelines documented with expectations of employee/employer.
5. Forecast of trends in patient population to deal with actual and potential problems.	5.1 Studies populations served. Makes attempts to learn clients' cultures, value systems, and expectations of health care delivery services.	5.1 Use of documented data from region. Data collection from region. Documented attendance of staff/self with community group(s) for input/output.
	5.2 Profiles nurses available; experiences, cultures, values. Tries to match patients with nurses available.	5.2 Documentation of profiles, assignments.
6. Fiscal responsibility.	6.1 Uses quantitative measurement system.	6.1 Documentation.
	6.2 Establishes norms of productivity.	6.2 Documentation of norms/variance.
	6.3 Conducts regular budget review.	6.3 Documented annual analysis.

	6.4 Has equal management input in budget planning.	6.4 Documented in budget-planning meeting.
7. Support of educational programs.	7.1 Gives active staff support for nursing students.	7.1 Students-Instructors feel staff helpful, knowledgeable role models.
	7.2 Provides community teaching programs for health promotion/maintenance as determined by needs of client population.	7.2 Documentation of educational programs.
8. Discharge planning and referral program.	8.1 Provides for discharge planning and referral as determined by client need and available community resources.	8.1 Documentation of outreach services; use of available resources.
9. Climate for growth and risk taking of staff.	9.1 Services are instituted from staff suggestions as well as nursing and hospital administrative and physician suggestions.	9.1 Documentation of services instituted, augmented in year.
10. Own continuing education in management.	10.1 Has knowledge of systems theory and application in practice.	10.1 Documentation of problem definition and exploration before Task Force organized to solve problem. Specific objectives with charge to chairperson. Able to measure Task Force

Continued

Standard Performance Factors	Indicators of Level of Performance	Specific Measurements Used
		effectiveness because charge is clear.
		Committee work more economical because duplication avoided.
		Task Force limited to specific task and time.
	10.2 The system interdigitates.	10.2 Documentation of projects set up in interdisciplinary teams demonstrates director's thinking in terms of total system, as others are included where appropriate.
	10.3 Uses power constructively.	10.3 Gains cooperation in meeting objectives within time limits set mutually.
		Documentation of M.B.O. Expectations to track priorities, deadlines.
		Documented: things to do; list of some type.

	10.4 How does power structure work?	10.4 Describe power structure: formal or informal? Documentation: Director is on committees with power to make changes.
11. Political astuteness.	11.1 Knowledge of local, state, national political influences affecting health care delivery.	11.1 Documentation.
12. Communication system.	12.1 Parameters are set.	12.1 How measure effect?
13. Clinical knowledge.	13.1 Has knowledge in depth required as determined by scope of responsibility, hospital size, kind of agency, number of students.	13.1 Effective communication documented. Subjective feeling of comfort when talking to various clinic groups.
14. Style of leadership.	14.1 Adopts a distinctive style.	14.1 Utilized in accomplishing goals.
		14.2 Utilizes resources and staff available.
15. Creative and innovative accomplishments.	15.1 Participates in research projects.	15.1 Evidence of use of results of research.
	15.2 Institutes new approaches to care which are effective in improvements, cost saving, staff saving.	15.2 Evidence of care projects.

Continued

Standard Performance Factors	Indicators of Level of Performance	Specific Measurements Used
16. Philosophy, standards, and objectives.	16.1 All staff are included in establishing and effecting written and visible philosophy, standards, and objectives.	16.1 Documentation of participation of staff in committees to develop these.
	16.2 Orientees are provided information upon entry to work system.	16.2 Documentation of orientee receipts and understanding.
	16.3 Planning for the future incorporates these.	16.3 Documentation of planning utilizing philosophy.
	16.4 Philosophy, standards, and objectives are viable and updated on a regular basis.	16.4 Revision dates noted.

12. Weekly Nursing Assignment

NURSING SERVICE DEPARTMENT

Policy

Nursing assignment sheets are posted weekly on the bulletin board
in the nursing station.

Purpose

1. Serve as a work plan to assure the assignment of all duties.
2. Assist to clearly fix responsibilities with no overlapping of duties.

Procedure

1. Each Friday the Head Nurse
   is to record and post the
   assigned team leader and
   team members of each
   team for each tour of duty
   for the following week.
2. Each day the current team
   leader records for the following day the assignments of
   patient care and the special
   duties of each team
   member.

3. Each morning the team leader
   revises the team members'
   assignments and makes the
   necessary adjustments.

Key Points

1. A separate form is to be used
   for each team.

2. The patient assignment is
   indicated by room number
   and the patient's name.
   The following code indicates:
   S.A. = Special Assignment as
      shown on the code list.
   B = Break period.
   L/S = Lunch or supper
      period.

TEAM MEMBERS' DAILY PATIENT CARE ASSIGNMENTS
AND SPECIAL DUTIES
NURSING SERVICE DEPARTMENT

Policy

The weekly assignment sheets are posted weekly on the nursing unit
bulletin board.

Purpose

1. Serve as a work plan to assure the assignment of patient care and
   other unit duties.
2. Assist in identifying responsibilities with no overlapping of duties.
3. Assist in coordinating nursing care activities.

Procedure	*Key Points*
1. Each Friday the Charge Nurse is to record and post the assigned team leader and team members of each team for each tour of duty for the following week.	1. A separate form is to be used for each team within the nursing unit.
2. Each day the current team leader records for the following day the assignments of patient care and the special duties of each team member.	2. The patient assignment is indicated by room number and the patient's name. The following code indicates: S.A. = Special Assignment as shown on the code list. B = Break period. L/S = Lunch or supper period.
3. Each morning the team leader revises the team member's assignment and makes the necessary adjustments.	

TEAM MEMBERS' DAILY PATIENT CARE ASSIGNMENTS AND SPECIAL DUTIES

Team _____   Nursing Unit _____

		MON.	TUE.	WED.	THUR.	FRI.	SAT.	SUN.
Name _____								
Position _____								
	S.A.							
	B-L/S							
Name _____								
Position _____								
	S.A.							
	B-L/S							
Name _____								
Position _____								
	S.A.							
	B-L/S							
Name _____								
Position _____								
	S.A.							
	B-L/S							

Policy

Each team member is to be given a written assignment for each tour of duty.

Purpose

1. Serves as a guide to assure that no part of the assignment is omitted.
2. Serves as note paper to add incidental directions given after the initial assignment has been presented and explained.
3. Serves as note paper to write reminders for a report to the team leader.

Procedure

1. The team leader is to complete an individual assignment for each team member.

2. Each individual assignment form is to be presented to the team leader prior to Team Conference #2.

Key Points

1. The team member is to receive this form during Team Conference #1.
   The team member is to use this form during Team Conference #1 to make notes relating to her responsibilities. The term S.A. = Special Assignment as indicated on the code list.

TEAM MEMBER PATIENT CARE ASSIGNMENT
NURSING SERVICE DEPARTMENT

Policy

Each team member receives a written patient care assignment for each tour of duty.

Purpose

1. Assures that no part of the assignment is omitted.
2. Incidental directions can be given after the initial assignment has been presented and explained.
3. Serves as note paper to write reminders for a report to the team leader.

Procedure

1. The team leader is to complete an individual assignment for each team member.

2. Each individual assignment patient care form is to be presented to the team leader prior to Team Conference #2.

Key Points

1. The team member is to receive this form during Team Conference #1. The team member is to use this form during Team Conference #1 to make notes relating to her responsibilities. The term S.A. = Special Assignment as indicated on the code list.

TEAM MEMBER PATIENT CARE ASSIGNMENT SHEET

NAME _____   S.A. _____

POSITION _____   DATE _____

TEAM LEADER _____   TEAM _____

ROOM NO.	NAME OF PATIENT	LEVEL OF CARE	ACTIVITY	SPECIAL NOTES

INDIVIDUAL NURSING CARE PLAN PROCEDURE
NURSING SERVICE DEPARTMENT

Purpose

1. The individual written care plans are guides used by members of the health team to provide continuity of effective, comprehensive care for the individual patient.
2. Written care plans provide a means of communication that safeguards and promotes continuity of nursing care.

Responsibility

Every nurse is required to check all treatment cards with Kardex at the beginning of the tour of duty.

Requisites

1. Nursing Care Plan Kardex Card.
2. Ink pen to fill in permanent data.
3. Pencil to fill in transcription of treatments, x-rays, lab., other diagnostic tests, and daily notes. Pencil is also used for objectives, needs and the nursing approach.
4. Pencil is used for the "General Nursing Care Plan."
5. Allergies — red pencil.
6. Kardex card holder.
7. Flag cards when indicated.
   (a) Red used in withhold on diet or fluids.
   (b) Yellow used for IVs.
   (c) Green used for surgery.
   (d) Brown used for lab. procedure.
   (e) Blue used for x-ray procedure.
   (f) Black indicates critical.

Procedure

1. Admission of patient, identifying data.

Key Points

1. All information is filled in with ink by nurse or unit clerk, except the age and

Procedure	*Key Points*
	diagnosis where pencil is used.
2. Special need identified: physical, spiritual, emotional, social.	2. Professional nurse interviews patient. It is her responsibility to enter in pencil the individual's special need that affects nursing care or the personnel-patient relationship. Confidential information about patient is not included.
3. Develop objectives of nursing for each individual patient depending on his specific needs and condition.	3. After the patient's needs are identified, the nursing objectives are formulated. Nursing objectives will change according to patient needs.
4. Development of plan by members of the health team.	4. All members of the health team having contact with patient share in the development of plan. The regular period for developing and revising nursing care plan is during team conference. Evaluation is made of nursing care being provided. Special needs are identified. Nursing approach plan is then developed, as to how, when, and by whom the team will meet the identified needs.
5. All nursing employees are responsible for making a contribution toward keeping the care plan up to date.	5. All members of the team should keep the team leader informed of changes in the patient's condition and/or needs. The team leader is to

Procedure

Key Points

keep the team members informed of changes in condition, doctor's orders, and procedures and suggested methods.

6. General nursing care includes what, how, and when procedures are to be done.

6. This is a written guide for the care of the patient according to his/her specific illness. Such information should be made available at all times to the nursing employees.

7. Transcription of treatment orders to be placed in treatment column.

7. To be done in pencil; should include the following information: Type of treatment (use only accepted abbreviation when transcribing). Interval treatment to be done, day, hours. Any additional instructions needed.

8. When a treatment is discontinued it is to be erased.

9. General Nursing Care Plan to be kept up to date as orders and the patient's needs change.

9. This area may be used to indicate treatments, e.g., writing the time(s) beside the word "Clinitest," or indicating how frequently the patient may be catheterized beside the word "catheterize."

10. Responsibility of keeping Kardex card up to date.

10. Night nurse will change hospital and P.O. days, and insert flag cards as needed. The person who transcribes orders is responsible for making changes on Kardex. This includes filling in the

Procedure	*Key Points*
	type of surgery when the post-operative orders are transcribed.
11. Condition of patient is evaluated by charge nurse (if in question, ask attending physician) and may be changed as necessary. Therefore, it should be written in pencil.	11. *Satisfactory* — meets medical expectations and progress good. *Fair* — questionable, slow progress. *Serious* — outcome questionable. *Critical* — recovery doubtful, death imminent.
12. Treatment and Nursing Care Kardex may be ordered from Purchasing Department.	12. Form number 641-044.

NURSING CARE PLANS

Purpose

1. Provide a systematic plan for individualized patient care.
2. Communicate relevant data to other members of the nursing and health teams regarding method of care.
3. Promote continuity of patient care.

Requisites

1. Nursing Care Plan Kardex Card.
2. Ink pen to fill in permanent data.
3. Pencil to fill in transcription of treatments, x-rays, lab., other diagnostic tests, and daily notes. Pencil is also used for objectives, needs and the nursing approach.
4. Pencil is used for the "General Nursing Care Plan."
5. Allergies — red pencil.
6. Kardex card holder.
7. Flag cards when indicated.

(a) Red used in withhold on diet or fluids.
(b) Yellow used for IVs.
(c) Green used for surgery.
(d) Brown used for lab. procedure.
(e) Blue used for x-ray procedure.
(f) Black indicates critical.

Procedure	*Key Points*
1. Admission of patient, identifying data.	1. All information is filled in with ink by nurse or unit clerk, except the age and diagnosis where pencil is used.
2. Special need identified: physical, spiritual, emotional, social.	2. Professional nurse interviews patient. It is her responsibility to enter in pencil the individual's special need that affects nursing care or the personnel-pencil the individual's fidential information about patient is not included.
3. Develop objectives of nursing for each individual patient depending on his/her specific needs and condition.	3. After the patient's needs are identified, the nursing objectives are formulated. Nursing objectives will change according to patient needs.
4. Development of plan by members of the health team.	4. All members of the health team having contact with patient share in the development of plan. The regular period for developing and revising nursing care plan is during team conference. Evaluation is made of nursing care being provided. Special needs are identified. Nursing approach plan is

Procedure	*Key Points*
	then developed, as to how, when, and by whom the team will meet the identified needs.
5. The nursing team members are responsible for making a contribution toward keeping the care plan up to date.	5. All members of the team should keep the team leader informed of changes in the patient's condition and/or needs. The team leader is to keep the team members informed of changes in condition, doctor's orders, and procedures and suggested methods.
6. General nursing care includes what, how, and when procedures are to be done.	6. This is a written guide for the care of the patient according to his/her specific illness. Such information should be made available at all times to the nursing team members.
7. Transcription of medical orders to be placed in treatment column.	7. To be done in pencil; should include the following information: Type of treatment (use only accepted abbreviation when transcribing). Interval treatment to be done, day, hours. Any additional instructions needed.
8. When a treatment is discontinued it is to be erased.	
9. General Nursing Care Plan to be kept up to date as orders and the patient's needs change.	9. This area may be used to indicate treatments, e.g., writing the time(s) beside the word "Clinitest," or indicating how frequently the patient may be cathe-

Procedure	*Key Points*
	terized beside the word "catheterize."
10. Responsibility of keeping Kardex card up to date.	10. Night nurse will change hospital and P.O. days, and insert flag cards as needed. The person who transcribes orders is responsible for making changes on Kardex. This includes filling in the type of surgery when the postoperative orders are transcribed.
11. Condition of patient is evaluated by charge nurse (if in question, ask attending physician) and may be changed as necessary. Therefore, it should be written in pencil.	11. *Satisfactory* — meets medical expectations and progress good. *Fair* — questionable, slow progress. *Serious* — outcome questionable. *Critical* — recovery doubtful, death imminent.
12. Treatment and Nursing Care Kardex may be ordered from Purchasing Department.	12. Form number 641-044.

Hospital   City, State

GENERAL PATIENT INFORMATION

Admission Date _____ Ht. _____ Wt. _____   Address _____ Phone _____

Hospital Day _____   Relative _____ Relationship _____

Adm'tting Diagnosis _____   Address _____ Phone _____

_____   Occupation _____ Religion _____

Admitting Service _____   Previous Hospitalization _____

_____   Disabilities _____

Surgery Day _____   Allergies: Medication _____ Food _____ Other _____

P.O. Day _____   _____

Type of Surgery _____   Other _____

_____

NURSING CARE PLAN

Activity	Hygiene	Diet	Elimination
Comp. bedrest _____	Bed _____	N.P.O. _____	Ck. Voiding _____
Bedrest _____	Partial _____	Reg. _____	Catheterize _____
Dangle _____	Self Adm. _____	Other _____	Foley _____
B.R.P. _____	Tub _____	_____	Irrigate cath. _____
Up in chair _____	Shower _____	_____	Change Foley (date) _____
Up ad lib _____	Sitz _____	Feed _____	Needs enema (date) _____
As ordered: _____	_____	Partial Help _____	Needs laxative _____
_____	_____	Eats Alone _____	B.M. (date) _____

Mouth Care

Denture _____   Other _____

Intake and Output	Temperature	Safety Factors
Intake _____ Output _____	Oral _____	Siderails _____ Full _____ Partial _____
Clinitest _____	Rectal _____	Other _____
Acetest _____	Axillary _____	_____

OBJECTIVE FOR PATIENT CARE

D*te	Nursing Problem	Expected Outcome	Time	Nursing Action

Room No.	Name	Hospital — Day	Condition	Doctor	Sex	Age

ROOM NO.

PATIENT
NAME

HOSPITAL NO.   PHYSICIAN

SEX

AGE

            DATE

PHYSICIAN'S ORDERS

DATE	Medications Treatment	Time	Date	Diagnostic Test	
				Type	Time
				Lab.	
				Other Diagnostic Tests	
	Daily Notes:				

NURSING PRACTICE COMMITTEE

Purpose

To establish standards of performance for safe, effective nursing care.

Objectives

1. To review procedures for simplification, make adjustments to meet new needs and draft new procedures as necessary.
2. To evaluate new supplies and equipment as they relate to nursing procedure.
3. To submit recommendations to the Director of Nursing regarding the practice of nursing and its procedures.

Membership

The Nursing Practice Committee shall consist of eight members:

1. Supervisor, Chairman
2. Supervisor
3. Head Nurse
4. Head Nurse, Central Service
5. Staff Nurse
6. Nursing Assistant
7. Staff Education Instructor
8. Physician, Medical Staff

Procedure for Appointment

1. Supervisors shall be appointed by the Director of Nursing. A supervisor shall serve as chairman for a period of two years.
2. The chairman shall appoint a head nurse, staff nurse, and nursing assistant to serve on the Nursing Practice Committee for a period of one year; they may be appointed for a second term.
3. The head nurse in Central Service and a staff education instructor shall be permanent members.
4. The physician appointment shall be made by the Chief of the Medical Staff for a period of one year.

NURSING PRACTICE COMMITTEE

Purpose

To establish standards for nursing performance as a means of quality assurance care.

Objectives

1. To identify standards for nursing practice that reflect the department's definition of nursing and the scope of nursing care.
2. To utilize the ANA standards of nursing practice, the JCAH standards for practice, and state nurse practice act as guides for nursing care.
3. To provide standards for nursing practice as a means of assessing the quality of nursing care provided to people.
4. To make recommendations through administrative channels.

Membership

The Nursing Practice Committee shall consist of eight members:

1. Supervisor, Chairman
2. Supervisor
3. Head Nurse
4. Head Nurse
5. Clinical Nurse Specialist
6. Nursing Assistant
7. Staff Education Instructor
8. Physician
9. Other resource persons as needed

Procedure for Appointment

1. Supervisors shall be appointed by the Director of Nursing. A supervisor shall serve as chairman for a period of two years.
2. The chairman shall appoint a head nurse, staff nurse, and nursing assistant to serve on the Nursing Practice Committee for a period of one year, possibly to be appointed for a second term.

3. The head nurse in Central Service and a staff education instructor shall be permanent members.
4. The physician appointment shall be made by the Chief of the Medical Staff for a period of one year.

New members shall be appointed each year during the month of September.

A recorder shall be elected during the first meeting in October.

Subcommittees may be appointed by the chairman.

Meetings

The Nursing Practice Committee shall meet on the fourth Wednesday (2:00–3:00 P.M.) of each placement — every four weeks — and subject to call.

All meetings shall be held in the Nursing Service Educational Unit.

Responsibilities of Chairman, Supervisor

A notice of the Nursing Practice Committee meetings shall be sent out to the members a week in advance.

The objectives and agenda of the meetings shall be determined in advance and stated in the notice of the meeting.

A copy of notice and agenda shall be sent to the Director of Nursing.

The committee's proceedings shall be recorded in the form of minutes and placed in a loose-leaf binder in Nursing Service Office.

Communicate to the Director of Nursing the committee's deliberations and submit in writing any recommendations that shall be made.

POLICY COMMITTEE

Purpose

To establish guides or policies for the personnel of the Nursing Service Department that delineate responsibilities and prescribe the action to be taken under a given set of circumstances.

Objectives

1. To periodically appraise nursing policies, followed by a revision, if indicated.
2. To develop new policies to meet present and future needs.
3. To review and make any recommendations on policies requiring collaboration with other departments.
4. To submit recommendations to the Director of Nursing regarding the development, revision or modification of policies.

Membership

The Policy Committee shall consist of six members:

1. Supervisor — Day Tour of Duty
2. Supervisor — Evening Tour of Duty
3. Supervisor — Night Tour of Duty
4. Head Nurse
5. Staff Nurse
6. Clinical Nurse Specialist

Procedure for Appointment

1. Supervisors shall be appointed by the Director of Nursing. A supervisor shall serve as chairman for a period of two years.
2. The chairman shall appoint members to serve on the committee.

New members shall be appointed each year during the month of September.

A recorder shall be elected at the first meeting in October. Subcommittees may be appointed by the chairman.

Meetings

The Policy Committee shall meet on the first Wednesday (2:00–3:30 P.M.) of each four-week placement schedule and subject to call.

All meetings shall be held in the Nursing Service Conference Room.

Responsibilities of Chairman

A notice of the Policy Committee meetings shall be sent out to the members a week in advance.

The objectives and agenda of the meetings shall be determined in advance and stated in the notice of the meeting.

A copy of the notice and agenda shall be sent to the Director of Nursing.

The committee's proceedings shall be recorded in the form of minutes and placed in a loose-leaf binder in the Nursing Service Office.

Communicate to the Director of Nursing the committee's deliberations and submit in writing any recommendations that shall be made.

JOB DESCRIPTION COMMITTEE

Purpose

The purpose of the Job Description Committee is to carefully determine the scope of work to be done for each level of nursing personnel as it relates to the total organization of the Nursing Service Department.

Objectives

1. To have available an accurate written description of the various jobs done, together with an assessment of the abilities required in an individual to perform them satisfactorily.
2. To periodically appraise job descriptions and make adjustments to meet new needs.
3. To submit recommendations through administrative channels.

Membership

The Job Description Committee shall consist of five members:

1. Supervisor, Chairman
2. Supervisor

3. Head Nurse
4. Staff Nurse
5. Representative of Personnel Department

Procedure for Appointment

A supervisor shall be appointed by the Director of Nursing and shall serve as chairman for a period of two years.

New members shall be appointed each year during the month of September.

A recorder shall be elected during the first meeting in October. Subcommittees may be appointed by the chairman.

Meetings

The Job Description Committee shall meet on the third Wednesday (1:00–2:00 P.M.) of each four-week placement schedule and subject to call.

All meetings shall be held in the Nursing Service Conference Room.

Responsibilities of Chairman

A notice of the Job Description Committee meetings shall be sent to the members a week in advance.

The objectives and agenda of the meetings shall be determined in advance and stated in the notice of the meetings.

A copy of notice and agenda shall be sent to the Director of Nursing.

The committee's proceedings shall be recorded in the form of minutes and placed in a loose-leaf binder in the Nursing Service Office.

Communicate to the Director of Nursing the committee's deliberations and submit in writing any recommendations that shall be made.

NURSING AUDIT COMMITTEE

Purpose

To review the care rendered to patients as evidenced in the nursing records for the purpose of evaluation, verification, and rendering of quality care.

Objectives

1. To provide a systematic review of the nursing records of patients discharged from the hospital.
2. To provide maintenance of a record of performance of each professional nurse on the staff.
3. To provide a biographical index of the quality of nursing received by each patient.
4. To provide a means for self-evaluation of nursing care.
5. To provide clinical data for use in research and education.
6. To provide a basis of communication between the physician and other health team members contributing to patient care.

Membership

The Nursing Audit Committee shall consist of eight members:

1. Associate Director of Nursing Service
2. Supervisor
3. Head Nurse
4. Staff Nurse
5. Clinical Nurse Specialist
6. Medical Records Librarian
7. Staff Education Instructor
8. Unit Clerk

Procedure for Appointment

1. The supervisor shall be appointed by the Director of Nursing for a period of one year and may be appointed for a second term.
2. The Associate Director shall be a permanent member of the committee.
3. The chairman shall be appointed annually by the Director.
4. The chairman shall select the members to serve on the committee for a period of one year; may be appointed for a second term.

5. New members shall be appointed each year during the month of September.
6. A recorder shall be elected during the first meeting in October.
7. Subcommittees may be appointed by the chairman.

Meetings

The Nursing Audit Committee shall meet on the second Wednesday (1:00–2:00 P.M.) of each four-week placement schedule.

All meetings shall be held in the Nursing Service Conference Room.

Responsibilities of Chairman

A notice of the Nursing Audit Committee meetings shall be sent out to members a week in advance.

The objectives and agenda of the meetings shall be determined in advance and stated in the notice of the meeting.

A copy of notice and agenda shall be sent to the Director of Nursing.

The Committee's proceedings shall be recorded in the form of minutes and placed in a loose-leaf binder in the Nursing Service Office.

Communicate to the Director of Nursing the Committee's deliberations and submit in writing any recommendations that shall be made.

SAFETY COMMITTEE

Purpose

To contribute toward the overall safety program of the hospital. To provide a safe environment for patients and all other persons entering the hospital.

Objectives

1. To review past incidents, discuss preventive measures, and make suggestions for improving the department's safety record.
2. To develop educational opportunities for employees that can be utilized in developing safe as well as productive work habits.

3. To conduct a monthly safety survey or inspection within the Nursing Service Department.
   a. Check facilities, operations and practices throughout the department.
   b. Locate items in need of routine repair or maintenance.
   c. Eliminate all unsafe conditions and unsafe acts.
4. To interpret Fire Plan and Disaster Plan.
5. To keep employees informed of the Safety Committee and of their vital part in the overall safety program of the hospital.
6. To be aware of the guidelines set by the Occupational Health and Safety Act (OSHA).
7. To submit recommendations to the Director regarding safety practices.

Membership

The Safety Committee shall consist of eight members:

1. Supervisor, Chairman
2. Head Nurse
3. Staff Nurse
4. Licensed Practical Nurse
5. Nursing Assistant
6. Staff Education Instructor
7. Unit Clerk
8. Representative from Maintenance Department

Procedure for Appointment

1. Supervisors shall be appointed by the Director of Nursing. A supervisor shall serve as chairman of the Safety Committee for a period of two years.
2. A Staff Education Instructor shall serve as a permanent member of the committee.
3. The chairman shall select members to serve on the committee for a period of one year. Members may be appointed for a second term.
4. New members shall be appointed each year during the month of September.
5. A recorder shall be elected during the month of October.

6. Subcommittees may be appointed by the chairman as needed.

Meetings

The Safety Committee shall meet on the first Wednesday (1:00–2:00 P.M.) of each month and subject to call.

All meetings shall be held in the Nursing Service Conference Room.

Responsibilities of Chairman, Supervisor

A notice of the Safety Committee meetings shall be sent out to the members a week in advance.

The objectives and agenda of the meetings shall be determined in advance and stated in the notice of the meeting.

A copy of notice and agenda shall be sent to the Director of Nursing.

The Committee's proceedings shall be recorded in the form of minutes and placed in a loose-leaf binder in the Nursing Service Office.

Communicate to the Director of Nursing the Committee's deliberations and submit in writing any recommendations that shall be made.

IN-SERVICE COMMITTEE FOR CONTINUING EDUCATION

Purpose

To assist nursing personnel in achieving and maintaining competence in providing nursing.

Objectives

1. To establish continuous and flexible programs based on the need of nursing service personnel.
2. To stimulate interest in learning as a continuous process.
3. To provide selected learning experiences for nursing personnel that meet changing patterns of delivery of nursing.
4. To stimulate interest in nursing studies and research.
5. To submit recommendations to the Staff Education Coordinator for program development.

Membership

The In-service Committee for Continuing Education shall consist of seven members:

1. Supervisor, Chairman
2. Staff Instructor
3. Head Nurse
4. Staff Nurse
5. Practical Nurse
6. Nursing Assistant
7. Faculty Member

Procedure for Appointment

1. A supervisor shall be appointed by the Director of Nursing Service to serve as chairman for a period of two years.
2. With the exception of the chairman, committee appointments shall be for one year. Members may be appointed for a second term.
3. The chairman shall appoint new members to the committee as needed for planning.
4. New members shall be appointed each year during the month of September.
5. A recorder shall be elected at the first meeting in October.
6. Subcommittees may be appointed by the chairman.

Meetings

The In-service Committee for Continuing Education shall meet on the first Wednesday (11:00–12:00) of each four-week placement schedule and subject to call.

All meetings shall be held in the Nursing Service Conference Room.

Responsibilities of Chairman, Supervisor

1. A notice of the In-service Committee meetings shall be sent out to the members a week in advance.
2. The objectives and agenda of the meetings shall be determined in advance and stated in the notice of the meeting.

3. A copy of notice and agenda shall be sent to the Director of Nursing Service.
4. The committee's proceedings shall be recorded in the form of minutes and placed in a loose-leaf binder in the Nursing Service Office.

PATIENT CARE COMMITTEE

Purpose

To improve patient care by analyzing critical incidents, analyzing patient care and health trends and reviewing nursing unit needs for providing care — staffing, equipment, physical facilities.

Objectives

1. To promote the team approach to nursing care planning and patient care.
2. To identify areas of patient care that should be developed and/or strengthened.
3. To determine methods of improving care.
4. To evaluate patient care.
5. To make recommendations through administrative channels.

Membership

The Committee shall consist of nine members:

1. Assistant Director
2. Supervisor
3. Head Nurse
4. Assistant Head Nurse
5. Staff Nurse
6. Licensed Practical Nurse
7. Nursing Assistant
8. Other resource persons as needed (patients, families, health team members)
9. Unit Clerk

Subcommittees of similar composition will be appointed on evening and night tours of duty. The chairman of each subcommittee will report to the Chairman of the committee.

Procedure for Appointment

1. Supervisors shall be appointed by the Director of Nursing Service. A supervisor shall serve as chairman for a period of two years.
2. The Assistant Director shall be a permanent member of the committee.
3. The chairman shall be appointed annually by the Director.
4. The chairman shall select the other members of the committee for a period of one year and members may be appointed for a second term.
5. New members shall be appointed each year during the month of September.
6. A recorder shall be elected during the first meeting in October.

Meetings

The Patient Care Committee shall meet on the first Wednesday of each four-week placement schedule at 11:00 A.M.

RECRUITMENT COMMITTEE

Purpose

To recruit qualified nursing personnel for nursing services.

Objectives

1. To stimulate interest that will encourage people to seek employment at the hospital.
2. To develop recruitment programs in conjunction with the Personnel Department.
3. To participate in community activities that supply information about nursing roles at the hospital.

Membership

The Recruitment Committee shall consist of eight members:

1. Supervisor, Chairman
2. Head Nurse
3. Assistant Head Nurse
4. General Duty Nurse
5. Clinical Nurse Specialist
6. Licensed Practical Nurse
7. Staff Education Instructor
8. Personnel Department (one representative)

Procedure for Appointment

1. A supervisor shall be appointed chairman by the Director of Nursing and shall serve for a period of two years.
2. Committee members shall be appointed at the beginning of each fiscal year.
3. A nursing service secretary shall be appointed to take minutes of the meetings.

Meetings

The Recruitment Committee shall meet four times a year, as notified by the Chairman.

Responsibilities of Chairman

1. A notice of the Recruitment Committee meetings shall be sent to the members a week in advance.
2. The objectives and agenda of the meetings shall be determined in advance and stated in the notice of the meeting.
3. A copy of the notice and agenda shall be sent to the Director of Nursing.
4. The committee's proceedings shall be recorded in the form of minutes and placed in a loose-leaf binder maintained in the Nursing Service Office.
5. Communicate to the Director of Nursing the committee's deliberations and submit in writing any recommendations that shall be made.

THE WESTERN PENNSYLVANIA HOSPITAL*
Department of Nursing
Staff Development
Overview

Staff Development is an on-going program of education with developed programs to assist employees' adjustment to their role in the total hospital organization, to develop manual and behavioral skills and to develop the employee's abilities to function effectively in caring for patients or directing patient care in the hospital.

Staff Development is developed around four areas of personnel needs:

1. Orientation — Introduce the employee to her/his position and responsibilities and the environment in which she or he will be functioning.
2. Skill Training — Training in manual and behavioral skills.
3. Special Courses — Meet the employees' need for advancement and prepare those qualified for management and supervisory positions.
4. Continuing Education — Stimulate interest and add to knowledge previously gained to keep up with the changes and newer concepts in the health field.

*Reprinted by permission of The Western Pennsylvania Hospital, Pittsburgh, Pennsylvania.

THE WESTERN PENNSYLVANIA HOSPITAL
DEPARTMENT OF NURSING
STAFF DEVELOPMENT

Frame of Action

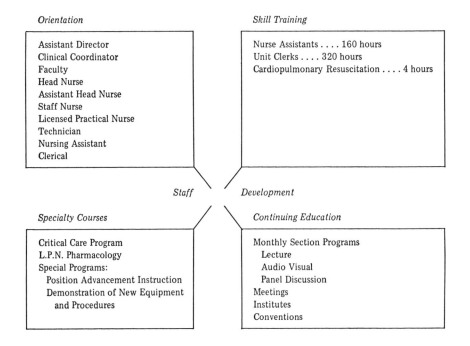

Orientation

Assistant Director
Clinical Coordinator
Faculty
Head Nurse
Assistant Head Nurse
Staff Nurse
Licensed Practical Nurse
Technician
Nursing Assistant
Clerical

Skill Training

Nurse Assistants . . . . 160 hours
Unit Clerks . . . . 320 hours
Cardiopulmonary Resuscitation . . . . 4 hours

Staff   *Development*

Specialty Courses

Critical Care Program
L.P.N. Pharmacology
Special Programs:
  Position Advancement Instruction
  Demonstration of New Equipment
    and Procedures

Continuing Education

Monthly Section Programs
  Lecture
  Audio Visual
  Panel Discussion
Meetings
Institutes
Conventions

ST. MARY'S HOSPITAL*
Milwaukee, Wisconsin
Nursing Service Inservice Education

Nursing Education

Nursing Education is an integral part of the Nursing Department organization. It has a major role in developing, monitoring and teaching nursing policy and procedures. It coordinates staff development for the department and has decentralized as well a centralized

*Reprinted by permission of St. Mary's Hospital, Milwaukee, Wisconsin, and the Catholic Hospital Association, St. Louis, Missouri.

focus. The nursing instructors based on each unit evaluate and meet specific learning needs of the personnel.

Records. Inservice and continuing education sessions are recorded for all nursing personnel on cards kept in the Nursing Education office. These records are available to the supervisor or the individual employee for reference. Inservice education hours are transferred from attendance sheets. The individual employee is responsible for supplying proof of outside continuing education hours for inclusion on cards.

Certification. Any procedure outside basic position expectations requires documentation of education and approval by supervisor or instructor. Such procedures include IV therapy for RNs, medication administration for LPNs, transcription of orders for Unit Secretaries, and intra-aortic balloon pump for RNs. Certificates are filed in the Nursing Education office and are sent to employee's file upon termination.

Programs

1. RN/LPN Initial Staff Development Program. A four-week program for all new RN and LPN employees includes orientation and clinical content, e.g., IV workshop and physical assessment and recognition-of-acute-emergencies workshop. A condensed two-week orientation is given for groups of five or fewer. IV certification is required of an RN's first six months of employment for a merit increase to be effective.
2. LPN Medication Course. Successful completion of this six-week course is necessary for LPN certification for medical administration. An LPN may challenge the course by passing a written exam and taking class in injection technique and LPN role in IV therapy. Eight hours' supervised practice is required of all LPNs. Certification is required in the first six months of employment for a merit increase to be effective.
3. Unit Secretary Training Program. A three-to-four-week class program with intense supervisory follow-up is utilized to train inexperienced individuals for the position of Unit Secretary. Certification is required in the first three months of employment for any merit increase to be effective.
4. Leadership Development. An ongoing program stresses managerial content as related to positions of supervisor and clinician.
5. Nurse Internship Program. A nine-week program (following three weeks of orientation) for new professional nurse graduates emphasizes assessment, clinical decision making, skill development, and nursing management.
6. Nursing Grand Rounds. Monthly case conferences are held to develop standardized care plans. Case presentation rotates by nursing unit.
7. Code 4 Team Classes. This 8- to 10-hour course prepares nurses for roles on the Code 4 Team. Enrollment is open to any employee in departments involved in Code 4.
8. Basic Cardiopulmonary Resuscitation. A three-hour program on CPR is presented in line with Wisconsin Heart Association guidelines. The program is open to any hospital employee and leads to Basic CPR Certification.

9. Fire, Disaster, and Safety. All nursing personnel are scheduled to participate in hospital-wide programs for fire, disaster, and safety.
10. Clinical Teaching Course. This 10-hour course for Nursing Instructors applies teaching-learning theory to the clinical teaching setting. It is open to any employee with major teaching responsibilities.
11. Staff Nurse Workshop. Day-long workshops for staff nurses focus on advanced clinical content.
12. Clinical Nursing Courses. A 4- to 15-week course on selected clinical nursing topics is presented once a year, e.g., critical care, cancer nursing, diabetes nursing.
13. Affiliating Agencies Orientation. A two-hour program is held for faculty and students of affiliating educational agencies early in the spring and fall semesters.
14. Patient Education Programs. A patient education instructor designs and implements new programs in collaboration with nursing and other staff. Ongoing programs include childbirth preparation and diabetes self-care classes.

Philosophy *

Mercy Hospital Department of Education is based on a hospital-wide concept, directed toward the improvement of hospital services, operation, and economy through the training strategy available to all personnel.

All activities of the Department support the Christian philosophy, which recognizes the existence of God, man's unique composition of body and soul, and the dignity of the human person. All activities of the Department also support the Hospital philosophy, its objectives and current goals.

The Education Department believes that the individual administrator, department head, manager, or supervisor has final responsibility for the orientation, training, job performance, and motivation of his personnel. The Education Department, as a staff function, provides educational services to assist managers at all levels to fulfill these responsibilities.

The Education Department believes that employees are motivated by an opportunity to be well informed and to achieve high performance standards. Therefore, programs should be continuing and flexible, need-based and realistic, and employee-involved.

*Reprinted by permission of Mercy Hospital, Department of Education, New Orleans, Louisiana.

The Education Department believes that all hospital personnel, the Medical Staff, patients and their families and visitors, and the community in general are integral elements in education for health and prevention of, or optimal recovery from, illness and injury. To the extent feasible, these elements are considered in educational programming.

The Education Department believes that effective teaching or learning is based on characteristics and goals of learners and on application of teaching or learning principles, methods, and technology.

I. Goals for 1976–77 Fiscal Year
   A. Continue improving physical facilities for a pleasant, healthy working environment that is conducive to adult learning.
   B. Support the Nursing Service division by continuing to provide in-service and continuing education programs and orientation programs for all Nursing Service personnel (ongoing).
   C. Pursue these joint goals with Nursing Service:
      1. Conduct two nurse refresher courses during the year.
      2. Implement an extended orientation plan for the new Louisiana State University (LSU) Associate Degree graduates, if the plan is desired by these graduates.
      3. Plan and conduct evening seminars in clinical nursing (general medical-surgical nursing topics).
      4. Seek funding through Orleans Parish School Board for a coronary care course, a course in neurological and neurosurgical nursing, and a course in cancer nursing.
      5. Attempt to obtain Continuing Education Recognition Points for continuing education activities.
   D. Special Projects (operational):
      1. Conduct training course for nurses in ICU and other areas such as Emergency Department, OR, and PAR, and general nursing units.
      2. Support the faith community and pastoral care.
      3. Expand patient education activities through:
         a. development of patient teaching modules;
         b. utilization of closed circuit television for regular programming of educational films.
      4. Continue to build A-V library on hospital safety.

5. Build A-V library on management aids.
6. Support Personnel Department in orientation, interviewing, standards appraisal, and pre-retirement counseling.

E. Offer educational programs for the community such as diabetic teaching, one or two pediatric orientations, hypertension (detection and treatment), and cancer.

INTRODUCTION TO NURSING SERVICE DEPARTMENT

Objectives

1. To acquaint new personnel with the scope of the hospital nursing service department's activities.
2. To gain an understanding of other hospital departments that are closely allied to nursing service.
3. To assist new personnel to see their role in relation to the hospital and the community.
4. To become aware of the many resources that are available to patients within the hospital.
5. To see total patient care as a cooperative, interdisciplinary effort.

Nursing Department
Nursing Service Educational Unit
Introduction to Nursing Service — Orientation Program

Objectives	Contents	Methods	Resources	Activities
I. Welcome to Nursing Service				
To introduce the key administrative Nursing Service personnel To make new personnel feel welcome to their positions	Welcome to all new personnel Introduction of Supervisors Purpose of Introduction to Nursing Service Importance of being flexible on the job Importance of individual jobs Individual learning and growth on the job Golden Rule as applied to patient care	Lecture Question and answer period	Director of Nursing or her representative Supervisors Administrative Assistant	None
II. Philosophy of Nursing Service				
To develop an awareness of the scope of Nursing Practice To understand the beliefs of Nursing Service regarding patient care To help the individual formulate her/his own understanding of the Nursing Service Philosophy	The most important person in our hospital Scope of Nursing Care Nursing Team Concept What every patient has a right to expect Additional responsibilities of Nursing Service Employee's responsibilities	Lecture Question and answer period	Nursing Service Administrative Staff Material: Philosophy of Nursing Service "10 Commandments of a Good Hospital"	None

To realize the importance of the patient to the existence of a hospital

III. Staffing Nursing Service Department

Objective	Content	Method	Responsible	Resources
To gain an appreciation of the problems involved in staffing a hospital To develop a sense of individual responsibility toward one's job	Master Staffing Plan How it is developed Float list Scheduling tours of duty Basis of employment Absenteeism Employee responsibilities	Lecture Question and answer period	Nursing Service Administrative Staff	Tour Nursing Office See Master Staffing Plan

IV. Dietary Department

Objective	Content	Method	Responsible	Resources
To gain an understanding of the operation of the Dietary Department To gain an understanding of the responsibility of nursing personnel in relation to patient's dietary needs	Patients' diets Cafeteria Selective menus Number of meals served daily Diet manuals Dietary Department trucks Handling diabetic trays Kitchen operations Meals on wheels Employee responsibilities	Lecture Question and answer period	Director of Dietary Department	Tour

V. Social Service Department

Objective	Content	Method	Responsible	Resources
To develop an appreciation of some of the problems faced by patients and the resources available to help solve them	Limitations of Medicare-Medicaid Welfare Private insurance companies Inter-agency referral	Lecture Question and answer period	Director of Social Social Department	None

Continued

Objectives	Contents	Methods	Resources	Activities
To gain an understanding of the role of the employee	Nursing homes Employee responsibilities			
To develop a deeper understanding of the problems of modern society as presented by patients and how they can be approached	The unwed mother Pre-natal clinic Legal aspects of the battered/neglected child Functioning of department in the hospital			

VI. Religious Life Department

Objectives	Contents	Methods	Resources	Activities
To develop an appreciation of the patient's spiritual needs	Introduction of Religious Life personnel and location of department How to reach Chaplain Chapel services	Lecture	Religious	Tour
To understand how the employee can cooperate with the Religious Life Department in meeting the spiritual needs of patients	Religious customs a. Jewish — dietary laws, circumcision b. Catholic — sacrament of the sick, communion, infant baptism c. Protestant — baptism, communion Feelings of various religions re: death, burial, cremation, autopsies Employee responsibilities			

VII. Fire Safety and Evacuation

Objectives	Content	Method	Resources	Activity
To learn about the use of fire extinguishers and the various methods of evacuating patients in the event of fire To enable Nursing Service personnel to function in an organized manner both during practice fire drills and in the event of fire	Basic review of hospital fire code What to do before the Fire Department arrives Methods of evacuation: a. Hip carry b. Packstrap carry c. Cradle drop d. Fireman's carry Classes of fires Use of extinguishers according to class of fire a. Soda-acid-water b. CO_2 Employee responsibilities	Lecture Demonstration a. Evacuation methods b. Extinguishers	Evansville City Fire Department Representative Fire plan Hospital Nursing units Safety leaflets	Return demonstration of: a. Evacuation methods b. Extinguishers Observe location of extinguishers in hospital and on nursing units

VIII. Housekeeping and Laundry Department

Objectives	Content	Method	Resources	Activity
To learn about the scope of housekeeping and laundry activities To increase cooperation between Nursing Service and Housekeeping/Laundry Departments	Cleaning schedules Furnishing rooms Housekeeping as opposed to nursing responsibility on the units Problems of maintaining a relatively germ-free environment: a. Disinfection methods b. Cultures Sewing Room Laundry Repair of torn linen Typical daily work load Employee responsibilities	Lecture Question and answer period	Housekeeping and Laundry Department Director	Tour areas

Continued

Objectives	Contents	Methods	Resources	Activities
IX. Central Service				
To gain an appreciation of the volume of supplies handled in Central Service	Methods of sterilization	Lecture	Central Service representative	Tour
	Type of equipment available in Central Service	Question and answer period		
To understand the vital importance of Central Service to the functioning of the hospital	Disposable equipment advantages and disadvantages			
	How to order from Central Service			
	Volume of work done in a typical day			
	Show examples of newest equipment available			
	Charges from Central Service			
	Stocking floor needs			
	Employee responsibilities			
X. Program Evaluation				
To assist in evaluating the orientation educational experience	Explain purpose of program evaluation	Lecture	Staff Education Instructors	Complete written evaluation
	Elicit comments, suggestions, reactions	Question and answer period	New Employees	
To understand purpose of evaluating the orientation program	Use of evaluation to improve program			

ADMINISTRATION OF A NURSING UNIT
(A Short Course for Hospital Personnel
Functioning in Head Nurse Roles)

Introduction

This course is designed to extend an understanding of the changing role of the head nurse today and tomorrow, thereby stimulating study of the head nurse role in the individual institutions for the ultimate purpose of increasing the contribution of these key persons in providing a climate for improved patient care. The title of Head Nurse may change with the role, but there will continue to be need for competent nurses to assume immediate responsibility for the nursing care of a group of patients and for the coordination of their total care. This approach emphasizes the study of the kinds of relationships the head nurse must have with other health personnel in order to achieve maximum effectiveness.

The course is divided into three units. The sequence of the units is as follows: (1) The head nurse in a modern hospital, which includes the organization of the hospital and the services it offers; (2) the head nurse's responsibility for nursing care administration, which includes quality of patient care, diagnosing and planning care, delegating responsibilities, supervision, and evaluation; and (3) the head nurse's responsibility for staff development, which entails supervision and evaluation of personnel as well as self-analysis and advancement.

Objectives

1. To identify concepts of the changing role of the head nurse.
2. To assume responsibility for providing an administrative climate conducive to good nursing care.
3. To apply knowledge of human behavior in the development of skill in maintaining effective relationships with other members of the health team.
4. To appreciate the need for continuous self-evaluation and experimentation leading to continual self-growth.

Unit I. The Head Nurse in Today's Hospital

Behavior	Content	Learning Activities

1. Understands organization of hospital and nursing service department.	I. Introduction
	  A. Get acquainted
	  B. Why are we here?
	  C. Management as an attitude of mind
	  D. Group participation
		Participants interview each other
		Lecture

2. Appreciates the importance of maintaining institutions that meet required standards of patient care.	II. Health Care in a Contemporary Society	Lecture (Resource Person)

3. Aware of the changing role of the Head Nurse.	III. Hospital Organization
	  A. Administration
	  B. Board of Directors
	  C. Accreditation
	  D. Patient Services
		Lecture (Resource Person)
		
		Question-Answer Period

	IV. Nursing Service Organization
	V. Changing Role of the Head Nurse
	  A. Historical Review
	  B. Present Trends
	  C. Future
		Take notes on own activities for a week — then evaluate as to what activities could be performed by other personnel.
		Lecture
		Discuss Nurse Practice Act. What are the legal limits of practice for the R.N. and L.P.N.?

	VI. Sound Organizational Planning for Hospital Nursing Service and the Head Nurse's Responsibility	Lecture Question-Answer Period

Unit II. The Head Nurse's Responsibility for Unit Administration

Behavior	Content	Learning Activities

4. Understands the principles of administration and their application.
5. Skilled in handling patient care on the unit.
6. Appreciates the importance of maintaining the integrity of personnel.
7. Enhances communication knowledge and skill.
	VII. Head Nurse
	  A. Dual Role
	    1. Manager
	    2. Clinical Practice
	VIII. Concepts and Principles of Management
	IX. Management Functions
	  A. Planning
	    1. Philosophy
	    2. Objectives
	  B. Organizing
	    1. Responsibility
	    2. Delegation
	    3. Consultation
	    4. Decision Making
	    5. Line and Staff
	    6. Centralization versus Decentralization
	    7. Committee and Group Leadership
	  C. Staffing
	    1. Selection
	    2. Interview
	    3. Appraisal
	    4. Promotion
	    5. Centralized versus Decentralized (Work Scheduling)
		Lecture
		Question-Answer Period
		Evaluate a Nursing Unit administration based on guide developed in text. To be done in class — discuss results.
		
		Resource Person
		
		Lecture
		Resource Person
		Question-Answer Period
		After reviewing material (hand-out) on staffing, identify which type

Continued

Unit II (Continued)

Behavior	Content	Learning Activities

	D. Directing
	  1. Giving Direction
	  2. Morale
	  3. Discipline
	  4. Motivation
	E. Controlling
	  1. Budget
	  2. Inventory
	F. Decision Making
	G. Communication
	H. Environment
		of scheduling would best fit your situation and justify position.
		Case Presentation — Group Discussion
		
		Resource Person

Unit III. The Head Nurse's Responsibility for Nursing Care Administration

Behavior	Content	Learning Activities
8. Understands the needs of patients during various phases of hospitalization.	X. Nursing Care Administration A. Quality of Patient Care 1. Needs	Lecture Question-Answer Period

9. Skilled in aiding nursing personnel to assess patient needs.
10. Skilled in delegating responsibility for planning patient care.
11. Appreciates the importance of supervision and evaluation of nursing care.

    a. Admission and discharge
    b. Acutely ill
    c. Convalescence and mild illness
    d. Referral
B. Admission of Patients
C. Diagnosing Nursing Needs
D. Planning Care
  1. Nursing Care Plans
    a. Objectives
    b. Areas of responsibility
    c. Therapeutic measures and rehabilitation
    d. Prevention and support
    e. Teaching
    f. Methods of transmitting
E. Delegating Responsibility for Nursing Care
  1. Knowledge of Patient Needs
  2. Qualifications of Personnel
  3. Making Assignments
    a. Personnel qualifications
    b. Amount of supervision available
    c. Needs of patients
    d. Continuity of patient care
  4. Philosophy of Team Nursing
  5. Supervision of Nursing Care
  6. Evaluation of Nursing Care

Unit IV. The Head Nurse's Responsibility for Personnel Development and Teaching Program

Behavior	Content	Learning Activities
12. Understands the importance of guided learning opportunities for nursing personnel.	XI. Personnel Development Inservice Education	Lecture Question-Answer Period
13. Skilled in assessing personnel performance.	A. Orientation B. Skill Training C. Continuing Education	
14. Appreciates the need for self-development as well as personnel development.	D. Leadership and Management	Panel: What Nursing Service Administrators Expect of a Head Nurse. (Resource Persons — Directors of Nursing Service)

19. Learning and Change*

A PATTERN OF LEARNING THAT LEADS TO CHANGE

1. This Is What Learners Often Have	2. This Is What Learners Often Do to Resolve Conflict
Conflict	*Defense*
Learner feels need for change, yet wishes to remain as he is when faced with ideas that threaten his present attitudes and behavior. This ambivalence is a conflict between "the old" and "the new." It creates tension in the learner. He becomes disturbed. He must resolve the conflict.	Learner defends himself against ideas that force him to admit his limitations; resists the will of someone else or something to change him. Defense may take some of the following forms:
NOTE: When the need for change is readily apparent, learners sometimes resolve this conflict by passing rapidly to Steps 3 and 4.	Projection — we defend our present ideas by asserting ourselves as we now are, by blaming somebody or some circumstances.
	Rationalization — we find reasons to justify our present feelings, opinions and behavior.
	Resistance — we become angry, we withdraw, or we don't listen actively in order to protect ourselves.
	NOTE: Productive change rarely comes about by a conflict of wills in the attempt to prove somebody right and somebody wrong.

*Source: Bergevin, P., and McKinley, J. *Adult Education for the Church.* St. Louis: Bethany Press, 1971. Page 57. Reprinted with permission.

433

3.
This Is What Learners
Should Do to Learn
Together Creatively

4.
This Is the Result
of Creative Learning

Resolve the Conflict

Learner struggles with himself —
the new way of thinking and
feeling vs. his habitual ways.

People can help each other in this
struggle to try to understand a
new idea objectively if they work
together as a team. The original
ambivalence is examined
objectively.

The learner himself must make the
decision to learn: the learner is
free to face the ambivalence within
himself (1) when no one insists on
changing him; (2) when he can
express himself freely; (3) when
he feels accepted regardless of his
attitude; (4) when he is not at-
tacked or put on the defensive as
a person.

The process of incorporation is aided
by the identification of individual
learners with the other members of
the learning team.

Incorporation

Learner understands, accepts
and assimilates the new
point of view.

Experiences Leading to Learning	*Resources for Learning Experiences*
Thinking	Textbooks
	Supplementary books
Discussing, conferring, speaking, reporting	Reference books, encyclopedias
Reading (words, pictures, symbols)	Magazines, newspapers
	Documents, clippings
Writing, editing	Duplicated materials
Listening	Programmed materials
Interviewing	(self-instructional)
Outlining, taking notes	
	Motion-picture films
Constructing, creating	Television programs
Drawing, painting, lettering	Radio programs
Photographing	Recordings (tape and disk)
Displaying, exhibiting	
Graphing, charting, mapping	Flat pictures
	Drawings and paintings
	Slides and transparencies
	Filmstrips
Demonstrating, showing	Microfilms, microcards
Experimenting, researching	Stereographs
Problem solving	
	Maps, globes
Collecting	Graphs, charts, diagrams
Observing, watching	Posters
Traveling	Cartoons
Exchanging	
Recording	Puppets
	Models, mockups
Dramatizing	Collections, specimens
Singing, dancing	
	Flannel-board materials
Imagining, visualizing	Chalkboard materials
Organizing, summarizing	Construction materials

*From *A-V Instruction — Materials and Methods* by J. Brown, R. Lewis, and F. Harclerood. Copyright 1964 by McGraw-Hill Book Company. Used with permission of McGraw-Hill Book Company.

Experiences Leading to Learning	*Resources for Learning Experiences*
Computing	Drawing materials
Judging, evaluating	Display materials
Working	

CHAPTER 5. NURSING RESEARCH*

5.01 Statement of Policy

Nursing research will be one of the processes used to improve the care of people in health and illness. Nursing Service staff will promote a climate receptive to nursing activities and application of research findings in a clinical setting.

5.02 General Provisions

VA nurses will be encouraged to initiate research directed toward development of relevant and reliable data in all patient care settings where nursing care will be given. In addition, nurses will be encouraged to publish their findings in order to communicate and implement new nursing knowledge. Application of research findings, whether from nursing research or from research of related health care disciplines, will be made through nursing administration, nursing education, or through clinical nursing staff. Nursing research protocols will be approved at the local level by:

a.   Nursing Service.
b.   Research and Development Committee.
c.   Subcommittee on Human Studies.

5.03 Scope

The scope of nursing research includes:

a.   Clinical nursing research that studies in depth patient needs, care, or aspects of illness.
b.   Studies relating to priority aspects of the VA mission or objectives critical to Nursing Service, e.g., studies of nurses' roles, investigations of expanded roles, projects related to problem-oriented medical records, and the care of the aging.
c.   Studies or projects designed to provide answers regarding nursing procedures, personnel, practices, and products.

*Used by courtesy of the Veterans Administration, Department of Medicine and Surgery, Washington, D.C., and Shreveport, Louisiana.

d. Projects, questionnaires, studies, and surveys that produce data of value to Nursing Service will be completed in conjunction with formal nursing programs, e.g., Chief, Nursing Service Training program.

e. Studies done by basic nursing students in conjunction with their clinical experience, or by graduate nursing students who have obtained permission to use the VA setting.

f. Medical research that has nursing implication, that is accomplished in patient care settings and supervised by nurses. It may be medical or interdisciplinary research that has nurses on the investigation teams.

g. Projects of nursing research that have been planned on a VA regionalization or medical district basis.

h. Cooperative nursing studies, that is, one protocol applied by nurse researchers at more than one VA setting after appropriate approval.

i. Surveys, projects, studies, questionnaires completed in conjunction with local, community, university, state, or national groups of nurses or other health professionals.

j. Evaluation teams with nurses as members.

k. Individual projects or investigations with approval by Research and Development Committees.

l. Individual or group projects that have been funded by Central Office, e.g., by Medical Research Service or Health Services Research and Development, cooperative studies, and health manpower.

m. Individual or group projects with national fundings, e.g., National Institutes of Health or National Institute of Mental Health.

5.04 Consultation Services Available for Nursing Research

Nursing research efforts will derive assistance from consultants, from collaboration with nurse researchers at local universities, and through group approaches to clinical nursing projects. Other informational support services will be available to nurse researchers through appropriate communication with:

a. VA Cooperative Studies Program Support Centers with statistical and computer resources.
b. Medline Bibliographic Retrieval Service. Librarians will forward requests to VA Central Office library.
c. National professional nursing organizations, e.g., American Nurses' Foundation, American Nurses' Association, Council of Nurse Researchers; and National Research Publications, e.g., Nursing Research International Nursing Index.
d. Central Office Nursing Service, where nursing research projects, newsletters, circulars, program guides, and published research studies will be available.

5.05 Nursing Research Personnel

a. All nurses with research preparation and experience will be encouraged to propose relevant research at health care facilities. At some hospitals, a position entitled Associate Chief, Nursing Service for Research, has been established. The nurse researchers, in addition to pursuing their own research, assist and guide the development of research in their own facility, work with others in the medical district, and will be available for nursing research assistance at other locales when specifically requested through Nursing Service.
b. Nursing research skills will be upgraded through joint courses held either at the university or the VA site, through VA-university consultation by nurse researchers, and through joint nursing research proposals. Because they focus on patients and their needs, these proposals will meet the objectives of VA Nursing Service and the expanding areas of interest by nursing faculty members in affiliated universities.

VETERANS ADMINISTRATION HOSPITAL*
Shreveport, Louisiana
Nursing Service Memorandum No. 74-1
March 1, 1974

Nursing Service Committees

1. Nursing Service committees are established to guide Nursing Service activities in achieving objectives.
2. Duties delegated to committees are as follows:
   a. *Planning and Coordinating Committee* will develop overall administrative and management plans for the functioning of Nursing Service, coordinate activities and duties of committees, and make final decisions on recommendations regarding policies and practices within Nursing Service.
   b. *Procedure Committee* will provide and stimulate use of procedures based upon scientific principles, policies, and currently accepted practices.
   c. *Safety Committee* will assist in providing safeguards for patients, visitors and personnel; and in formulating directives for nursing personnel to follow in order to prevent accidents and injuries.
   d. *Nursing Practice Committee* will be responsible for studying nursing care, developing standards and guidelines to upgrade quality of patient care, and systematically reviewing patients' records as a means to improve quality of patient care.
   e. *Research and Studies Committee* will foster inquiry and provide means for nurses to apply the scientific process in problem solving and develop a procedural framework that will enable them to use research findings in their daily work situations.
3. Committee members are appointed by the Chief, Nursing Service, upon recommendations of supervisors and the individual's expressed interest. Membership will be periodically rotated. Membership on a committee is to be considered a regular part of the employees' duties and attendance at all committee meetings during hours of duty is expected.
4. Replacements to committees will be appointed by Chief, Nursing Service, when requested by committee chairmen.

*Used by courtesy of the Veterans Administration, Department of Medicine and Surgery, Washington, D.C., and Shreveport, Louisiana.

5. Regular meetings will be held and written minutes prepared. The official file for minutes will be maintained in the Nursing Office. A copy of the minutes of the Safety Committee will be sent to the Safety Technician (138).
6. An annual evaluation of each committee's activities will be prepared by the chairman and forwarded to the Chief, Nursing Service, for use in preparing the Systematic Review report.
7. RESCISSION: Nursing Service Memorandum No. 73-1, dated January 17, 1973, and Nursing Service Memorandum No. 73-8, dated October 15, 1973.

VETERANS ADMiNISTRATION HOSPITAL*
Shreveport, Louisiana
Nursing Service Memorandum No. 75-3
December 1, 1975

Guidelines for Obtaining Approval for Nursing Studies

1. *Purpose:* To establish Nursing Service policy for submitting and obtaining approval for nursing studies and projects.
2. *Policy:* It is the policy of Nursing Service that studies must be approved before they are implemented. Nurses conducting approved studies may have designated times away from regular duties if necessary to carry out the project, with the approval of the Chief, Nursing Service.
3. *Responsibility:* The Chairman of the Research and Studies Committee will review all studies submitted with the committee members and make recommendations to the Chief Nurse. The Chief Nurse is responsible for final approval of a study or project.
4. *Procedures:*
   a. Nursing studies proposed are to be submitted in writing to the Chairman of the Research and Studies Committee. This initial submission need only contain the topic and proposed method of study.
   b. Study will be routed by the Chairman to members of the Research and Studies Committee for comments.
   c. Studies approved by the committee will be sent to the Chief Nurse for his approval.
   d. A nurse who has an approved study will be assisted by an assigned committee member in developing design and methodology and conducting the project.
   e. Members of the Research and Studies Committee are available for guiding the writing of proposals, through the Chairman.
   f. Studies not approved will be returned to the writer with suggestions for re-working the project or the rationale for disapproval.
5. *Rescission:* None.

*Used by permission of the Veterans Administration, Department of Medicine and Surgery, Washington, D.C., and Shreveport, Louisiana.

Guide for Writing Study or Research Proposal

The following guide should be used in writing up a proposal and for the completed study. (For brief studies the sections under Introduction and Conceptual Framework may be combined if more convenient.)

   I. Introduction
      A. Relation of study to needs of field or present practice, etc. (one paragraph will do)
      B. Significance of study to nursing and/or other fields (one or two paragraphs will do)
      C. Statement of general area of concern
  II. Conceptual Framework
      A. Discussion of concepts involved in study (one paragraph on literature relevant to each concept involved in the study will do)
      B. Review of relevant research (one paragraph on each study will do)
      C. Definition of terms
      D. Summary statement
 III. Methodology
      A. Statement of research problems
      B. Statement of hypotheses
         1. Assumptions
         2. Rationale and deduced consequences
      C. Research design
         1. Type of design
            a. Research method
            b. Data collection
               (1) Nature of data
               (2) Technique of data collection (instrument development or selection)
               (3) Administration of observation technique or instrument
         2. Sampling
            a. Sample space
            b. Sample (full description)
         3. Ethics (one paragraph will do)

        D. Analysis
           1. Qualitative: categorizations
           2. Quantitative: statistics
        E. Study limitations
  IV. Administrative Planning
        A. Timetable
        B. Budget
           1. Personnel
           2. Material
           3. Equipment
   V. Appendixes
        A. Instrument(s)
  VI. Bibliography

Involvement

Involve all who are to be affected by the change in the planning for it from the very beginning. Together, discuss what should be changed and what strategies should be used to effect it. People will usually adopt innovations which they perceive will be benefitial to themselves.

Motivation

One needs to understand that feelings and emotions govern behavior in order to motivate people. To do this, advocates of change create an openness of communications, a trust, and reduce status barriers. Motivation involves honesty in recognizing one's feelings as well as caring for and respecting those of others. It means knowing and practicing the art of a helping relationship.

Planning

This is the *sine qua non* for effecting permanent and productive change. Planning means considering the inputs and constraints that are "givens"; it means considering inputs that should be sought. It means communicating and arranging the physical, social and emotional environment so that all needed resources are available.

Legitimation

For change to be permanent, it must be sanctioned by society and legitimized. For the expanded nurse role to be sanctioned, all who will be affected by it must see the new role as a desirable and legitimate one. The idea of expanded nursing practice must be sold to the power structure in the occupational setting and in the community, both medical and nonmedical, for it to be accepted.

Education

To implement change, one re-educates, using principles of "people" and "thing" technology. "People" technology refers to techniques one uses in relation to the behavior of man. "Thing" technology refers to techniques involved in implementing ideas. In order for administrators to educate those who will be involved in the movement, knowledge of both human behavior and the functions and responsibilities of the expanded nursing role is vital.

*Source: Talbot, Dorothy.   Social change and occupational health nursing. *Occupational Health Nursing,* April, 1974, p. 11.

Management
Practice is required in striking a balance between the two aspects of management, that of maximizing freedom for those at the grass roots level and enforcing agency policy and authority. This is the art of management. Nurse administrators use techniques for changing people's attitudes; they also use strategies of power. How to be flexible with power is the most important aspect of management.

Expectations
In implementing change, one holds many expectations. One expects resistance; expects only a few adopters in the beginning; expects problems. There will always be some who will not accept the new. There will always be problems when change is introduced. According to the theory of cultural lag, problems occur when change is implemented before people's customs and environment are adapted in order to accommodate the change.

Nurturance
One must nurture those who change, the adopters. They have much resistance to overcome, from patients, nurse colleagues, and physicians. They need support, both emotional and administrative. The best way to obtain early adopters is to locate those dissatisfied with the *status quo*, those who want to change. These are often the young and most highly educated, those desiring status and prestige, and willing to take risks; they have less to lose in their professional lifetimes.

Trust
Trust is the crux for effectively changing people's ways of doing things. Trust people to do what is right for themselves. Be trustworthy, for administrators have power.

Index

Accident and incident reports in
personnel file, 181
Accountability
delegation of, 50
quality assurance program and,
137–147. *See also* Quality
assurance program (QAP)
Administration, 15. *See also* Administrators, hospital; Management; Nurse director
capital expenditure budget, guidelines for, 117
committees, 164–166
communication effectiveness and,
95–97, 278–279, 279–282
facilities and, 251
interaction of nursing service department with, 273–287. *See
also* Nursing service department,
interactions with administration
meetings of, 163–164
of nursing units, program of education, 427–432
objectives of, 95–97
performance standards and, 136, 137
philosophy and, 82–83, 84
policy communication to, 107–108
responsibility for equipment and
supplies, 263, 264, 266
safety and, 253, 258, 259
support of nursing care plans by, 160
Administrators, hospital, 29–30, 297–
300
functions of, 297–298
nurse director and, 297–298, 298–
299, 299–300
personal characteristics of effective,
299
problems of, 299
public and, 298
Admission to hospital, 16
Adult education. *See* Education
American Hospital Association Quality
Assurance Program for Medical
Care in Hospitals, 138, 140
American Medical Association
code of ethics, 305
on nurses and health care, 304

American Nurses' Association
peer review guidelines and philosophy, 147, 363–373
personnel services of, 218
Annual report of nursing department,
169–170
Appeal of peer review decisions, 373
Application blank in personnel folder,
179
Assessment in nursing process, 156,
158
Assignment methods, 149–151
assignment sheets, 150–151
examples, 383–385, 387–389
primary nursing, 150
types of, 149–150
Audio-visual instruction, 214–215
Audit. *See* Nursing audit
Authority
delegation of, 46, 49, 50
leadership vs., 55–56
Autocratic leadership, described,
57, 58–59

Behavioral sciences, 273–278
defined, 273
human needs hierarchy, 273–275
motivation, 273–278. *See also*
Motivation
Benefits, union and, 290, 292
Budgets, 113–124
advantages of establishing, 114
capital expenditures, 116–117, 121,
351. *See also* Capital expenditure budget
cash, described, 117–118
control of, 123
defined, 113
equipment and supplies in, 116–117,
121, 351
importance of, 113
of nursing service department
budget committee, 119–120, 121
calendar for, 355–357
factors and needs in, 118–119
operating, described, 115–116
preparation of, 120, 121–122,
355–357

Budgets, of nursing service department — *Continued*
  presentation of, 122
  review of, 123
  operating, 115-116, 121, 347-349. *See also* Operating budget
  preparation, 119-120, 120-122
    analysis of past operations in, 120
    calendars for, 353-357
    equipment and supply needs and, 121
    new activities and, 120
    nursing budget committee in, 119-120, 121
    nursing care quality and, 120-121
    units and departments and, 121-122
  prerequisites for, 114-115
  presentation of, 122
  review of, 121, 123
  for staff education program, 197, 198

Capital expenditure budget
  described, 116-117
  equipment and supplies in, 116-117, 121, 351
  review of, 121
Case-functional method of assignment, 149
Case method of assignment, 149
Cash budget, described, 117-118
Change, 297, 310-322
  agents of, 316-317
  approaches to, 312-314, 315-316
  conflict and, 319-320
  defined, 311-312
  deliberate and collaborative nature of, 314-315
  implementing
    elements in, 320-321
    guidelines for, 321-322, 447-448
  importance of, 311
  learning patterns and, 433-434
  managed, described, 313, 314
  nurse director and, 310-311, 317-318, 319, 320-321, 322

  by "organizational drift," 314
  planned
    approaches to, 315-316
    described, 314-315
  process of, described, 312
  rate and significance of, 311
  resistance to, 317-319
  understanding, attitude and, 318-319
Clinical nurse specialist, 32-33
Command
  chain of, in organizational chart, 102
  span of control, 48-49
  unity of, 48
Committees, 164-166
  advantages of, 164-165
  on equipment and supplies
    for nursing practice, 266-267
    standardization of, 264-265
  on in-service education, 410-412
  on job description, 405-406
  on nursing audit, 406-408
  on nursing budget, 119-120, 121
  on nursing practice, 266-267, 441
    meetings, 403
    membership, 40, 402-403
    objectives, 401, 402
    responsibilities of chairman, 403
  on nursing service department
    philosophy and policies, 83-84, 107, 403-405, 441-442
  on patient care, 412-413
  on peer review, 364, 367-373. *See also* Peer review, committees
  permanent, 367-373
  on planning and coordination, 441
  on policy development, 106-107
  on procedures, 441
  in quality assurance program, 142
  on recruitment, 129, 218, 413-414
  on research, 229-230
    nursing service research, 228, 230, 441
  on safety, 253-254, 408-410, 441
    infection control, 255-256
    meetings, 410

membership, 409
objectives, 408-409
responsibilities of chairman, 410
selection of members, 165-166. *See also under specific committees*
standing, described, 165, 166. *See also specific topic, e.g.,* Safety, committees
temporary, 366-367
Communication, 278-282
administrative meetings and, 163
of educational program plans, 197
effective
establishment of, 280-282
factors in, 278-279
flexibility and organizational change, 279-280
importance of, 278, 279-280
improving, 280
nurse call system, 246, 254
nurse director and, 278-279, 280, 281, 301
nursing care plans and, 159
of nursing service philosophy, 88-89
of objectives, 95-97
of policies, 107-108
questions and problem definition in, 281-282
of rules of conduct, 285
system in nurses' station, 247
Community
health care delivery and, 8, 9, 309
health maintenance organization (HMO) and, 309-310
hospital response to needs of, 13
participation in activities of, 197, 206
role of service agencies, 309
sharing education with, 22
Conference rooms, 248
Confidentiality
of medical records, 17
of personnel files, 181
as right of patient, 17
Conflict, 319-320
Consultation services for research, 438-439

Control, 41, 42, 60-63
basic guidelines for, 61-62
comprehension of objectives and, 95
discipline and, 284-285. *See also* Discipline
maintenance of, 62
planning and, 60
responses to, 62
span of, in command, 48-49
Continuing education programs, 205-206, 415, 416

Decision making, 63-67
alternative choices in, 63
as creative process, 64
deadlines in, 66-67
delaying decisions, 65-66
involving others in, 64-65
management and, 41
organization and, 46
planning and, 43, 44, 45
policy development and repeated, 106
risks in, 66
steps in, 63-64
Delegation, 46, 49-51, 150
of authority, 49, 50
defined, 49
effective, described, 50-51
of responsibility, 49-50
for meeting attendance, 164
for policy application, 107
in quality assurance program, 142-143
Democratic leadership, described, 57-58
Department directors. *See also* Nurse director
coordination of activities of, 300-303
described, 29-30
Diagnostic services, 16
Diet and nutrition, 19
Director of nursing. *See* Nurse director
Discharge of patients, 22, 379

Discipline, 284-287. *See also* Control
fairness of, 286
handling problems, 285-286
importance of, 284
nurse director and administration
of, 286-287
origin of, 284-285
in quality control program, 146
record of action in personnel file,
180
system of progressive, 285
unions and, 292
Discrimination in employment, legislation on, 219, 295

Education, 195-216
achievements in personnel file,
181
activities in, 195, 198-199
audio-visual instruction, 214-215
budget for, 197, 198
change and, 447
committee on in-service, 410-412
in communication concepts, 278-
279
conference rooms for, 248
continuing education programs,
205-206, 415, 416
in equipment maintenance and use,
267-268
evaluation of programs, 197, 210-
212
examples of programs, 415-419,
421-427, 427-432
follow-up of programs, 212
future trends in, 215-216, 307-
309
head nurse development program,
427-432
as hospital function, 22
importance of, 308
interest and needs in, 197, 208-210
in leadership and management, 207
learning and
adult learning, 212-214
environment for, 87-88, 307,
308

patterns leading to change, 433-
434
resources for, 435-436
motivation and, 197, 199, 206, 208
nurse director and, 41, 196-197,
307-309, 379, 411, 412
objectives of, 95, 195, 417-418,
419, 421
opportunities for, unions and, 293
orientation programs, 199-202, 415,
416, 421, 422-426. *See also*
Orientation programs
in hospital and nursing service
philosophy, 307, 416-417,
418-419
planning programs, 197, 207-208
in problem-oriented nursing, 174
quality assurance and, 146
for return to nursing, 220-221
in rules of conduct, 285
sharing with community, 22
skill training, 202-205, 415, 416
special courses, 415, 416
supervisory, by nurse director, 41
training vs., 195-196
work simplification programs, 277-
278
Electrical hazards, 254
Emergency services, 15, 250
Environment. *See specific topic, e.g.,*
Learning, environment favor-
able for; Rooms
Equipment and supplies, 263-268
in budgets, 116-117, 121, 351
education on maintenance and
control of, 267-268
equipment, defined, 263-264
evaluation of, 265-266
guidelines for management of, 267
for learning, 435-436
new and experimental, 266, 268
nurse director and, 263, 265, 266-
267
nursing practice committee and,
266-267
nursing unit maintenance system,
264

procurement department, 263-264, 265

safety and adequacy of, 17

selection of, establishment of system for, 265-268

standardization committee on, 264-265

supplies, defined, 263

Ethics

AMA code of, 305

research and, 229-230

Evaluation in nursing process, 156-157, 158

Exit interview, 223-224

Expectations of patient, 23

nursing service philosophy and, 86, 87

quality assurance and, 138

Facilities. *See specific topic, e.g.*, Nursing unit; Rooms

Families of patients, room for, 248

Federal government

chronology of major health legislation, 333-334

hospitals and health care and, 9-10

Firing, 285, 286

exit interview, 223-224

unions and, 290, 292

Free-rein (laissez-faire) leadership, described, 57, 59-60

Functional method of assignment, 149

Goals. *See* Objectives and goals

Governing body, functions of, 29

Grievance procedures

peer review decisions, 373

unions and, 291, 292, 293

Group-participation training, 203-205

Handbooks. *See* Manuals

Head nurse

authority of, 31

education program for, 427-432

Health care. *See also specific topic*

changing social values and, 8, 9

community and, 8, 9, 309

comprehensive approach to, 10-12

continuity of, 22-23

dehumanization and depersonalization of, 5-6

expectations in, 3-4

federal government and, 9-10, 333-334

health maintenance organization (HMO), 309-310

as inherent right, 7

issues of concern in, 5-6

participation in delivery of, 6-7, 7-10, 303-307

perceptions on, 4

pressures for change in, 158

primary focus of, 11-12

staff education and, 195

trends in, 3-14, 250-252, 297-300

change and, 310-322

hospital role and, 12-14, 297-300, 300-303

national philosophy of, 4-5

nurse-physician cooperation, 303-307

Health maintenance organization (HMO), 309-310

Health status in personnel file, 180

Homogeneous assignments in organization, 49

Hospital. *See also specific topic, e.g.*, Administration. Nursing unit

changing role in health care, 12-14

educational contributions of, 87-88, 215-216

environment of, 241

expansion and maintenance of facilities, 250-252

objectives in design of, 249, 250, 251-252

federal health care programs and, 10

orientation programs on, 201

philosophy of, 82-83

response to community needs, 13

Implementation

of nursing care plans, 159

in nursing process, 156, 158

Infection control, 255-257
  committee for, 255-256
  isolation for, 256
  prevention of infection transmission
    in, 257
Informed consent concept, 230
In-service education. *See* Education
Interdisciplinary approach
  hospital environment and, 241
  management and, 41
  need for, 7-8
  nursing service philosophy and,
    83-84, 89
  physician-nurse cooperation, 303-
    307
  quality assurance and, 141
  team method of assignment, 149,
    383-385, 387-389
Interviews
  exit, 223-224
  form in personnel folder, 179-180

Job description
  committee on, 405-406
  described, 186, 187, 188, 190
Job evaluation, 183-193
  accuracy of, 188-189
  analysis of jobs, 184-186
    defined, 184
    items in, 185-186, 187
    records of, 186-189
  defined, 183
  functions of, 183
  job description, 186, 187, 188, 190,
    405-406
  job specifications, 186, 187, 188
  types of, 183
  wage and salary program and, 183-
    184
Joint Commission on the Accredita-
    tion of Hospitals
  performance standards of, 137, 138,
    140
  on records, 109

Ladder organizational structure, 102,
    103

Leadership, 41, 42, 53-60
  authority vs., 55-56
  autocratic, described, 57, 58-59
  climate of, performance appraisal
    and, 189-190
  democratic, described, 57-58
  of education programs, 197
  free-rein (laissez-faire), described,
    57, 59-60
  interpersonal relations and, 53-54
  personal, by nurse director, 53-54
  principles of effective, 56-57
  qualities for, 54-57
  quality assurance programs and,
    141, 142
  for research, 227
  training in, 207
Learning
  adult, nature of, 212-214
  environment favorable for, 87-88,
    215, 307, 308
  experiences, resources and, 435-436
  facilitation and interpersonal
    relations, 307, 308
  patterns leading to change, 433-434
Legal factors
  antidiscrimination legislation, 219,
    295
  definition of nursing practice and,
    136
  employment practices, 218-219
  legal liability and peer review com-
    mittees, 371
  major federal health legislation,
    333-334
  management-union relations and,
    293-295
  nurse-patient relations and, 230
  Occupational Safety and Health
    Act (OSHA), 257-259
  records of policies and procedures
    and, 108-109
Line responsibilities, staff and, 51, 52
Lounge for visitors, 248

Management, 39-75
  as art and science, 39-41

change and, 448
control function of, 41, 42, 60-63
decision making and, 41, 63-67.
    See also Decision making
defined, 39
departments of hospital, 300-303
improvement and development of,
    41
interdepartmental coordination and,
    300-303
leadership, 41, 42, 53-60. *See also*
    Leadership
management-union relations, 293-
    296
  legal framework of, 293-295
by objectives, 93-100. *See also*
    Objectives and goals
organization and, 41, 42, 46-53,
    81-92. *See also* Organization
organizational chart and, 101-104
organizational philosophy and, 81-
    92
planning function and, 41, 42-46.
    See also Planning
policies and procedures, 105-112.
    See also Philosophy; Policies and
    procedures
scientific, for determining personnel
    requirements, 126
success as test of, 40-41
systems approach, 67-75. *See also*
    Systems approach
training in, 207
trends in, 297-307
  change and, 310-322
  health maintenance organization,
    309-310
  hospital administrator, 297-300
  hospital departments, 300-303
  medical staff, 303-307
turnover rate and, 223
Manuals
  conduct rules and, 285
  on nursing department practice,
    136-137
  on nursing policies and procedures,
    109-112

format of, 109
maintenance and revision of, 111-
    112
organization of, 110-111
problems in development of, 111
topics in, 109-110
usefulness of, 109, 112
of nursing unit, 201
orientation programs and, 201
on safety, 253
Master staffing plan, 128-131, 132
defined, 129-130
development and approval of, 130
scheduling and, 133-134
staffing board, described, 130-131,
    132
use of, 130-131
Medical care
defined, 12
staff organization and, 15
Medical records
confidentiality of, 17
defined, 21
function and importance of, 21, 170
nursing audit, 175-179. *See also*
    Nursing audit
problem-oriented, 170-175
  applications to nursing, 172-173
  described, 170-171
  development of, 171-172, 172-
    173
  education in, 174
  nurse director and, 173-174
  storing patient charts, 247
Medical records librarian, 175-176,
    177, 178
Medical staff
  attitudes of nurses toward, 306-307
  cooperation with nurses, 303-307
Medication room, 247
Meetings
  administrative, 163-164
  committee, 165, 166
    in-service education, 411
    job description, 406
    nursing audit, 408
    nursing practice, 403

Meetings, committee — *Continued*
    nursing service department policy,
      404
    patient care, 413
    recruitment, 414
    safety, 410
Minutes
    of administrative meetings, 163-164
    of committee meetings, 165, 166
Morale, 282-284
    defined, 282
    equilibrium nature of, 283-284
    good, described, 284
    nurse director and, 283, 284
    problems relating to, 282-283
Motivation, 273-278
    change and, 447
    defined, 273-274
    education and, 197, 199, 206, 208
    to join unions, 290-291
    motivation hygiene theory, 276-277
    productivity and, 273, 275-276
    work simplification programs and,
      277-278

Noise control, 247, 259-261
Nurse call system, 246, 254
Nurse director, *See also specific topic*
    American Hospital Association on,
      34-35
    change and, 310-311, 317-318,
      319, 320-321, 322
    changing role of hospital and, 13-14
    community service agencies and, 309
    conflict and, 319-320
    coordination of activities with other
      departments, 300-303
    criteria for progressive, 3
    education and, 41, 196-197, 307-
      309, 379, 411, 412
    supervisory training by, 41
    effectiveness strengthening, 297-
      298, 323
    employer-employee relations and,
      289
    equipment and supplies and, 263,
      265, 266-267
    facilities and, 250-251, 252

future challenges of, 297, 323-325
general functions and responsibilities
    of, 35-37, 39
hospital administrator and, 297-
    298, 298-299, 299-300
ideals and philosophy of, 81-82,
    82-83
importance of, 33-34
interpersonal relations and, 273, 377
medical records and, 173-174
morale and, 283, 284
negative qualities of, 300
nursing audit committee and, 407,
    408
nursing service department policy
    committee and, 404, 405
organization of nursing service de-
    partment and, 33-37
patient care committee and, 413
peer review guidelines and tools for,
    375-382
perceptions of health care by, 4
performance standard evaluation
    guidelines and tools for, 376-
    382
physician-nurse cooperation and,
    305, 306-307
planning function of, 42, 43, 44, 45,
    46
quality assurance program and, 140-
    141, 141-143, 145-146
recruitment and, 218, 221, 414
research and, 227-229, 230, 234
responsibility delegation by, 30-31
safety committee and, 409, 410
trends and issues in health care and,
    6, 7
Nurse practitioners, 32-33
    in health care, 32-33, 323-324
    in research, 230, 234
Nurses' station, 246-247, 255
Nursing, definitions of, 135-137, 359-
    361
Nursing audit, 175-179
    committee, 406-408
    defined, 176
    departments and staff performing,
      177

essential elements of, 177
functions of, 175
initiation of
  permanent, 178-179
  preliminary, 177-178
medical records librarian and, 175-
  176, 177, 178
nurse director and, 377
retrospective, 179
Nursing care
corrective action and, 146
evaluation of responsibilities in, 6-7
focus of nursing activity, 18
management on nursing unit, 90,
  91-92
nursing assignment examples, 383-
  385, 387-389
nursing definitions and, 135-137,
  359-361
nursing process concept, 153-158.
  See also Nursing process
nursing service philosophy and, 86-
  90
nursing service vs., 30
objectives of, 153
peer review. *See* Peer review
plans, 158-160, 391-399. *See also*
  Nursing care plans
primary nursing, defined, 150
qualifications of staff for, 86
quality of. *See also* Performance
  standards; Quality assurance
  program (QAP)
  budget preparation and, 120-121
  defined, 139-141
  nursing audit and, 175-179. *See
    also* Nursing audit
  nursing process application and,
    154-155
  staffing by requirements for,
    126, 127
rounds, 160-162
Nursing care plans, 158-160
charts of, 398, 399
defined, 159
implementation and objectives of,
  159
procedures in, 391-399

purpose of, 391, 394
requirements for, 391, 394-395
responsibility for, 391
Nursing Performance Review, 365,368
Nursing practice
committees, 441
  on equipment and supplies, 266-
    267
  meetings, 403
  membership, 401, 402-403
  objectives, 40, 402
  responsibility of chairman, 403
emerging roles in, 323-324
future trends in, 297, 308-309
need for research in, 225, 226-227
nursing definition and, 359-361
problem-oriented approach to, 172-
  173, 173-175
  challenge of, 175
  education on, 174
  nurse director and, 173-174
  scientific basis of, 226-227
Nursing process, 153-158
assessment in, 156, 158
benefits of, 153
evaluation in, 156-157, 158
evaluation of, 154, 155
future of, 158
general properties of, 153-154
implementation in, 156, 158
meaning and definitions of, 154-156
nursing goal and, 153
phases of, 157-158
planning in, 156
as problem-solving process, 155
quality of nursing care and, 154-155
research and, 233-234
sense of accomplishment and, 157
Nursing Professional Standards Review, 364-365, 368
Nursing research. *See* Research
Nursing rounds
function of, 160
outline guide to, 160-162
Nursing service department. *See also*
  Nurse director; Nursing unit;
  and specific topic, e.g., Communication

Nursing service department — *Continued*
  activation of, 301
  administration of, 273
    interactions of administration
  budget
    budget committee, 119-120, 121
    calendar, 355-357
    factors and needs in, 118-119
    operating, described, 115-116
    preparation of, 120, 121-122,
      355-357
    presentation of, 122
    review of, 123
  community service agencies and,
    309
  interactions with administration,
    273-287
    behavioral science concepts and,
      273-278
    communication and, 278-282
    coordination with other depart-
      ments, 300-303
    discipline and, 284-287
    importance of, 273
    morale and, 282-284
    motivation and, 273-274, 275-
      278
  objectives, form illustrating, 344-
    345
  organization of, 30-36
    authority of head nurse, 31
    clinical nurse specialist and, 33
    nurse director and, 33-37
    service unit management (SUM),
      31-32
  orientation program for, 201, 421,
    422-426
  performance standards, 135, 136-
    137. *See also* Performance
    standards
  performing duties of other depart-
    ments, 302-303
  philosophy of, 81-82, 83-92
    application as test of, 85-88
    common concepts in, 84-85
    communication of, 88-89
    defined, 83
    development of, 83-84

    examples of, 335-342
    revision of, 89-90
  policies and procedures manuals,
    109-112
    format of, 109
    maintenance and revision of, 111-
      112
    organization of, 110-111
    problems in developing, 111
    topics in, 109-110
    usefulness of, 109, 112
  policy committee, 83-84, 107,
    403-405, 441-442
  records and reports, 166-170
    administrative, 167
    annual, 169-170
    importance of, 166-167
    statistical information in, 168
  sample nursing assignments, 383-
    385, 387-389
Nursing unit, 243-248
  administration of, education
    program for, 427-432
  budget preparation, 121-122
  design of, 249
    objective in, 243
    size and shape, 243-244
  employee facilities, 248
  expansion and maintenance of facili-
    ties, 250-251
  general regulations in, 243
  maintenance system for equipment
    and supplies, 264
  management of care in, 90
  manuals, 110, 201
  nurse call system, 246, 254
  nurses' station, 246-247
  nursing audit, 175-179. *See also*
    Nursing audit
  objective of, 90-92, 95
  orientation program, 201-202
  patient's room, 244-245. *See also*
    Patient's room
  philosophy of, 90-92
  primary nursing organization of,
    150
  provision of good working environ-
    ment, 250

special rooms, 247

Objectives and goals, 93–100
    administrative staff and achievement
        of, 95
    attitudes of staff and attaining, 94–95
    as basis for policies and procedures,
        105
    classification of, 93–94
    common interdepartmental, 302
    establishment and communication
        of, 95–97
    evaluation and review of, 95, 96
    general vs. specific, 93
    of head nurse education program,
        427
    of hospital design, 249, 250, 251–
        252
    of in-service education committee,
        410
    of job description committee, 405
    management process related to,
        99, 100
    of nursing audit committee, 406–
        407
    nursing care plan and, 159
    of nursing practice committee,
        401, 402
    nursing process related to, 153, 156–
        157
    of nursing service department
        form illustrating, 344–345
        policy committee, 404
    of nursing unit, 90–92, 95
        design, 243
    of orientation programs, 199
    past experience and establishing,
        98–100
    of patient care committee, 412
    of performance appraisal, 143, 156–
        157, 190, 191
    principles in developing, 94
    programming into action, 97
    progress review of, 98
    of quality assurance program, 143
    of recruitment committee, 413
    of research, 228
    of safety committee, 408–409

    of staff education, 95, 195, 199,
        417–418, 419, 421
    in staffing, 127–128
    of unions, 291–293
    usefulness of, 93
Occupational Safety and Health Act
        (OSHA) of 1970, 257–259
Operating budget
    described, 115–116
    items in, 347–349
    review of, 121
Organization, 29–36, 41, 42, 46–53.
        See also specific topic
    basic structural concepts of, 46,
        48–51
    delegation, 49–51
        homogeneous assignment, 49
        span of control and, 48–49
        unity of command and, 48
    department directors and, 29–30
    friction and, 46
    governing body and, 29
    hospital administration in, 29–30.
        See also Administration; Ad-
        ministrators, hospital
    implication of cooperation in, 52
    levels of executives in, 30
    line and staff responsibilities and,
        51–52
    medical care delivery and, 15
    of nursing service, 30–36. See also
        Nurse director; Nursing service
        department
    organizational chart, 101–104
    philosophy of, 81–82
        of hospital, 82–83
        of nursing service, 83–92
        of nursing units, 90–92
    procedure, 53
        steps in, 46–48
    purpose of planning structure in,
        44–45
    of quality assurance program, 142–
        143
    structural types of, 102–104
        ladder, 102, 103
        pyramidal, 102-, 103–104
        supergriddle, 102, 103

Organization — *Continued*
  structural vs. procedural compo-
    nents of, 47–48
  systems approach to, 67–75. *See
    also* Systems approach
Organizational chart, 101–104
  department functions in, 101–102
  guidelines for, 101–102
  organizational structures in, 102–
    104
Orientation programs, 199–202, 415,
    416
  to hospital, 201
  to nursing service department, 201,
    421, 422–426
  to nursing unit, 201–202
  objectives of, 199
  strengthening experiences with,
    200
  support for, 199–200
Outpatient care, 16, 250

Participation training, 203–205
Part-time staff, use of, 220
Pathology department, 16
Patient. *See specific topic, e.g.,*
    Patient's room; Protection of
    patient
Patient care
  assignment, example of, 383–385,
    387-389
  committee of, 412–413
  defined, 12
  patient's bill of rights, 331–332
Patient's bill of rights, 331–332
Patient's room, 244–246, 249–250
  design of, 244–245, 249
  facilities, 245–246, 249
  nurse call system, 246, 254
  privacy and, 249–250
Peer review, 141, 146, 147, 179,
    363–373, 375–382
  committees, 364, 365–373
    authority of, 370–371
    composition and representation
      on, 368–369
    functions and purpose of, 368
    legal liability and, 371

  membership selection policies,
    369–370
  permanent, guidelines for, 367–
    373
  policy development by, 371–372
  protocol, 372–373
  size of, 370
  subcommittees, 370
  temporary, guidelines for, 366–367
  nurse director's guidelines and
    tools for, 375–382
  Nursing Performance Review, 365,
    368
  Nursing Professional Standards Re-
    view, 364–365, 368
  process of, 364
  purposes of, 363–364
  referral lines and appeal of decisions,
    373
Performance appraisal, 189–193. *See
    also* Job evaluation; Peer review;
    Performance standards, appraisal
    of
Performance standards, 135–137
  appraisal of, 189–193. *See also* Job
    evaluation; Peer review
  advantages of, 192
  defined, 189
  leadership climate and, 189–190
  nurse director in, tools and guide-
    lines for, 376–382
  objectivity of, 190, 191
  planning, 190–192
  records of, 192–193
  associations developing organized,
    137
  auditing, 138, 140, 175–179. *See
    also* Nursing audit
  committee in revision, review and
    development of, 136
  as criteria, 136
  needs in, 136
  nursing definition and, 135–137
  nursing service department policies
    and, 135, 136–137
  peer review, 141, 146, 147, 179,
    363–373, 375–382
  quality assurance program and,

137-147. *See also* Quality assurance program (QAP)
records of, 180, 192-193
responsibility for establishing, 135
unions and, 292
Personnel. *See* Staff; *and specific topic, e.g.,* Nurse director
Personnel records, 179-182
contents, 179-181
file storage of, 181-182
Pharmacy department, 17
Philosophy
as basis for policies and procedures, 105
educational, 307, 416-417, 418-419
of hospital, 82-83
nursing care delivery and, 86-89
of nursing service department, 81-82, 83-92, 335-342. *See also* Nursing service department, philosophy of
communication of, 88-89
organizational aspects of, 81-92
staff and development of, 83-84
of nursing units, 90-92
of organization, 81-92
of hospital, 82-83
of nursing service, 83-92
of nursing units, 90-92
of peer review, 363-373
predetermined objectives and, 93
of research, 228
Physical medicine department, 22
Planning, 41, 42-46. *See also* Decision making
alternative solutions in, 42, 43, 44
analysis and comparison of alternatives in, 43, 44
change and, 447
committee on, 441
control and, 60
difficulties in, 45-46
elements and activities in, 42-43
nursing care, 158-160
in nursing process, 156
nursing service philosophy and, 87
performance appraisal, 190-192
plan selection in, 43, 44

problem diagnosis and, 42-43
purposes of, 44-45
staff education program, 197, 207-208
systems approach and, 71
time required for, 45
Plant operations department, 252
Policies and procedures, 105-112. *See also specific topic, e.g.,* Nursing service department; Records and reports
committee on, 441
nursing care plans and, 160
organizing procedures, described, 53. *See also* Organization
peer review committee, 368, 371-372
philosophy and objectives as basis of, 105
policy communication, 107-108
policy development, 106-107
policy vs. procedure, defined, 105
on records
legal aspects of, 108-109
manuals, 109-112. *See also* Manuals
on research, 228, 230, 437
on safety, 253
on staffing, 127
on supplies and equipment, 264
usefulness of policies, 105-106
Postmortem examinations, 16
Primary nursing, defined, 150
Privacy
of patient
rights in, 17
room and facilities and, 249-250
protection of, in research, 229-230
Procedures. *See* Policies and procedures
Procurement (purchasing) department, 263-264, 265
Professional organizations. *See also specific organization*
interest and participation in, 197, 206
joining, vs joining unions, 291
quality assurance programs and, 138, 140

Professional Standards Review Organizations (PSROs), 138
Promotions
  policies on, 217
  unions and, 290, 292, 293
Protection of patient
  hospital responsibility in, 17-18
  infection control, 225-257
    isolation for, 256
  patient's bill of rights, 331-332
  privacy, 17, 249-250
  property, 17
  in research, 229-230
  safety measures, 254, 255. *See also*
    Safety
Pyramidal organizational structure,
  102-103, 103-104

Quality assurance program (QAP),
  137-147, 179
  benefits of, 146-147
  corrective action and, 146
  criteria development for, 143-144
  defined, 137
  development of, 144-146
    characteristics of, 144-145
    model program, 145-146
    steps in, 145
  functions of, 141-142
  need for, 137-138
  nurse director and nursing staff's
    role in, 140-141, 141-143, 145-
    146
  objectives of, 143
  organization of, 142-143
  peer review and, 141, 146, 147, 179
  professional organizations and, 137,
    138, 140
  quality nursing care, defined, 139-
    141
  as system, 143-144
  tools for evaluating, 140-141

Radiology department, 16
Records and reports, 166-182. *See
  also* Manuals
  on job evaluation, 186-189
  medical. *See* Medical record(s)

minutes of meetings
  administrative, 163-164
  committee, 165, 166
  nursing audit, 175-179. *See also*
    Nursing audit
  nursing personnel, 179-182
    contents, 179-181
    file storage, 181-182
  nursing service department, 166-
    170
    administrative, 167
    annual, 169-170
    importance of, 166-167
    statistical information in, 168
  of performance, 180, 192-193
  of policies and procedures, legal
    implications of, 108-109
  recording areas in nurses' station,
    246
  of staff education program, 197
  of staffing data, 128
Recreational service, 20
Recruitment, 217-224
  committee for, 129, 218, 413-414
  legislation and, 218-219, 295
  nurse director and, 218, 221
  promotion policies and, 217
  sources of staff, 217-218
  staff shortages and, 219-221
  turnover of nurses and, 219, 221-
    223
Referral lines from peer review, 373
Referral of patients, 22, 379
Refresher courses, 220-221
Rehabilitation services, 22
Reports. *See* Records and reports
Research, 225-234, 437-439
  application to education programs,
    197
  consultation services available for,
    438-439
  defined, 225
  environment for, 227
  guidelines for approval of, 228, 230,
    443
  guidelines for writing, 445-446
  human rights and, 229-230
  identification of research problems

in nursing, 225, 233–234
informed consent concept, 230
leadership for, 227
as method, 225–226
need for nursing, 225, 226–227
nurse director and, 227–229, 230, 234
nurses' role in, 231–234
nursing process and, 233–234
nursing service committee and, 228, 230, 441
objectives of, 228
personnel in, 439
philosophy and policies on, 228, 230, 437
process of, 231
promotion of, 228–229
research proposal, 231
  guidelines for approval, 443–444
  guidelines for writing, 445–446
review committee, 229–230
scope of, 437–438
Responsibility
  delegation
    for attending meetings, 164
    described, 46, 49–50
    in quality assurance program, 142–143
  line vs. staff, 51–52
  of nurses, in nursing service philosophy, 86–87
  for policy application, 107
Rights of patient, 9, 331–332. *See also* Protection of patient
  confidentiality, 17
  privacy, 17, 249–250
  spiritual care, 18
Rooms
  for educational programs, 248
  patient's, 244–246, 249–250. *See also* Patient's room
  medication, 247
  safety and security of, 17
  treatment, 248
  workrooms, 247–248

Safety, 253–261
  administration and, 253

committees, 253–254, 408–410, 441
  infection control and, 255–256
  meetings, 410
  membership, 409
  objectives, 408–409
  responsibilities of chairman, 410
electrical hazards, 254
of equipment, 17
fire protection, 253, 254
infection control, 255–257
noise control, 247, 259–261
Occupational Safety and Health Act (OSHA), 257–259
policy statements on, 253
preventive and corrective maintenance program for, 254
of rooms, 17
smoking regulations, 254–255
Salaries and wages, 183–184
  legislation and, 219
  in personnel file, 180
  unions and, 290, 291–292, 293
Scheduling, 131, 133–134
  centralized staffing and, 131
  checking suitability of, 131, 133
  cyclical staffing and, 133
  decentralized staffing and, 133
  master staffing plan and, 133–134
  policies, effective staffing and, 134
  unions and, 290, 292
Service unit management (SUM) of nursing service, 31–32
Shortage of nurses, 129, 219–221
Skill training program, 202–205, 415, 416
Small-group activities, 203, 205
Smoking regulations, 254–255
Social service program, 19–20
Solarium, 248
Specialist nurses, 32–33. *See also* Nurse practitioners
Spiritual care of patients, 18
Staff. *See also* Scheduling; Staffing; *and specific topic, e.g.*, Recruitment; Salaries and wages
  attitudes, attaining objectives and, 94–95

Staff — *Continued*
  changing role of hospital and,
    13-14, 195
  command, 48-49. *See also* Command
  discipline, 284-287. *See also* Discipline
  education programs, 195-216. *See also* Education
  estimation, in budget preparation,
    120, 121
  evaluation. *See* Job evaluation; Peer review; Performance standards
  legal protection for, 218-219, 257-258
  line vs. staff responsibilities, 51-52
  morale, 282-284
  motivation. *See* Motivation
  organizational friction and, 46
  part-time, 220
  personnel records, 179-182
    contents, 179-181
    file storage of, 181-182
  philosophy of nursing service department and, 83-84
  policies and procedures manual and,
    109, 112
  proportion involved in direct patient care, 127
  role in quality assurance program,
    140-141, 141-143
  scientific management and, 40
  unions and, 289-296. *See also* Unions
  volunteer, 17, 20
  work simplification programs, 277-278
Staff responsibility, defined, 51-52
Staffing, 125-134. *See also* Recruitment; Scheduling
  activities in, 125
  assignment methods, 149-151, 383-385, 387-389
  availability of personnel and, 129
  centralized, 131
  cyclical, 133
  decentralized, 133
  effective, scheduling and, 134
  master staffing plan, 128-131, 132.
    See also Master staffing plan
  medical care delivery and, 15
  objectives of, 127-128
  personnel requirement determination, 125-127
    empirical subjective method, 125-126
    nursing care requirements in, 126, 127
  problems in, 128-129
  promotion policies and, 217, 290, 292, 293
  for quality, 126, 127
  scientific management and, 126
  selection criteria for, 17-18
  shortages and, 129, 219-221
  turnover and, 219, 221-223
Staffing board, described, 130-131, 132
Standards of performance. *See* Performance standards
Standing committees. *See* Committees
Supergriddle organizational structure,
  102, 103
Supplies, defined, 263. *See also* Equipment and supplies
Systems approach, 67-75
  concepts from systems theory and,
    73-74
  description of system and, 69
  environment of system and, 70, 72-73
  goals and objectives and, 69-70
  as guideline, 68-69
  implications for nurse director,
    74-75
  importance and value of, 67-68, 75
  interactions of components of, 70-71
  management of system, 71
  nursing process, 155
  open vs. closed systems, 71-72
  planning and, 71
  property characteristics of system and, 72-73

quality assurance program as, 143–144
resources of system and, 70, 72
system definition and, 68

Teaching. *See* Education
Team method of assignment, 149, 383–385, 387–389
Team work. *See* Interdisciplinary approach
Termination
exit interview, 223–224
handling, 285, 286
turnover of nurses and, 219, 221–223
unions and, 290, 292
Therapeutic environment, described, 21
Training. *See* Education
Transfers
opportunities, unions and, 290, 292, 293
in personnel file, 180

Treatment rooms, 248, 250
Turnover of nurses, 219, 221–223

Unions, 289–296
collective bargaining by, 291, 294, 295
election of, management and, 295–296
management-union relations, 293–296
legal framework of, 293–295
objectives of, 291–293
reasons for joining, 289–291
reasons for rejecting, 291

Volunteers, 17, 20

Wages. *See* Salaries and wages
Work simplification programs, 277–278
Workrooms, 247–248